Prostate MRI Essentials

Temel Tirkes
Editor

Prostate MRI Essentials

A Practical Guide for Radiologists

Springer

Editor
Temel Tirkes
Department of Radiology and Imaging Sciences
Indiana University School of Medicine
Indianapolis, IN
USA

ISBN 978-3-030-45934-5 ISBN 978-3-030-45935-2 (eBook)
https://doi.org/10.1007/978-3-030-45935-2

This Springer imprint is published by the registered company Springer Nature Switzerland AG
The registered company address is: Gewerbestrasse 11, 6330 Cham, Switzerland

Dedicated to my children

John and Katherine

Preface

A dramatic shift in clinical practice has occurred over the last decade, from the radical treatment of virtually all newly diagnosed prostate cancer patients to a much more selective approach, incorporating expectant management, or active surveillance, for the roughly 40% of patients with low-risk disease. Prostate imaging became a centerpiece of prostate cancer management after switching the target of the therapy from the entire prostate to the localized cancer. Within a short period of time, a number of multi-parametric MRI (mp-MRI) examinations logarithmically increased across the academic centers and peripheral imaging centers alike.

The PI-RADS committee was established and tasked to provide a standardized reporting system for the radiologists so that we can all speak the same language in our reports. There has been insufficient guidance to the technologists about how to perform these examinations. Similarly, most radiologists have been caught unprepared to the mpMRI, which requires an independent workstation to do post-processing. As of today, mpMRI of the prostate has been established in almost all of the academic centers in the USA.

The primary aim for this handbook style textbook is to provide a practical guideline to the radiologists, radiology residents, and fellows who are new to prostate imaging and interpretation. It covers anatomy, pathology, imaging techniques, and interpretation standards based on PI-RADS v2.1, post-processing for targeted biopsies, molecular imaging, and ablation treatments. Technologists will find useful imaging protocols (planning and prescription) and parameters with representative images for each MRI sequence.

This textbook is a collaboration of radiologists, pathologist, urologists, and radiation oncologists. I am honored and grateful to all the authors for their efforts. I hope you will find it to be useful for your practice.

Thank you.

Indianapolis, IN, USA　　　　Temel Tirkes, MD, FACR

Contents

Contributors

Oguz Akin, MD Memorial Sloan Kettering Cancer Center, Department of Radiology, New York, NY, USA

Joyce G. R. Bomers, PhD Radboud University Medical Center, Department of Radiology and Nuclear Medicine, Nijmegen, The Netherlands

Adam C. Calaway, MD, MPH Case Western University/University Hospitals, Department of Urology, Cleveland, OH, USA

Aritrick Chatterjee, PhD University of Chicago, Department of Radiology, Chicago, IL, USA

University of Chicago, Sanford J. Grossman Center of Excellence in Prostate Imaging and Image Guided Therapy, Chicago, IL, USA

Liang Cheng, MD Department of Pathology and Laboratory Medicine, Indiana University School of Medicine, Indianapolis, IN, USA

Peter L. Choyke, MD NCI, NIH, Molecular Imaging Program, Bethesda, MD, USA

Alessia Cimadamore, MD Polytechnic University of the Marche Region (Ancona), School of Medicine, United Hospitals, Institute of Pathological Anatomy and Histopathology, Ancona, Marche, Italy

Mehmet Coskun, MD Health Science University Dr. Behçet Uz Child Disease and Surgery Training and Research Hospital, Department of Radiology, İzmir, Turkey

Marcin B. Czarniecki, MD MedStar Georgetown University Hospital, Department of Radiology, Washington, DC, USA

Steven C. Eberhardt, MD University of New Mexico Hospital, Department of Radiology, Albuquerque, NM, USA

University of New Mexico, Albuquerque, NM, USA

Bryan R. Foster, MD Oregon Health & Science University, Department of Diagnostic Radiology, Portland, OR, USA

Jurgen J. Fütterer, MD, PhD Radboud University Medical Center, Department of Radiology and Nuclear Medicine, Nijmegen, The Netherlands

Gordon Guo, MD Indiana University Simon Cancer Center, Department of Radiation Oncology, Indianapolis, IN, USA

Melina Hosseiny, MD Ronald Reagan UCLA Medical Center, Department of Radiology: Abdominal Imaging and Cross Sectional IR, Los Angeles, CA, USA

Sunil Jeph, MD Weill Cornell Imaging/New York Presbyterian Hospital, Department of Radiology, New York, NY, USA

Gregory S. Karczmar, PhD University of Chicago, Department of Radiology, Chicago, IL, USA

University of Chicago, Sanford J. Grossman Center of Excellence in Prostate Imaging and Image Guided Therapy, Chicago, IL, USA

Michael O. Koch, MD Indiana University Health, Department of Urology, Indianapolis, IN, USA

Antonio Lopez-Beltran, MD Faculty of Medicine, University of Cordoba, Unit of Anatomic Pathology, Cordoba, Spain

Daniel J. A. Margolis, MD Weill Cornell Imaging/New York Presbyterian Hospital, Department of Radiology, New York, NY, USA

Yousef Mazaheri, PhD Memorial Sloan Kettering Cancer Center, Department of Medical Physics and Radiology, New York, NY, USA

Roberta Mazzucchelli, MD Polytechnic University of the Marche Region (Ancona), School of Medicine, United Hospitals, Institute of Pathological Anatomy and Histopathology, Ancona, Marche, Italy

Esther Mena, MD NCI, NIH, Molecular Imaging Program, Bethesda, MD, USA

Rodolfo Montironi, MD Polytechnic University of the Marche Region (Ancona), School of Medicine, United Hospitals, Institute of Pathological Anatomy and Histopathology, Ancona, Marche, Italy

Moozhan Nikpanah, MD NIH, Clinical Center, Radiology and Imaging Sciences, Bethesda, MD, USA

Aytekin Oto, MD, MBA University of Chicago, Department of Radiology, Chicago, IL, USA

University of Chicago, Sanford J. Grossman Center of Excellence in Prostate Imaging and Image Guided Therapy, Chicago, IL, USA

Federico Pineda, PhD University of Chicago, Department of Radiology, Chicago, IL, USA

Andrei S. Purysko, MD Cleveland Clinic, Section of Abdominal Imaging and Nuclear Radiology Department, Cleveland, OH, USA

Steven S. Raman, MD, FSIR, FSAR Ronald Reagan UCLA Medical Center, Department of Radiology: Abdominal Imaging and Cross Sectional IR, Los Angeles, CA, USA

Marina Scarpelli, MD Polytechnic University of the Marche Region (Ancona), School of Medicine, United Hospitals, Institute of Pathological Anatomy and Histopathology, Ancona, Marche, Italy

Ryan W. Speir, MD Indiana University, Department of Urology, Indianapolis, IN, USA

Martha F. Terrazas, MD University of New Mexico Hospital, Department of Radiology, Albuquerque, NM, USA

University of New Mexico, Albuquerque, NM, USA

Baris Turkbey, MD National Cancer Institute (NIH), Center of Cancer Research, Molecular Imaging Program, Bethesda, MD, USA

Annemarijke van Luijtelaar, MD Radboud University Medical Center, Department of Radiology and Nuclear Medicine, Nijmegen, The Netherlands

Ryan D. Ward, MD Massachusetts General Hospital, Division of Abdominal Imaging, Boston, MA, USA

Natasha E. Wehrli, MD Weill Cornell Imaging/New York Presbyterian Hospital, Department of Radiology, New York, NY, USA

Antonio C. Westphalen, MD, FSAR University of California, San Francisco, Department of Radiology and Biomedical Imaging, and Urology, San Francisco, CA, USA

Joseph H. Yacoub, MD MedStar Georgetown University Hospital, Department of Radiology, Washington, DC, USA

Editor Biography

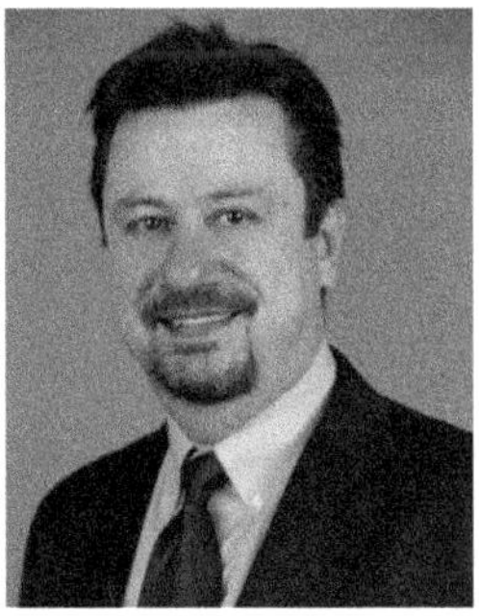

Temel Tirkes, MD, FACR is an associate professor of radiology, urology, and imaging Sciences; a Fellow of the American College of Radiology; and Diplomate of the American Board of Radiology since 2001. He is serving as Director of Genitourinary Radiology at Indiana University Health. His external academic responsibilities include serving as a member of the Genitourinary Scientific Committee of the Radiological Society of North America, Chairman of the Pancreatitis Disease Focus Group and a member of the Scientific Program Committee of the Society of Abdominal Radiologists. Dr. Tirkes has been practicing academic radiology since he completed his Abdominal Imaging Fellowship at the University of Pennsylvania in 2002. He was a member of Abdominal Imaging Faculty at University of Texas Southwestern Medical Center for 6 years until joining the Indiana University School of Medicine in 2008.

Dr. Tirkes is a subspecialized diagnostic radiologist and his focus has been on MR imaging of the pancreas and prostate. He is participating in the Consortium for the Study of Chronic Pancreatitis, Diabetes, and Pancreatic Cancer (CPDPC) and serves as Chair of the Imaging Committee. Dr. Tirkes is currently the PI of the "Magnetic Resonance Imaging as a Non-Invasive Method for the Assessment of Pancreatic Fibrosis" (MINIMAP) study. This is a multi-institutional prospective study funded by the NIDDK (R01DK116963) aiming to demonstrate that magnetic resonance imaging (MRI) can detect parenchymal abnormalities related to chronic pancreatitis and may serve as a biomarker of pancreatic fibrosis and disease progression. He is also a co-investigator for Prospective Evaluation of Chronic Pancreatitis for Epidemiologic and Translational Studies (The PROCEED Study). Dr. Tirkes has been highly innovative in quantitative MRI of the pancreas, publishing the first MR relaxometry and radiomics imaging for the early diagnosis of chronic pancreatitis. He is one of the first investigators to show that pancreatic steatosis is closely associated with diabetes and chronic pancreatitis and MRI is the optimal tool to quantify pancreatic steatosis in this context. Dr. Tirkes has published a consensus paper as the first author about reporting standards of chronic pancreatitis by CT and MRI.

As a result of his close collaboration with urologists, IU Health is currently offering the latest diagnostic and minimally invasive therapeutic interventions to prostate cancer patients. IU became one of the first ten centers in the USA to offer high-frequency ultrasound ablation (HIFU). Dr. Tirkes was a co-investigator for a transurethral approach MRI-guided ultrasound ablation phase II clinical trial, which was successful, receiving FDA approval. He is currently a site PI of Multiparametric MRI for Preoperative Staging and Treatment Planning for Newly-Diagnosed Prostate Cancer (ECOG-ACRIN EA8171). This study aims to develop a risk prediction model by incorporating overall PI-RADS, PSA, Gleason score, and clinical stage to predict the presence of aggressive prostate cancer.

Author Biographies

Oguz Akin, MD is Director of Body MRI at MSKCC. He is particularly interested in using imaging to provide timely and accurate information for diagnosis, staging, treatment planning, and seeing how a therapy is working. His research focuses on MRI in cancer imaging with a special interest in genitourinary cancers. Dr. Akin has published research studies on the appropriate use of imaging for people with cancer and novel imaging techniques that provide both anatomical and functional information about tumors. He is also very involved in medical education through training and mentoring other doctors, both in their work with patients and in their research. Dr. Akin has published several books, book chapters, and scholarly articles in oncologic imaging.

Joyce Bomers, PhD is Technical Physician at the Department of Radiology at the Radboudumc and allied to the Medical Innovation and Technology expert Center (MITeC) and the Prostate MRI Expert Center (PMRC).

Dr. Bomers was one of the first pioneers obtaining her Master's degree in Technical Medicine from the University of Twente in Enschede in 2009. She started as a PhD candidate in the department of Radiology at the Radboudumc and completed her doctoral research entitled "MRI-guided focal therapy in patients with localized (recurrent) prostate cancer" in 2017. Simultaneously, Dr. Bomers completed a 2-year fellowship in Technical Medicine in 2016.

Her main focus is on diagnostics and treatment of prostate cancer with the help of MR imaging. With particular interest, she is implementing and performing MR-guided oncological prostate interventions such as MR-guided cryosurgery (clinical), focal laser ablation (clinical), focused ultrasound ablation (pre-clinical and clinical), and in-bore biopsy.

Adam C. Calaway, MD, MPH completed his Urology training at Indiana University in 2017. He then remained at Indiana University where he completed the Urologic Oncology Fellowship in 2019. He also earned a Master of Public Health in Epidemiology from the Richard Fairbanks School of Public Health at Indiana University Purdue University Indianapolis during his fellowship. He currently serves as an Assistant Professor in the Department of Urology at Case Western Reserve University/University Hospitals in Cleveland, Ohio.

Aritrick Chatterjee, PhD is a Research Assistant Professor in the Department of Radiology, University of Chicago. His current research focuses on the improved diagnosis of prostate cancer using MRI, including the development of new MRI acquisition, analysis, and interpretation methods to provide reliable information such as cancer localization, volume, and aggressiveness for deciding the optimal treatment option.

His work focuses on estimating prostate tissue composition non-invasively using Hybrid Multidimensional MRI and developing CAD risk analysis tools that effectively detect prostate cancer. His other projects involve using pretreatment quantitative multi-parametric MRI and determining its association with biochemical outcome in men treated with radiation therapy for prostate cancer, investigating the feasibility of dynamic contrast enhanced MRI using low doses of contrast agent (Gadolinium), and ultrafast DCE-MRI for diagnosis of prostate cancer.

Dr. Chatterjee has a wide range of expertise in medical imaging, especially MRI. He received his PhD from the University of Sydney, focusing on understanding the biophysical basis of diffusion in prostate MRI, and received his MSc degree from University College London, where he worked on imaging the microstructure of the brain using oscillating gradients on MRI.

Liang Cheng, MD is the inaugural Virgil H. Moon Endowed Professor of Pathology and Urology at Indiana University School of Medicine, Indianapolis, Indiana, USA. Currently, he is Chief of the Genitourinary Pathology Service, Director of the Urologic Pathology Fellowship, and Director of Molecular Diagnostics and Molecular Pathology Laboratories. Dr. Cheng is board certified in Molecular Genetic Pathology as well as Anatomic and Clinical Pathology by the American Board of Pathology. Dr. Cheng has received numerous prestigious awards including the Stowell-Orbison Award from the United States and Canadian Academy of Pathology and the Koss Medal Award from the International Society of Urological Pathology (ISUP). Dr. Cheng received the Arthur Purdy Stout Prize from the Arthur Purdy Stout Society of Surgical Pathologists in recognition of outstanding contributions to the field of surgical pathology for a surgical pathologist less than 45 years old. Dr. Cheng has published over 900 peer-reviewed SCI articles in high-impact scientific journals. His published work has been cited more than 40,000 times (ISI Web of Science *h-index*: 101). He is also the author of over 100 book chapters and several books, including *Bladder Pathology*, *Urologic Surgical Pathology*, *Essentials of Anatomic Pathology*, *Molecular Genetic Pathology*, *Molecular Surgical Pathology*, and *Atlas of Anatomic Pathology* (Series Editor). Currently, he is an active member of over 30 Editorial Boards, including *Molecular Cancer* (Associate Editor), *Human Pathology* (Senior Associate Editor), *American Journal of Surgical Pathology, Modern Pathology, Urologic Oncology.* He is currently the Editor-in-Chief of *Expert Review of Precision Medicine and Drug Development.*

Peter L. Choyke, MD is a Senior Investigator and Chief of the Molecular Imaging Program of the National Cancer Institute. He received his medical degree from Jefferson Medical College and trained at Yale and Penn. His research has focused on the development of novel targeted imaging and treatment agents, based on optical, MRI, and radionuclide techniques, for oncologic imaging. He has focused on cancers of the genitourinary tract including prostate, renal, bladder, and malignancies of the bone marrow.

Alessia Cimadamore, MD is Pathologist at the Pathological Anatomy and Histopathology at United Hospitals, Ancona, Italy. She obtained her medical degree from the Medical School of the University of Ancona, Italy, in 2014.

During her residency, she received advanced training in the field of genitourinary pathology being involved in important research projects and collaborations with world leaders in the field, in particular with Professors Rodolfo Montironi, Antonio Lopez-Beltran, and Liang Cheng.

Dr. Cimadamore research work is centered in genitourinary tumor pathology, with particular interest in PD-L1 expression in bladder and kidney cancers in relation with prognosis, predictive value, and immunotherapy response. In 2018, as part of her PhD, she has started a research project on genetic alterations in renal cell carcinoma and their application in liquid biopsy.

During her 4 years of research activity, she contributed as author or co-author to complete more than 50 publications in peer-reviewed international journals and more than 30 book chapters in the field of genitourinary tumor pathology. Dr. Cimadamore has been invited as speaker at national and international pathology meetings. She is a member of several international societies of pathology and of urology, including the European Society of Pathology and Genitourinary Pathology Society.

Mehmet Coskun, MD is a radiologist and board certified in Diagnostic Radiology by the Turkish Society of Radiology and European Board of Radiology since 2018.

He graduated from Hacettepe University Faculty of Medicine in 2012. He completed radiology training program at İzmir Katip Çelebi University Atatürk Training and Research Hospital in 2018. His fields of expertise are prostate MRI and physics principles of diagnostic imaging systems.

Marcin B. Czarniecki, MD is a fellow at MedStar Georgetown University Hospital. He was previously affiliated with the Molecular Imaging Program at the National Institutes of Health, where he was engaged in multiple research projects on prostate imaging. Dr. Czarniecki's research interests include PI-RADS reporting, large international collaborative initiatives, and image perception. He has numerous publications in the field, including original articles, reviews and book chapters. He previously trained in Warsaw, Poland and Addenbrooke's Hospital in Cambridge, UK, and is a diplomate of the European Board of Radiology.

Steven C. Eberhardt, MD is a Clinical Professor, Vice Chair for Clinical Operations, and Chief of Abdominal and Oncologic Imaging at University of New Mexico Radiology and The UNM Cancer Center. He came to UNM in 2004 following Body Imaging fellowship and 3 years as an attending radiologist at Memorial Sloan-Kettering Cancer Center in New York. Clinical activities have centered on oncology imaging with CT and MRI, with particular expertise in GU radiology. Educational and research activities include subjects in abdominal and oncology radiology with prostate cancer imaging with MRI a particular focus. Dr. Eberhardt has served on numerous national committees and panels, including leadership roles, namely the American College of Radiology Appropriateness Criteria panel on genitourinary radiology, the editorial board of the journal *Radiology*, panel chair for genitourinary imaging for the editorial board of the journal *RadioGraphics*, and Chair of the Clinical Practice Subcommittee for the SAR Disease Focused Panel for Prostate Cancer. He has been a Fellow of the Society of Abdominal Radiology since 2015.

Bryan R. Foster, MD is an Associate Professor of Diagnostic Radiology at Oregon Health & Science University in Portland, Oregon. He joined the faculty in 2011 and works in the body imaging section. Dr. Foster attended medical school and residency at Boston University, where he was chief resident. His fellowship training was in abdominal imaging at the University of Utah. Dr. Foster's clinical interests include oncologic, hepatobiliary, pancreatic, prostate, and small bowel imaging. Dr. Foster also serves as the Director of Ultrasound where he enjoys performing complex image-guided biopsies and is one of only two radiologists in the region performing MRI-guided prostate biopsies. Recently he was selected as an Honored Educator for the Radiological Society of North America and in the past has been named Teacher of the Year by the radiology residents.

Jurgen J. Fütterer, MD, PhD is Interventional-Radiologist at Radboudumc and full professor at the Robotics and Mechatronics group, University of Twente.

His role focuses on imaging techniques in cancer, image-guided interventions, and robotics. With particular interest, he is implementing and performing oncological interventions with special focus on MR-guided interventions, such as MR-guided cryosurgery (clinical), focal laser ablation (clinical), and focused ultrasound surgery (pre-clinical and clinical).

Dr. Fütterer qualified at Radboud University, Nijmegen, in 2001, and completed his PhD on MRI techniques in the localization and staging of prostate cancer in 2006. He was a radiology resident at the University Medical Centre, Nijmegen, in 2003, and completed a fellowship in interventional radiology/body MRI in 2009.

Dr. Fütterer has published extensively on MRI in prostate cancer in various journals and book chapters. He has also introduced a robotic device for MRI-guided biopsy of the prostate, which has been established as a novel prostate intervention.

Gordon Guo, MD is a practicing radiation oncologist and assistant professor of radiation oncology at Indiana University Simon Cancer Center, a National Cancer Institute designated comprehensive cancer center. He went to medical school at the University of Toronto, completed residency training at the

University of Manitoba, then went on to receive specialized training in a brachytherapy fellowship in the Mount Sinai Health system in NYC. Dr. Guo led the radiation oncology service in genitourinary and gynecological oncology tumor sites at Indiana University since August 2016.

Dr. Guo is a member of the NRG Oncology Scientific Committee, American Society for Radiation Oncology, and American Brachytherapy Society. He has authored over 20 manuscripts and abstracts in peer-reviewed journals and conference proceedings.

Dr. Guo believes that radiation oncology is a rapidly evolving field of medicine that takes full advantage of therapeutic radiation and advancement of computer-based treatment planning and imaging. His clinical interests include prostate brachytherapy, genitourinary, and gynecological malignancies. Quality and safety are his priorities.

Melina Hosseiny, MD is a postdoctoral research fellow in Department of Radiological Sciences at the University of California, Los Angeles (UCLA), under supervision of Dr. Steven S. Raman. After entering medical school, she completed her clinical rotations and internship at the Tehran University of Medical Sciences (TUMS), Iran, followed by extra clinical training at St Mary's hospital in United Kingdom. She has been a dynamic and productive member of prostate and kidney IDx (integrated diagnostics) groups at UCLA. She pioneered the creation of the ever-growing database for in-bore MR-guided biopsy of prostate at UCLA, which she has presented at several national radiology meetings. Her current research interests include applications of in-bore MR-guided biopsy of prostate, technical measures to improve the image quality of prostate MRI, and investigation of artificial intelligence models for prediction of renal tumors microenvironment on cross-sectional imaging.

Sunil Jeph, MD is a Body Imaging fellow at Weill Cornell Imaging – New York Presbyterian Hospital. He completed his radiology residency from Geisinger medical center. He was awarded the Roentgen Resident/Fellow Research Award for 2019. Dr. Jeph finished his medical school and residency in Nuclear Medicine from All India Institute of Medical Sciences, India. He has served as a visiting scientist at MD Anderson Cancer center in 2013. Dr. Jeph's research interest includes the role of PET and MRI in abdominal tumors.

Gregory S. Karczmar, PhD received his bachelor's degree from Reed College and master's degree and PhD from the University of California at Berkeley. He has developed and validated new approaches to functional and anatomic magnetic resonance imaging for over 30 years. Dr. Karczmar has applied these methods to improve detection and diagnosis of cancer and monitor cancer response to therapy. He is a Professor of Radiology, Medical Physics and the College at the University of Chicago, Director of Magnetic Resonance Imaging Research at the University of Chicago, and Co-Director of the Advanced Imaging Program of the University of Chicago Comprehensive Cancer center. He and his collaborators in the body and breast imaging groups at UChicago made pioneering contributions to the development of ultrafast DCE-MRI and to the development of specialized image reconstruction and analysis methods for ultrafast sampling. Dr. Karczmar pioneered new methods to improve prostate and breast cancer diagnosis and understanding of prostate and breast cancer biology.

Michael O. Koch, MD has served as the Chairman of the Department of Urology at Indiana University School of Medicine since 1998. He had previously been a member of the faculty at Vanderbilt University for 12 years. Dr. Koch has served in many roles for urology nationally. Dr. Koch is a former trustee and past-President of the American Board of Urology, past-Chairman of the Examination Committee for the American Board of Urology, past-President of the Society of Urology Chairpersons, past-President of the Society of University Chairpersons, Chair of the Residency Review Committee for urology training programs, and a member of the honorary societies of the GU Surgeons and the Clinical Society of GU Surgeons. In 2015, he was honored by the American Urologic Association's Distinguished Contribution Award. In 2017, Dr. Koch was awarded the Health Care Hero award by the *Indianapolis Business Journal* for his involvement in the development of High Intensity Ultrasound for the treatment of prostate cancer.

Antonio Lopez-Beltran, MD is currently the Director of Anatomic Pathology Service for Champalimaud Clinical Center, in Lisbon, Portugal. He served as the Director of Anatomic Pathology for Althia Health in Barcelona and Full Professor of Anatomic Pathology at the University of Cordoba where he designed and implemented novel molecular technics to evaluate prognostic features of bladder and prostate cancer. Through the years he discovered and/or validated some biomarkers of clinical utility, mostly tissue and urine related. Studies from his lab have granted him to be a "Highly Cited Author" by the Institute of Scientific Information with h-index of 61. He received the medical degree, at the University of Seville in 1979, completed the residency program in Anatomic Pathology until 1982 and received a PhD in Experimental Pathology at the University of Cordoba in 1984. He has been a visiting physician pathologist at the pathology service of the University College (London, UK, 1986 (6 months), Roswell Park Cancer Institute (Buffalo, NY, 1987–1989, 2 years), and Mayo Clinic (Rochester, MN, 1995, 6 months). He is a member of several international pathological organizations and the current Chair of the European Working Group on Urologic Pathology of the European Society of Pathology.

Daniel J. A. Margolis, MD is a board-certified radiologist specializing in Body Imaging. He is Assistant Professor of Radiology at Weill Cornell Medical College and Assistant Attending Radiologist at New York Presbyterian Hospital-Weill Cornell Campus. Dr. Margolis is a graduate of the University of California, Berkeley, earning his BSc in Biochemistry with honors in 1992. Dr. Margolis earned his MD degree from University of Southern California in 1998.

Following a transitional internship year at Los Angeles VA Healthcare System, Dr. Margolis served as a resident in Diagnostic Radiology from 1999 to2003 at David Geffen School of Medicine at UCLA. Dr. Margolis then completed a fellowship in Advanced Imaging at Stanford University Medical Center.

While at UCLA, Dr. Margolis completed the K30 Graduate Training Program in Translational Investigation and was principal investigator or co-principal investigator on numerous research projects. His primary focus was the use of MRI for the detection and characterization of prostate cancer, with over 50 publications in this field. He also serves as a member of the American College of Radiology Prostate Imaging Reporting and Data Systems committee, setting the standard for prostate MRI worldwide. He has given invited talks on prostate imaging in three continents and looks to continue his success collaborating with urologists, radiation oncologists, and medical oncologists to continue the fight against prostate cancer.

In addition to prostate imaging, Dr. Margolis participated in research or clinical programs on pancreas cancer, liver disease, and inflammatory bowel disease, and was director for virtual colonography, a screening test for early colon cancer.

Dr. Margolis was recruited to the full-time faculty of Weill Cornell Medical College and was appointed Assistant Professor of Radiology and Assistant Attending Radiology at the New York Presbyterian Hospital Weill-Cornell Campus in September 2016.

Yousef Mazaheri, PhD is an Associate Attending in the Departments of Medical Physics at Memorial Sloan Kettering Cancer Center (MSKCC) with a joint appointment in the Department of Radiology. He has extensive experience in the technical development and clinical implementation of novel MRI sequences and data modeling techniques. His areas of research include medical image analysis, advanced MRI techniques to develop imaging techniques capable of predicting tumor growth, response to cancer treatment, and transport properties within tumors. Dr. Mazaheri also serves as a resource for department physicians, fellows, and residents who wish to incorporate MRI techniques into their research.

Roberta Mazzucchelli, MD, PhD is assistant professor of pathology at the Medical School of the Polytechnic University of the Marche Region, Italy.

Dr. Mazzucchelli obtained her medical degree from the Medical School of the University of Ancona, Italy, in 1994 and the board certificate in pathology from the Polytechnic University of the Marche Region in 1999. She received her PhD from the University of Siena, Italy, in 2004.

Dr. Mazzucchelli's work is centered on genitourinary tumor pathology. She is an author or co-author of more than 150 publications in peer-reviewed international journals.

Esther Mena, MD is a Board-Certified physician in the field of Nuclear Medicine. She is a Staff Clinician in the Molecular Imaging Program (MIP) at the National Cancer Institute (NCI), National Institutes of Health (NIH) in Bethesda, Maryland. Born in Barcelona, Spain, Dr. Mena went to medical school at the UAB, Barcelona, completing a Nuclear Medicine residency at Sant Pau Hospital, Barcelona, and worked as an attending Nuclear Medicine physician in the UDIAT.CD. Barcelona. Dr. Mena joined the Molecular Imaging Program at the National Cancer Institute as a Clinical Research Fellow in 2009. She subsequently completed her residency in Nuclear Medicine at Johns Hopkins University in Baltimore, Maryland, followed by a fellowship program in PET imaging at Johns Hopkins. Dr. Mena re-joined NIH as a Staff Clinician in 2016 within the Molecular Imaging Program. Dr. Mena's ongoing research involves the use of novel PET/CT imaging for diagnosis and management of prostate cancer, with the goal of using molecular imaging to understand the tumor biology and to further improve clinical outcome. She is also interested in the use of systemic, targeted radionuclides or conjugates as a treatment modality for cancer.

Rodolfo Montironi, MD is Professor of Pathology at the Medical School of the Polytechnic University of the Marche Region and Director of the Uropathology Program, United Hospitals, Ancona, Italy

Dr. Montironi, MD, and IFCAP, obtained his medical degree from the Medical School of the University of Ancona, Italy, in 1976; the board certificate in pathology and laboratory medicine at the University of Parma, Italy, in 1979; and the board certificate in clinical oncology at the University of Ancona in 1982. He received his advanced training in pathology in several British institutions under the supervision of world leaders in pathology, in particular at Hammersmith Hospital, London, UK, with Dr. John G. Azzopardi in 1979.

Dr. Montironi is International Fellow of the College of American Pathologists. He is Professor of Pathology at the Medical School of the Polytechnic University of the Marche Region and Director of the Uropathology Program, United Hospitals, Ancona, Italy. Dr. Montironi is a Past President of the International Society of Urological Pathology. He is the Chairman of the ESUP (EAU Section of Uropathology). Dr. Montironi is a member of different international societies of pathology and of urology, including the European Society of Pathology and European Association of Urology.

Dr. Montironi's work is centered in genitourinary tumor pathology. He is an author or co-author of more than 800 publications in peer-reviewed international journals and of more than 30 chapters in books in the field of genitourinary tumor pathology. He has been a regular invited speaker at all major national and international pathology meetings. He organized and co-organized several international courses on genitourinary tumor pathology. Rodolfo serves on the editorial boards of several international pathology and urology journals, including *European Urology*, *European Urology Focus*, and *European Urology Oncology*

Moozhan Nikpanah, MD earned her Doctorate in Medicine from Iran University of Medical Sciences in 2015. While in medical school, she conducted research on the expression of putative cancer stem cell markers in prostate carcinomas at the Oncopathology Research Center, Iran University of Medical Sciences.

Dr. Nikpanah joined the Radiology and Imaging Sciences, NIH Clinical Center, in 2016.

Her main research areas include imaging characterization of genitourinary cancers (utilizing multiparametric MRI, CT, and PET/CT) and radiological manifestations of Erdheim-Chester Disease. Dr. Nikpanah has ongoing collaborations with the National Cancer Institute (NCI) and National Human Genome Research Institute (NHGRI) on numerous research projects.

Aytekin Oto, MD, MBA is Professor of Radiology and Surgery and Chair of Radiology at the University of Chicago. Dr. Oto has a wide range of experience and expertise in the imaging of diseases affecting abdomen and pelvis. His research interest focus is development and clinical application of novel prostate MRI acquisition and interpretation so as to facilitate and improve the efficiency of prostate cancer and develop image-guided prostate therapy options for the appropriate patients diagnosed with prostate cancer.

Dr. Oto's research has resulted in more than 200 publications and over 150 scientific exhibits at national and international meetings. The two overarching aims of his research are "non-invasive and accurate diagnosis of aggressive prostate cancer using MR imaging" and "eradication of localized prostate cancer with minimal complications using minimally invasive treatment methods." Dr. Oto's group has developed new MR sequences, pilot CAD software for prostate MRI, and tested MR-guided therapy methods such as laser and focused ultrasound ablation in clinical and pre-clinical studies. He has several industry, foundation, and NIH grants and serves at the Editorial Board of *Radiology*. Dr. Oto received numerous awards including Distinguished Investigator Award, RSNA Honored Educator Award, and Distinguished Senior Clinician Award.

Federico Pineda, PhD received a BS in Physics from Carnegie Mellon University and his PhD in Medical Physics from the University of Chicago, where he is currently a Research Assistant Professor in the Department of Radiology. His research focuses on the development of acquisition, reconstruction, and analysis methods of dynamic contrast-enhanced MRI, specifically for breast and prostate imaging applications. Recently Dr. Pineda has been involved in the development of ultrafast breast DCE-MRI protocols and their translation into clinical use.

Andrei S. Purysko, MD is a staff physician of the section of Abdominal Imaging and Nuclear Radiology Department at Cleveland Clinic. He is also a member of the Glickman Urological and Kidney Institute at Cleveland Clinic and a Clinical Assistant Professor of Radiology at Case Western Reserve University School of Medicine. Dr. Purysko graduated from the Faculdade de Medicina de Petrópolis in Rio de Janeiro and completed his residency training in Radiology at the Hospital Beneficência Portuguesa in São Paulo, Brazil. He then joined Cleveland Clinic in 2009, where he completed his fellowship training in Radiology. Dr. Purysko has led the prostate MRI program at Cleveland Clinic since 2014. He assisted in developing the MRI/US fusion biopsy service line at Cleveland Clinic's main campus and in several other facilities in northeast Ohio, Florida, and Nevada. Dr. Purysko serves as a member of the ACR prostate MRI accreditation working group and of the Appropriateness Criteria expert panel in Uroradiology.

Steven S. Raman, MD, FSAR, FSIR is a Professor of Radiology, Urology, and Surgery at University of California, Los Angeles (UCLA). He has been an attending radiologist at David Geffen School of Medicine at UCLA since 1999, after completing his radiology residency at the University of California San Diego (UCSD) and Abdominal Imaging fellowship at the Department of Radiological Sciences at UCLA. Currently, Dr. Raman is director of abdominal imaging fellowship program at UCLA, Director of GI-GU Core Lab (MedQIA) Abdominal Imaging, Co-Director of Prostate MR Imaging and Research Group, and Co-Director of UCLA Prostate SPORE Imaging Core Lab. He has served on genitourinary scientific committees of RSNA and SAR, has published more than 200 peer-reviewed scientific papers and review articles, has co-authored 20 book chapters on body imaging, and has lectured in more than 100 national and international meetings and conferences. Dr. Raman has mentored and inspired hundreds of medical students, residents, postdoctoral research fellows, and body imaging fellows throughout his carrier at UCLA abdominal radiology. His current research focuses are prostate multiparametric MRI and MR-targeted biopsy, liver and renal tumor imaging, image-guided tumor ablation, and application of machine and deep learning for cancer detection.

Marina Scarpelli, MD is currently the Director of the Pathological Anatomy Service, United Hospital, Ancona, Italy. Her postgraduate training and professional experience includes the Institute of Neurological Sciences, Department of Neuropathology, University Of Glasgow; Department of Paediatrics and Neonatal Medicine, Jerry Lewis Muscle Centre Laboratories, Royal Postgraduate Medical School, Hammersmith Hospital, London; Histopathology Department Royal Postgraduate Medical School, Hammersmith Hospital, London; University of Arizona, Optical Sciences Center, Tucson, Arizona; and University of Turku, Finland. Dr. Scarpelli's previous positions include Full Professor of Pathology, Department. of Biomedical Sciences and Public Health, Polytechnic University of the Marche Region; Assistant Pathologist, University of Ancona, Italy, 1987–2003; Associate Professor of Pathology, University of Ancona; and Assistant Neurosurgeon, Department of Neurosurgery, Ancona, Italy. She received her Medical Doctor (cum laude) degree in 1976 from University of Ancona, School of Medicine, Italy, with a specialty in Pathology and Laboratory Techniques. Dr. Scarpelli's field of interest includes neuropathology with a focus on CNS tumors and the development of new diagnostic and prognostic markers that can be utilized in the clinical management; uropathology, in particular carcinoma of the prostate and urinary bladder; and endocrine pathology with a special interest in adrenal gland and thyroid tumors.

Ryan W. Speir, MD completed his Urology training in 2015 at Madigan Army Medical Center in Tacoma, WA. He served as a faculty for 3 years at Tripler Army Medical Center in Honolulu, HI from 2015 to 2018. He returned to training in 2018 and is currently a urologic oncology fellow at Indiana University.

Martha F. Terrazas, MD is an Assistant Professor of Abdominal and Oncologic Imaging at the University of New Mexico Radiology and UNM Cancer Center. She completed her medical school training and radiology residency at the University of New Mexico, School of Medicine, and completed an MR Predominant Body Imaging Fellowship at Northwestern University in 2019. As a trainee, she has participated for the SAR Disease Focused Panel for Prostate Cancer. Dr. Terrazas is very passionate about resident education by creating a positive and collegial learning environment to provide quality patient care.

Baris Turkbey, MD is an Associate Research Physician at the Molecular Imaging Program, National Cancer Institute, NIH. He is a member of PI-RADS Steering Committee. Dr. Turkbey's main research areas include imaging of prostate cancer (multiparametric MRI, PET-CT), prostate biopsy techniques, focal therapy of prostate cancer, and artificial intelligence.

Annemarijke van Luijtelaar, MD is a medical doctor and PhD candidate in the Department of Radiology and Nuclear Medicine at the Radboudumc, Nijmegen.

Dr. van Luijtelaar studied medicine at the Radboud University Nijmegen. In 2016 she completed her research internship aimed at "Direct in-bore Magnetic Resonance Image-guided prostate biopsy in men with and without prior negative systematic Transrectal Ultrasound-guided biopsy" in the Department of Radiology and Nuclear Medicine of the Radboudumc. In July 2018, Dr. van Luijtelaar started her PhD under supervision of Jurgen Fütterer, Michiel Sedelaar, and Joyce Bomers. The project is focused on the effect of focal treatment of prostate cancer with Magnetic Resonance-guided focal laser ablation and Transurethral Ultrasound ablation (TULSA).

Ryan D. Ward, MD received his medical degree from the University of Tennessee and completed residency at The Cleveland Clinic Foundation where he served as chief resident and was the first Thomas F. Meaney research scholar. While there, he held the academic appointment of Clinical Instructor of Radiology with the Cleveland Clinic Lerner College of Medicine of Case Western Reserve University. Dr. Ward is currently completing an abdominal imaging fellowship at Massachusetts General Hospital in Boston, where he holds the Clinical Assistant of Abdominal Imaging academic appointment with MGH and the Harvard Medical School. His research focus is in imaging of the genitourinary tract with special interest in prostate MRI. Dr. Ward has authored or co-authored multiple manuscripts and presented at national meetings on these topics.

Natasha E. Wehrli, MD is a board-certified radiologist specializing in Body Imaging. She is an Assistant Professor of Radiology at Weill Cornell Medical College and Assistant Attending Radiologist at New York-Presbyterian Hospital – Weill Cornell Campus. Dr. Wehrli serves as the Director of the Body Imaging Fellowship and is a member of the Cornell Radiology Residency Education Committee. She earned her BA in Economics from the University of Pennsylvania School of Arts and Sciences in 2002 and was awarded her MD from the University of Pennsylvania School of Medicine in 2007. As a diagnostic imager, Dr. Wehrli specializes in CT, MRI, and ultrasound of the abdomen and pelvis and whole body PET-CT/PET-MRI. Her research interests include advanced MR imaging of the bowel, prostate, and liver; ultrasound elastography; and PET/MRI for evaluation of prostate cancer. Dr. Wehrli's non-radiology research interests include the role of dietary factors in the development of common disease processes and the benefits of evidence-based nutrition in restoring a healthy gut microbiome and in treating/reversing chronic disease.

Antonio C. Westphalen, MD, FSAR became interested in an academic career during medical school, when he first got involved with research, having received support for 2 years from the Brazilian National Council of Research, Scientific Initiation Institutional Program. During the next 2 years after graduation, Dr. Westphalen served the Brazilian military as a primary care physician and was an Internal Medicine post-doctoral scholar at the Federal University of Rio Grande do Sul School of Medicine, Brazil. He subsequently joined and completed his radiology residency in 2001 at the Institute of Cardiology of Rio Grande do Sul/Cardiology University Foundation and Moinhos de Vento Hospital in Porto Alegre, Brazil. In 2003 Dr. Westphalen came to UCSF as a visiting research scholar, and in 2005 he completed a Clinical Fellowship in Abdominal Imaging and then a 1-year Clinical Radiology Research Fellowship, after which he was recruited as a faculty member in the Department of Radiology. During this time, he intensified his academic activities, including research and teaching of trainees and practicing physicians. In 2011, he received his Master's Degree in Clinical Research from the UCSF Department of Epidemiology and Biostatistics, and in 2012 he completed his PhD in Surgical Sciences, Urology, through the Federal University of Rio Grande do Sul, Brazil. Dr. Westphalen has a shared appointment with the UCSF Department of Urology, directs the UCSF Department of Radiology Clinical Prostate MRI Program, and chairs the UCSF Department of Radiology MR Safety Committee.

Joseph H. Yacoub, MD is associate professor of radiology at Georgetown University. Dr. Yacoub completed his radiology residency at the University of Chicago and his fellowship training at Northwestern University. He joined the radiology department at Loyola University Medical Center in Chicago where he started the prostate imaging program. During his time there, he engaged in multiple research and quality improvement projects in prostate imaging where he particularly took interest in multidisciplinary collaboration with urology and radiation oncology colleagues. He then joined the radiology department at Medstar Georgetown University hospital where he continues to focus on teaching and education of prostate MRI. Dr. Yacoub has published multiple review articles on prostate imaging and imaging-guided interventions of the prostate including in *RadioGraphics* and *Radiologic Clinics of North America* and has spoken on the topic in multiple local and national meetings.

1 Pathology of the Benign and Malignant Diseases of the Prostate

Rodolfo Montironi, Roberta Mazzucchelli, Alessia Cimadamore, Marina Scarpelli, Antonio Lopez-Beltran, and Liang Cheng

1.1 Anatomy of the Prostate Gland

The prostate gland is a male reproductive organ whose main function is to secrete prostate fluid, one of the components of semen. It surrounds the urethra and is located posterior to the inferior aspect of symphysis pubis, superior to the urogenital diaphragm, and anterior to the rectum [1]. It lies below the urinary bladder and is in front of the rectum. It is a pyramid-shaped organ with the base located superiorly abutting the urinary bladder and apex pointing inferiorly. It measures approximately 5 cm × 4 cm × 3 cm and weighs 20 g between 20 and 50 years of age and then increases to 30 g between 60 and 80 years of age.

McNeal has identified three zones (Fig. 1.1). The transition zone surrounds the urethra between the colliculus and bladder neck. The central zone forms a funnel or ring-like zone and is located between the transition and peripheral zones. The ejaculatory ducts run through the central zone. The peripheral zone includes the peripheral sections of the prostate gland [1–4].

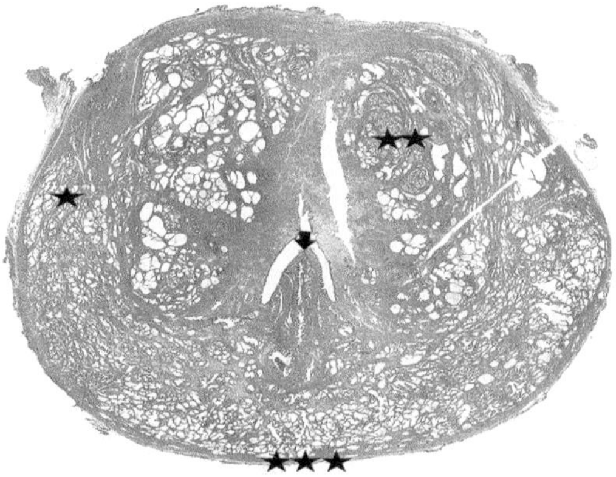

Fig. 1.1 Anatomy of the prostate gland as seen in a whole mount section (arrow = verumontanum; single star = peripheral zone; double star = transition zone; triple star = central zone)

R. Montironi (✉) · R. Mazzucchelli
A. Cimadamore · M. Scarpelli
Polytechnic University of the Marche Region (Ancona), School of Medicine, United Hospitals, Institute of Pathological Anatomy and Histopathology, Ancona, Marche, Italy
e-mail: r.montironi@univpm.it; r.mazzucchelli@univpm.it; m.scarpelli@univpm.it

A. Lopez-Beltran
Faculty of Medicine, University of Cordoba, Unit of Anatomic Pathology, Cordoba, Spain

L. Cheng
Department of Pathology and Laboratory Medicine, Indiana University School of Medicine, Indianapolis, IN, USA
e-mail: lcheng@iupui.edu

1.2 Benign Prostatic Hyperplasia

The size of the prostate gland increases as men get older, usually due to hormone imbalance as well as effects of several growth factors. Benign prostatic hyperplasia is a very common condition in older men [5]. It is defined as the increase in size of the prostatic tissue in the transitional area

T. Tirkes (ed.), *Prostate MRI Essentials*, https://doi.org/10.1007/978-3-030-45935-2_1

around the urethra (also called prostate adenoma) (Fig. 1.2). Over time, this condition causes difficulty in urinating [6, 7].

1.3 Prostatitis

Prostatitis is inflammation of the prostate and can affect any prostate zone. The prevalence of histologically proven prostatitis on autopsy studies is 6–44%. It can be seen at any age during adulthood. The macroscopic appearance is not specific and can mimic prostate cancer (PCa).

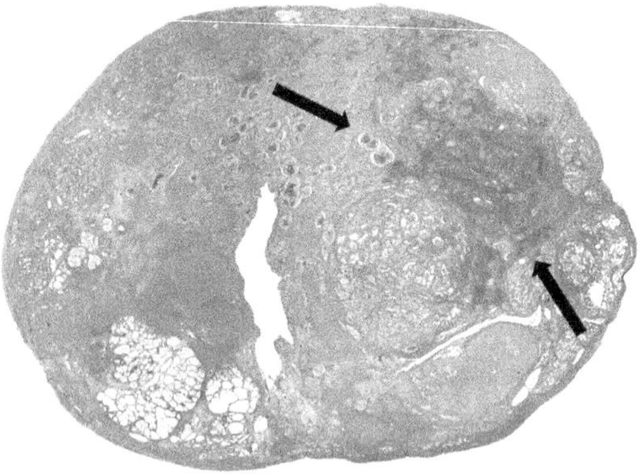

Fig. 1.2 Whole mount section of the transition zone with benign prostatic hyperplasia (arrows: infarction associated with BPH)

Microscopically, inflammation can involve the stroma, epithelium, and lumen of the glands.

Etiology and associated morphologic features include [8, 9]:

- *Acute bacterial prostatitis*: often intraluminal inflammation, showing anywhere from few scattered neutrophils to micro abscesses
- *Chronic prostatitis*: lymphocytic and plasmocytic inflammatory cell infiltration
  - Bacterial
  - Abacterial: this is subdivided into inflammatory and non-inflammatory or prostatodynia
- *Granulomatous prostatitis*: necrotizing or non-necrotizing granulomas may be seen in men who have undergone BCG treatment for bladder cancer; however, most cases are idiopathic (Fig. 1.3) [8].

The differential diagnosis for prostatitis includes (1) lymphocytic infiltration vs chronic lymphocytic lymphoma involving prostate; (2) reactive epithelial changes vs prostatic intraepithelial neoplasia (PIN); and (3) post-atrophic hyperplasia vs PCa. Concerning the outcome, proliferative inflammatory atrophy has been considered as a potential precursor to PIN and PCa [10].

Fig. 1.3 Granulomatous inflammation (arrow: giant cell)

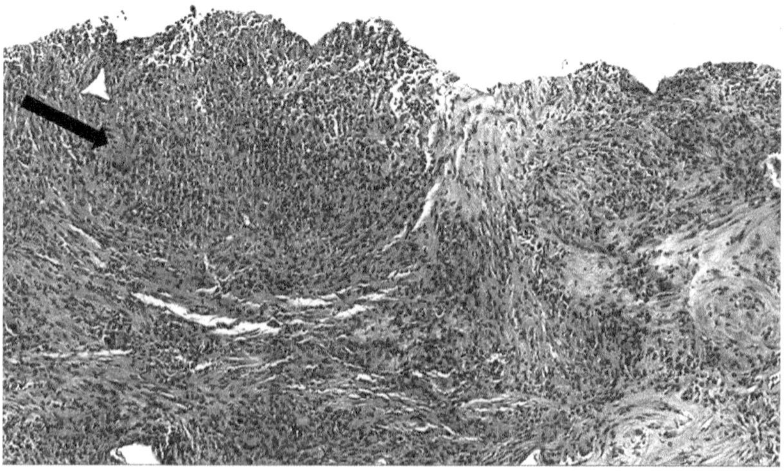

1.4 Putative Preneoplastic and Intra-acinar/Intraductal Neoplasms

1.4.1 Prostatic Intraepithelial Neoplasia (PIN)

PIN consists of preexisting prostatic ducts and acini lined by cytologically atypical cells and is dichotomized into low-grade and high-grade PIN (LGPIN and HGPIN, respectively). PIN is predominantly found in the peripheral zone (75–80%) and rarely in the transition zone (10–15%) or in the central zone (5%). The prevalence of HGPIN in needle biopsy ranges from 5% to 16%, whereas the prevalence of HGPIN in radical prostatectomy specimens is remarkably high (i.e., 85–100% of specimens), reflecting a strong association between this lesion and PCa [11]. HGPIN is identified at low magnification by three important findings: (1) the lining of the ductal structures is darker; (2) it is thicker than the surrounding normal ducts and acini; and (3) a complex intraluminal pattern of growth may be present. At high magnification, there are varying degrees of nuclear enlargement with nuclear stratification, hyperchromasia, and nucleolar prominence (Fig. 1.4) [12, 13].

The nuclei of cells composing LGPIN are enlarged, vary in size, have a normal or slightly increased chromatin content, and possess small or inconspicuous nucleoli. HGPIN is characterized by cells with large nuclei of relatively uniform size, an increased chromatin content, which may be irregularly distributed, and prominent nucleoli that are like those of carcinoma cells.

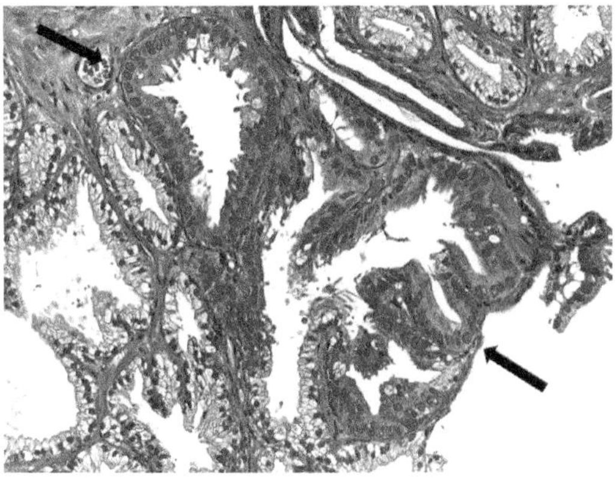

Fig. 1.4 High-grade prostatic intraepithelial neoplasia (HGPIN) (arrows) with adjacent normal ducts and acini

HGPIN is a precursor lesion to some carcinomas of the prostate [11–16]. Contemporary data report that the median risk of cancer following a diagnosis of HGPIN on biopsy is only 22% (the median risk of finding cancer in a repeat biopsy following a benign diagnosis is 15–19%). The number of cores involved by HGPIN is the pathological parameter that predicts a higher risk of subsequent carcinoma on re-biopsy. Finding HGPIN on more than three cores is associated with a higher risk of subsequent cancer and warrants repeating the biopsy within 1 year. For cases with one or two cores of HGPIN on needle biopsy, repeat needle biopsy is not recommended unless clinically indicated [11, 16]. In cases with HGPIN and adjacent small atypical glands, the risk of cancer is equivalent to that of "atypical glands suspicious for carcinoma" warranting a re-biopsy within 3–6 months of diagnosis [15].

1.4.2 Intraductal Carcinoma of the Prostate (IDC-P)

The 2016 WHO definition of intraductal carcinoma of the prostate is "intra-acinar and/or intraductal neoplastic epithelial proliferation that has some features of high-grade prostatic intraepithelial neoplasia (HGPIN) but exhibits much greater architectural and/or cytological atypia, typically associated with high-grade, high-stage prostate carcinoma" (Fig. 1.5) [17].

Intraductal carcinoma of the prostate (IDC-P) represents a late event in PCa evolution, with intraductal spread of aggressive prostatic carcinoma, i.e., invasion of preexisting ducts and acini by high-grade PCa [18]. A minority of cases, however, may be precursor lesions [19]. IDC-P is not assigned a Gleason grade [17, 20].

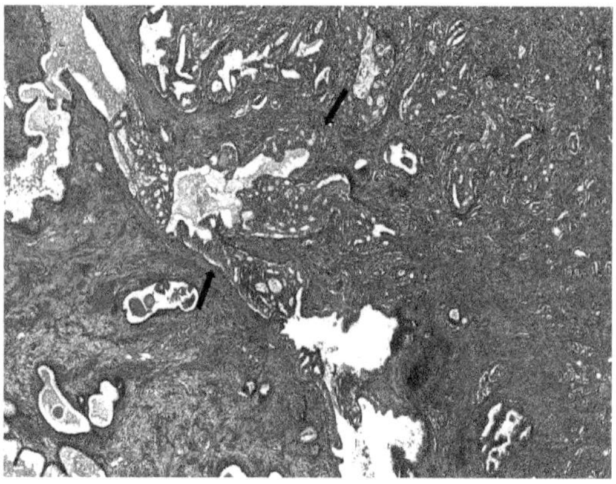

Fig. 1.5 Intraductal carcinoma of the prostate (arrows) showing intraductal spread of aggressive prostate carcinoma

Diagnostic separation of IDC-P from HGPIN is very important because of its association with an average Gleason score of 8 and stage pT3 prostatic PCa in the radical prostatectomy specimen [19, 21, 22]. In contrast to HGPIN, IDC-P exhibits a solid or dense cribriform pattern or a loose cribriform or micropapillary pattern with either marked nuclear atypia (i.e., nuclear size 6 greater than normal) or comedonecrosis [23–25]. IDC-P shows chromosomal translocations involving the PTEN loss and ERG expression, whereas PTEN loss is rare in HGPIN, and ERG expression is very uncommon [24, 26, 27].

Many genetic alterations have been described in IDC-P. ERG status is 100% concordant between IDC-P and adjacent invasive carcinoma. PTEN loss between IDC-P and adjacent acinar carcinoma is concordant in 92% of cases [26, 27].

Staining for basal cell markers should be considered if there is a concern for the presence of intraductal carcinoma only or invasive cancer or when the Gleason grade could change with the diagnosis of IDC-P [22–25]. Intraductal carcinoma is usually associated with high-grade and poor prognostic parameters at radical prostatectomy. Even when intraductal carcinoma is identified without concomitant invasive carcinoma in the prostate biopsy, definitive therapy may be indicated to the patient [18, 19].

1.4.3 Atypical Adenomatous Hyperplasia (Adenosis)

Atypical adenomatous hyperplasia (AAH) is characterized by circumscribed proliferation of closely packed small glands that tend to merge with histologically benign glands. AAH has been considered a premalignant lesion of the transition zone (Fig. 1.6). A direct transition from AAH to cancer has not been documented [28–30].

1.4.4 Atypical Small Acinar Proliferation

Atypical small acinar proliferation (ASAP; also called atypical focus, suspicious but not diagnostic of malignancy) is a diagnostic category rather than an entity. It represents a microscopic growth of small acini with insufficient cytological abnormalities to warrant the diagnosis of malignancy (Fig. 1.7). The incidence of ASAP is between 2% and 9% [15, 31].

The distinction between benign proliferations that mimic cancer and atypical glandular proliferations that are suspicious for, but not diagnostic of prostate carcinoma requires accurate histopathological assessment and use of immunohistochemistry. Most of the information is available on hematoxylin- and eosin-stained sections,

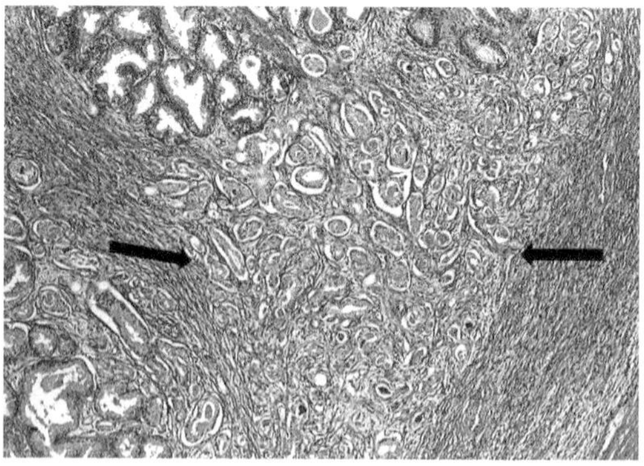

Fig. 1.6 Adenosis (atypical adenomatous hyperplasia) (arrows) is characterized by circumscribed proliferation of closely packed small glands that tends to merge with histologically benign glands

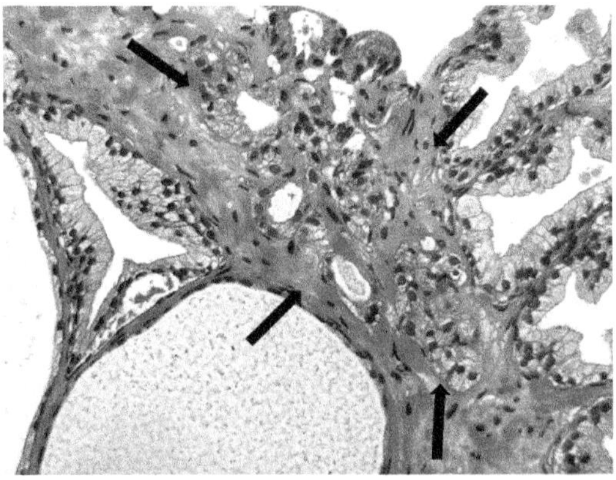

Fig. 1.7 Atypical small acinar proliferation (arrows). ASAP represents a microscopic growth of small acini with insufficient cytological abnormalities to warrant the diagnosis of malignancy

while immunohistochemical stains are used for confirmation.

Isolated ASAP has a predictive value of 37% for cancer [32]. This is only a slight decrease from 45% observed between 1989 and 1996 [15, 33]. Some of the decrease in predictive value of ASAP for cancer in recent studies is probably due to the use of extended biopsy techniques and advances in immunostaining.

Given the documented high risk of cancer in patients with ASAP, it is reasonable to consider repeating the biopsy within 3 to 4 months after the initial diagnosis. In subsequent biopsies, the chance of detecting cancer greatly increases, not only at the biopsy site but within the adjacent areas as well [34, 35]. Park et al. reported 65% probability of finding a cancer at the original ASAP site, which increases to 88% if it also involves the adjacent sites [36].

1.5 Prostate Cancer (PCa)

PCa is the most frequently diagnosed noncutaneous malignant neoplasm in men. In this chapter we discuss classification, grading, staging, and current definition of clinically significant PCa [37–39]. Tissue biomarkers predicting upgrading and/or significant disease and tissue-based genomic tests for diagnosis and prognosis are mentioned briefly.

1.5.1 New Variants of Acinar Adenocarcinoma

Some variants of acinar adenocarcinoma (Fig. 1.8) can be difficult to diagnose since they appear deceptively benign.

These variants include atrophic, microcystic, pseudohyperplastic, and foamy gland PCa [40, 41]. There are also variants characterized by worse prognosis when compared to usual acinar adenocarcinoma. These variants are signet ring-like, sarcomatoid, and pleomorphic giant cell PCa [39, 42–44]. The newly recognized acinar adenocarcinoma variants were added to the 2016 WHO classification. These are microcystic adenocarcinoma, pleomorphic giant cell adenocarcinoma, and large cell neuroendocrine carcinoma [39].

Microcystic adenocarcinoma is a deceptively benign appearing variant of acinar PCa, and the assigned Gleason pattern is 3. Since glands in PCa rarely show cystic changes, microcystic adenocarcinoma may be confused with cystic change in benign atrophic glands. The glands lack basal cells on immunohistochemistry using p63 and 34bE12 antibodies. Immunohistochemical expression of alpha-methylacyl-CoA racemase is present [40, 41] (Fig. 1.9).

Pleomorphic giant cell adenocarcinoma is a rare variant of PCa, characterized by the presence of giant, bizarre, anaplastic cells with pleomorphic nuclei. This variant is unusual in terms of the degree of nuclear atypia. In fact, even the highest grade of usual acinar adenocarcinoma

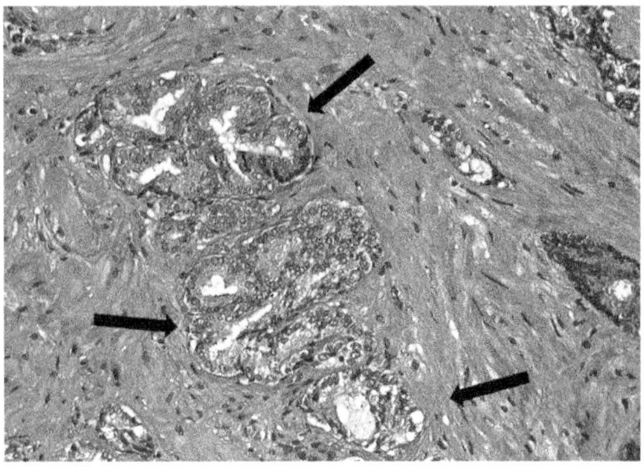

Fig. 1.8 Acinar adenocarcinoma, usual type (arrows)

typically displays nuclei that are relatively uniform. Some patients have a history of hormonal or radiation therapy. The clinical course is expected to be highly aggressive [42–44].

Large cell neuroendocrine carcinoma is a very rare neuroendocrine tumor variant of the PCa [45, 46]. Almost all cases are seen after hormonal therapy for PCa. The morphologic features are identical to those of large cell neuroendocrine carcinoma in other organs. Outcome is expected to be very poor with the mean survival being only 7 months even after platinum-based chemotherapy [45].

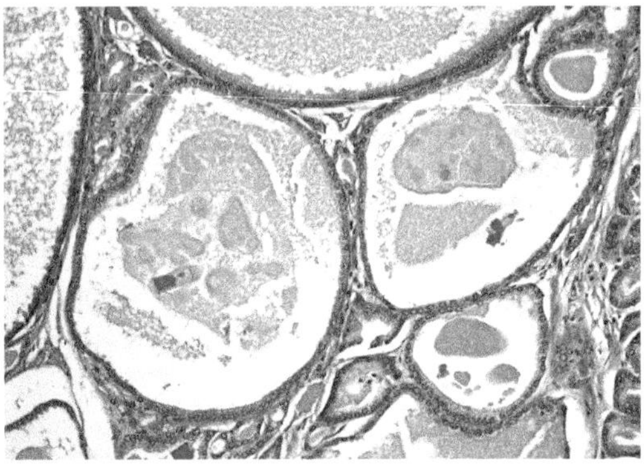

Fig. 1.9 Acinar adenocarcinoma with microcystic features (PCA glands with cystic changes)

1.5.2 Grading of Prostate Cancer

The Gleason grading system is one of the most important prognostic factors in PCa. In 1966 D.F. Gleason recognized heterogeneity of PCa by assigning two grades to the two most common patterns [47]. The Gleason system has undergone important and substantial changes since the original proposal following two ISUP conferences [48, 49]. The current assignment of the Gleason score (GS) is based on the 2014 ISUP consensus criteria [49]. The consensus addressed key areas including definitions of the grading patterns (GP) of usual and variants of PCa, exclusion of IDC-P from grading, and the support for the novel grade groups (GG) system. Only well-formed discrete glands are included in the modified GP 3. Cribriform glands (Fig. 1.10) are all considered GP 4, independent of size and histology. The morphologic spectrum of the current GP 4 pattern also includes fused, ill-defined, and glomeruloid glands, in addition to cribriform glands [49, 50].

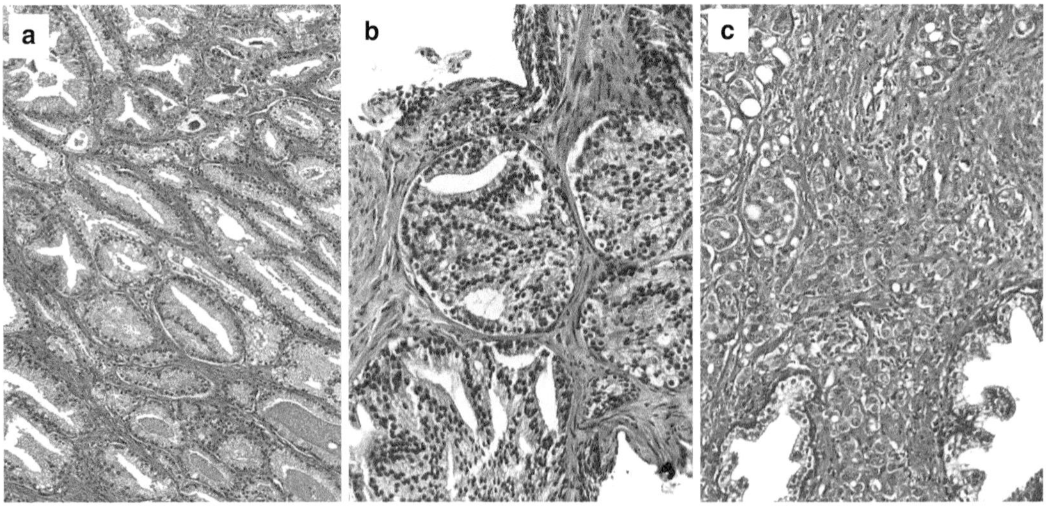

Fig. 1.10 Acinar adenocarcinoma (examples of a (**a**) Gleason pattern 3, well-formed discrete glands; (**b**) Gleason pattern 4, cribriform; and (**c**) Gleason pattern 5, lack of gland formation with or without poorly formed/fused/cribriform glands

1.5.3 5-Tiered Grading Prognostic System

The basis for the proposal was the five grade groups (GG) originally derived from data from Johns Hopkins Hospital [51, 52]. The GG, first described in 2013, equates the GS with the following prognostic groups: GG 1 (GS 6), GG 2 (GS 3 + 4 = 7), GG 3 (GS 4 + 3 = 7), GG 4 (GS 8), and GG 5 (GS 9 and 10) (Table 1.1).

The key contributions of using GG are as follows:

- GG 1 is designated as the lowest score in contrast to 6 in GS, which is at the middle of the scale (GS 2 to 10). This is a recurring problem when counseling patients for active surveillance.
- GS 7 is not a homogenous cancer and is split into GG 2 and GG 3, projecting different approaches in prognosis and management in trials and clinical practice.
- GS 8–10, often considered as one group of high-grade tumors, can be split prognostically and stratified into different treatment strategies in GG 4 and GG 5.

Table 1.1 Morphologic definition of the five prognostic grade groups (GG)

GG	Gleason score	Morphologic definition
1	≤ 6	Individual discrete well-formed glands only
2	3 + 4	Predominantly well-formed glands with lesser component of poorly formed/fused/cribriform glands
3	4 + 3	Predominantly poorly formed/fused/cribriform glands with lesser component of well-formed glands
4	4 + 4 *or* 3 + 5 *or* 5 + 3	Only poorly formed/fused/cribriform glands *or* Predominantly well-formed glands and lesser component lacking glands *or* Predominantly lacking glands and lesser component of well-formed glands
5	4 + 5 *or* 5 + 4 *or* 5 + 5	Lack gland formation (or with necrosis) with *or* without poorly formed/fused/cribriform glands [58]

The accurate prognostic stratification of GG has been validated in a large multi-institutional cohort including prostate biopsy and radical prostatectomies [51, 52]. The 2016 WHO guidelines adopted GG, updated CAP prostate cancer protocols, and clinical guidelines [39, 53–55]. GG will be used in combination with GS for the foreseeable future with its value analyzed over time [56].

1.5.4 Staging of Prostate Cancer

The American Joint Commission on Cancer (AJCC) guidelines modified staging and prognostic stage grouping for prostate cancer. In the eighth edition of these guidelines, T2 category (i.e., the pathologically organ confined cancers) is no longer substaged on the basis of bilaterality and extent of involvement (pT2a, pT2b, and pT2c) (Table 1.2) [37]. This decision was based on the lack of the prognostic evidence [57–61]. In addition to this, the previous pT2b was extremely rare, and small multifocal neoplasms could be assigned to a higher subcategory of pT2 [59, 61]. There are no clinical studies correlating the previous pT2 stage subgroupings with survival in localized PCa. There is emerging data suggesting that unlike the pT2 substaging, tumor volume has a higher prognostic value [62]. However, the 3-tiered T2 subclassification is still used for clini-

Table 1.2 Updates to the staging of prostate cancer by the American Joint Commission on Cancer (AJCC), eighth edition [63]. (Used from Paner et al. [63], with permission from Elsevier)

Category	Details
pT2	Pathologically organ-confined tumors no longer subcategorized based on bilaterality and extent of involvement
Histologic grade	Gleason score to be based on ISUP 2014 criteria Grade group to be reported in addition to Gleason
Prognostic stage group III	Includes select organ-confined disease tumors based on PSA and Gleason/grade group status
Statistical prediction models	Prognostic models that met all AJCC quality criteria added

cal practice of tumor staging and used in risk assessment and treatment [37].

1.5.4.1 Prognostic Stage Groups (Major Features)

With the incorporation of serum PSA levels and GG into the AJCC prognostic stage groups, organ-confined PCa (T1–T2) may be staged as prognostic stage group IIIA [37]. This is in distinction to lymph node negative, non-organ-confined prostate cancer (T3–T4) (Fig. 1.11), where GG1–GG4 is prognostic stage group IIIB, i.e., a stage group for which some clinicians would recommend adjuvant radiation. Adjustments in stage group selections were made in order to be consistent with the clinical risk groups in the guidelines, having similar treatment options for T3 or T4 and T1–T2 but with GG5 and PSA of >20 ng/ml. Stage group IIC was also added [64]. Stage groups III and IV were both subdivided into A and B. This modification has been validated recently in a large radical prostatectomy cohort [65].

1.5.4.2 Union of the International Cancer Control (UICC), Eighth Edition

Unlike the eighth edition AJCC, the eighth edition of the UICC retained the pT2 substaging (pT2a, pT2b, and pT2c) and adopted the GG. The designation of pNmi (mi stands for micrometastasis) for regional lymph node metastasis no larger than 2 mm has been added, although the clinical relevance of this subcategory in PCa remains to be validated. The eighth edition UICC also omitted prognostic stage groups (i.e., with PSA and GG incorporated), only including the anatomic stage grouping [66, 63].

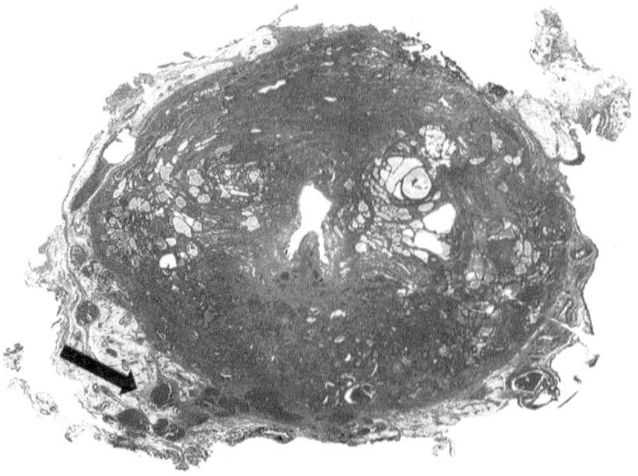

Fig. 1.11 Radical prostatectomy specimen with extraprostatic extension (arrow)

1.5.5 Clinically Significant Versus Insignificant Prostate Cancer

The definition of clinically significant versus insignificant PCa is an ongoing process that was initiated several years ago, when evidence was acquired that a great proportion of men with PCa discovered at autopsy did not have any clinical signs and symptoms [67–69]. Studies looking into radical prostatectomy specimens established the definition of significant cancer for PCa: tumor volume of 0.5 cm^3, GS 6 (GG 1), and organ-confined disease. Data from radical prostatectomy analysis were then used to develop prediction models for significant PCa in needle biopsies (Tables 1.3 and 1.4).

The first of such models was used to identify the first active surveillance criteria, known as the Epstein criteria, in which patients with a GS 6 (GG 1) PCa involving fewer than two cores, and < 50% of any given core, and a PSA density of <0.15 ng/ml per cm^3 had a minimal risk of significant cancer [68]. These criteria were then adopted in the definition of the "very-low-risk category" of the National Comprehensive Cancer Network guidelines. With the increase in the popularity of active surveillance, much research has

Table 1.3 Useful prognostic features in disease risk stratification on prostate biopsy

Prognostic features
Tumor histologic type (acinar, ductal, etc.)
Tumor grade (Gleason score and grade group)
Percentage of high-grade cancer
Number of cores involved by cancer
Percentage (or length in mm) of core involved by cancer
Unilateral vs bilateral disease
Perineural invasion
Extraprostatic extension
Seminal vesicle invasion

Table 1.4 Useful prognostic features in disease risk stratification on radical prostatectomy

Prognostic features
Tumor histologic type (acinar, ductal, etc.)
Tumor grade (Gleason score and grade group)
Pathologic stage
Extraprostatic extension
Seminal vesicle invasion
Margin status
Lymphovascular invasion
Tumor volume

been carried out to better define significant versus insignificant cancer, in order to be able to safely offer active surveillance to a larger proportion of patients without the risk of undertreatment [68].

1.5.6 Tissue Biomarkers

Morphologic findings associated with PCa have been the most useful in predicting tumor biology and disease prognosis. Recent investigations have demonstrated that genomic biomarkers can predict clinical outcomes in a manner that outperforms traditional morphology-based tumor grading and staging [70–76].

There is an increased need for biomarkers to improve upon conventional risk assessment tools to aid in decision-making. Several diagnostic and prognostic biomarker tests have been introduced recently. These tests include PHI, 4 K score, SelectMDx, ConfirmMDx, PCA3, MiPS, and ExoDX. ConfirmMDx is the only tissue-based assay. Prognostic tests that have been used to aid in treatment selection (i.e., definitive treatment vs active surveillance) include OncotypeDX GPS, Prolaris, ProMark, DNA-ploidy, and Decipher [77–79].

References

1. McNeal JE. Normal and pathologic anatomy of prostate. Urology. 1981;17:11–6.
2. Fine SW, Al-Ahmadie HA, Gopalan A, Tickoo SK, Scardino PT, Reuter VE. Anatomy of the anterior prostate and extraprostatic space. A contemporary surgical pathology analysis. Adv Anat Pathol. 2007;14:401–7.
3. Yossepowitch O, Briganti A, Eastham JA, Epstein JI, Graefen M, Montironi R, et al. Positive surgical margins after radical prostatectomy: a systematic review and contemporary update. Eur Urol. 2014;65:303–13.
4. Cheng L, MacLennan GT, Lopez-Beltran A, Montironi R. Anatomic, morphologic and genetic heterogeneity of prostate cancer: implications for clinical practice. Expert Rev Anticancer Ther. 2012;12:1371–4.
5. Roehrborn CG. Benign prostatic hyperplasia: an overview. Rev Urol. 2005;7(Suppl 9):S3–S14.
6. Ozayar A, Zumrutbas AE, Yaman O. The relationship between lower urinary tract symptoms (LUTS), diagnostic indicators of benign prostatic hyperplasia (BPH), and erectile dysfunction in patients with moderate to severely symptomatic BPH. Int Urol Nephrol. 2008;40(4):933–9.
7. Foster CS. Pathology of benign prostatic hyperplasia. Prostate Suppl. 2000;9:4–14.
8. Epstein JI, Hutchins GM. Granulomatous prostatitis: distinction among allergic, nonspecific, and post-transurethral resection lesions. Hum Pathol. 1984;15:818–25.
9. Magri V, Boltri M, Cai T, Colombo R, Cuzzocrea S, De Visschere P, et al. Multidisciplinary approach to prostatitis. Arch Ital Urol Androl. 2019;90:227–48.
10. De Marzo AM, Marchi VL, Epstein JI, Nelson WG. Proliferative inflammatory atrophy of the prostate: implications for prostatic carcinogenesis. Am J Pathol. 1999;155:1985–92.
11. Bostwick DG, Humphrey PA, Montironi R, Srigley JR. High-grade prostatic intraepithelial neoplasia. In: Moch H, Humphrey PA, Ulbrigh TM, Reuter VE, editors. WHO classification of tumours of the urinary system and male genital organs. Lyon: IARC; 2016. p. 162–3.
12. Bostwick DG, Amin MB, Dundore P, Marsh W, Schultz DS. Architectural patterns of high-grade prostatic intraepithelial neoplasia. Hum Pathol. 1993;24:298–310.
13. Montironi R, Mazzucchelli R, Lopez-Beltran A, Scarpelli M, Cheng L. Prostatic intraepithelial neoplasia: its morphological and molecular diagnosis and clinical significance. BJU Int. 2011;108:1394–401.
14. De Marzo AM, Haffner MC, Lotan TL, Yegnasubramanian S, Nelson WG. Premalignancy in prostate cancer: rethinking what we know. Cancer Prev Res. 2016;9:648–56.
15. Epstein JI, Herawi M. Prostate needle biopsies containing prostatic intraepithelial neoplasia or atypical foci suspicious for carcinoma: implications for patient care. J Urol. 2006;175:820–34.
16. Herawi M, Kahane H, Cavallo C, Epstein JI. Risk of prostate cancer on first re-biopsy within 1 year following a diagnosis of high grade prostatic intraepithelial neoplasia is related to the number of cores sampled. J Urol. 2006;175:121–4.
17. Epstein JI, Oxley J, Ro JY, Van der Kwast T, Zhou M. Intraductal carcinoma. In: Moch H, Humphrey PA, Ulbrigh TM, Reutere VE, editors. WHO classification

of tumours of the urinary system and male genital organs. Lyon: IARC; 2016. p. 164–5.
18. McNeal JE, Yemoto CE. Spread of adenocarcinoma within prostatic ducts and acini. Morphologic and clinical correlations. Am J Surg Pathol. 1996;20:802–14.
19. Robinson BD, Epstein JI. Intraductal carcinoma of the prostate without invasive carcinoma on needle biopsy: emphasis on radical prostatectomy findings. J Urol. 2010;184:1328–33.
20. Cohen RJ, Wheeler TM, Bonkhoff H, Rubin AM. A proposal on the identification, histologic reporting, and implications of intraductal prostatic carcinoma. Arch Pathol Lab Med. 2007;131:1103–9.
21. Guo CC, Epstein JI. Intraductal carcinoma of the prostate on needle biopsy: histologic features and clinical significance. Mod Pathol. 2006;19:1528–35.
22. Watts K, Li J, Magi-Galluzzi C, Zhou M. Incidence and clinicopathological characteristics of intraductal carcinoma detected in prostate biopsies: a prospective cohort study. Histopathology. 2013;63:574–9.
23. Shah RB, Magi-Galluzzi C, Han B, Zhou M. Atypical cribriform lesions of the prostate: relationship to prostatic carcinoma and implication for diagnosis in prostate biopsies. Am J Surg Pathol. 2010;34:470–7.
24. Shah RB, Zhou M. Atypical cribriform lesions of the prostate: clinical significance, differential diagnosis and current concept of intraductal carcinoma of the prostate. Adv Anat Pathol. 2012;19:270–8.
25. Zhou M. High-grade prostatic intraepithelial neoplasia, PIN-like carcinoma, ductal carcinoma, and intraductal carcinoma of the prostate. Mod Pathol. 2018;31:S71–9.
26. Han B, Suleman K, Wang L, Siddiqui J, Sercia L, Magi-Galluzzi C, et al. ETS gene aberrations in atypical cribriform lesions of the prostate: implications for the distinction between intraductal carcinoma of the prostate and cribriform high-grade prostatic intraepithelial neoplasia. Am J Surg Pathol. 2010;34:478–85.
27. Lotan TL, Gumuskaya B, Rahimi H, Hicks JL, Iwata T, Robinson BD, et al. Cytoplasmic PTEN protein loss distinguishes intraductal carcinoma of the prostate from high-grade prostatic intraepithelial neoplasia. Mod Pathol. 2013;26:587–603.
28. Cheng L, Montironi R, Davidson DD, Wang M, Lopez-Beltran A, Zhang S. Molecular evidence supporting the precursor nature of atypical adenomatous hyperplasia of the prostate. Mol Carcinog. 2019;58:1272–8.
29. Qian J, Bostwick DG. The extent and zonal location of prostatic intraepithelial neoplasia and atypical adenomatous hyperplasia: relationship with carcinoma in radical prostatectomy specimens. Pathol Res Pract. 1995;191:860–7.
30. Zhang C, Montironi R, MacLennan GT, Lopez-Beltran A, Li Y, Tan PH, et al. Is atypical adenomatous hyperplasia of the prostate a precursor lesion? Prostate. 2011;71:1746–51.
31. Montironi R, Scattoni V, Mazzucchelli R, Lopez-Beltran A, Bostwick DG, Montorsi F. Atypical foci suspicious but not diagnostic of malignancy in prostate needle biopsies (also referred to as "atypical small acinar proliferation suspicious for but not diagnostic of malignancy"). Eur Urol. 2006;50:666–74.
32. Schlesinger C, Bostwick DG, Iczkowski KA. High-grade prostatic intraepithelial neoplasia and atypical small acinar proliferation: predictive value for cancer in current practice. Am J Surg Pathol. 2005;29:1201–7.
33. Borboroglu PG, Sur RL, Roberts JL, Amling CL. Repeat biopsy strategy in patients with atypical small acinar proliferation or high grade prostatic intraepithelial neoplasia on initial prostate needle biopsy. J Urol. 2001;166:866–70.
34. Ericson KJ, Wenger HC, Rosen AM, Kiriluk KJ, Gerber GS, Paner GP, et al. Prostate cancer detection following diagnosis of atypical small acinar proliferation. Can J Urol. 2017;24:8714–20.
35. Merrick GS, Galbreath RW, Bennett A, Butler WM, Amamovich E. Incidence, grade and distribution of prostate cancer following transperineal template-guided mapping biopsy in patients with atypical small acinar proliferation. World J Urol. 2017;35:1009–13.
36. Park S, Shinohara K, Grossfeld GD, Carroll PR. Prostate cancer detection in men with prior high grade prostatic intraepithelial neoplasia or atypical prostate biopsy. J Urol. 2001;165:1409–14.
37. Buyyounouski MK, Choyke PL, Kattan MW. Prostate. In: Amin MB, Edge SB, Greene FL, et al., editors. AJCC cancer staging manual. 8th ed. New York: Springer; 2017. p. 715–26.
38. Epstein JI, Egevad L, Amin MB, Delahunt B, Srigley JR, Humphrey PA, et al. The 2014 international society of urological pathology (ISUP) consensus conference on Gleason grading of prostatic carcinoma: definition of grading patterns and proposal for a new grading system. Am J Surg Pathol. 2016;40:244–52.
39. Humphrey PA, Amin MB, Berney DM, et al. Acinar adenocarcinoma. In: Moch H, Humphrey PA, Ulbrigh TM, Reutere VE, editors. WHO classification of tumours of the urinary system and male genital organs. Lyon: IARC; 2016. p. 138–62.
40. Humphrey PA. Variants of acinar adenocarcinoma of the prostate mimicking benign conditions. Mod Pathol. 2018;31:S64–70.
41. Yaskiv O, Cao D, Humphrey PA. Microcystic adenocarcinoma of the prostate: a variant of pseudohyperplastic and atrophic patterns. Am J Surg Pathol. 2010;34:556–61.
42. Alharbi AM, De Marzo AM, Hicks JL, Lotan TL, Epstein JI. Prostatic adenocarcinoma with focal pleomorphic giant cell features: a series of 30 cases. Am J Surg Pathol. 2018;42:1286–96.
43. Lopez-Beltran A, Eble JN, Bostwick DG. Pleomorphic giant cell carcinoma of the prostate. Arch Pathol Lab Med. 2005;129:683–5.
44. Parwani AV, Herawi M, Epstein JI. Pleomorphic giant cell adenocarcinoma of the prostate: report of 6 cases. Am J Surg Pathol. 2006;30:1254–9.
45. Evans AJ, Humphrey PA, Belani J, van der Kwast TH, Srigley JR. Large cell neuroendocrine carcinoma of

prostate: a clinicopathologic summary of 7 cases of a rare manifestation of advanced prostate cancer. Am J Surg Pathol. 2006;30:684–93.
46. Fine SW. Neuroendocrine tumors of the prostate. Mod Pathol. 2018;31:S122–32.
47. Gleason DF. Classification of prostatic carcinomas. Cancer Chemother Rep. 1966;50:125–8.
48. Epstein JI, Allsbrook WC, Amin MB, Egevad LL, ISUP Grading Committee. The 2005 International Society of Urological Pathology (ISUP) consensus conference on Gleason grading of prostatic carcinoma. Am J Surg Pathol. 2005;29:1228–42.
49. Epstein JI, Amin MB, Reuter VE, Humphrey PA. Contemporary Gleason grading of prostatic carcinoma: an update with discussion on practical issues to implement the 2014 international society of urological pathology (ISUP) consensus conference on Gleason grading of prostatic carcinoma. Am J Surg Pathol. 2017;41:e1–7.
50. Montironi R, Cimadamore A, Cheng L, Lopez-Beltran A, Scarpelli M. Prostate cancer grading in 2018: limitations, implementations, cribriform morphology, and biological markers. Int J Biol Markers. 2018;33:331–4.
51. Pierorazio PM, Walsh PC, Partin AW, Epstein JI. Prognostic Gleason grade grouping: data based on the modified Gleason scoring system. BJU Int. 2013;111:753–60.
52. Epstein JI, Zelefsky MJ, Sjoberg DD, Nelson JB, Egevad L, Magi-Galluzzi C, et al. A contemporary prostate cancer grading system: a validated alternative to the Gleason score. Eur Urol. 2016;69:428–35.
53. CAP Cancer Protocol Templates. 2017. http://www.cap.org
54. NCCN Clinical practice guidelines in oncology (NCCN guidelines). 2017. https://www.nccn.org/professionals/physician_gls/f_guidelines.asp
55. Sanda MG, Chen RC, Crispino T, et al. Clinically localized prostate cancer. In: AUA/ASTRO/SUO Guideline. 2017. http://www.auanet.org/guidelines/clinically-localized-prostate-cancer-new-(aua/astro/suo-guideline-2017)
56. Montironi R, Cheng L, Cimadamore A, Lopez-Beltran A. Prostate cancer grading: are we heading towards grade grouping version 2? Eur Urol. 2019;75:32–4.
57. Chun FK, Briganti A, Lebeau T, Benayoun S, Lebeau T, Ramirez A, et al. The 2002 AJCC pT2 substages confer no prognostic information on the rate of biochemical recurrence after radical prostatectomy. Eur Urol. 2006;49:273–9.
58. Eichelberger LE, Cheng L. Does pT2b prostate carcinoma exist? Critical appraisal of the 2002 TNM classification of prostate carcinoma. Cancer. 2004;100:2573–6.
59. Ettel M, Kong M, Lee P, Zhou M, Melamed J, Deng FM. Modification of the pT2 substage classification in prostate adenocarcinoma. Hum Pathol. 2016;56:57–63.
60. Kordan Y, Chang SS, Salem S, Cookson MS, Clark PE, Davis R, et al. Pathological stage T2 subgroups to predict biochemical recurrence after prostatectomy. J Urol. 2009;182:2291–5.
61. van der Kwast TH, Amin MB, Billis A, Epstein JI, Griffiths D, Humphrey PA, et al. International society of urological pathology (ISUP) consensus conference on handling and staging of radical prostatectomy specimens. Working group 2: T2 substaging and prostate cancer volume. Mod Pathol. 2011;24:16–25.
62. Epstein JI. Prognostic significance of tumor volume in radical prostatectomy and needle biopsy specimens. J Urol. 2011;186:790–7.
63. Paner GP, Stadler WM, Hansel DE, Montironi R, Lin DW, Amin MB. Updates in the eighth edition of the tumor-node-metastasis staging classification for urologic cancers. Eur Urol. 2018;73:560–9.
64. Bhindi B, Karnes RJ, Rangel LJ, Mason RJ, Gettman MT, Frank I, et al. Independent validation of the American joint committee on cancer 8th edition prostate cancer staging classification. J Urol. 2017;198:1286–94.
65. Buyyounouski MK, Choyke PL, McKenney JK, Sartor O, Sandler HM, Amin MB, et al. Prostate cancer-major changes in the American joint committee on cancer eighth edition cancer staging manual. CA Cancer J Clin. 2017;67:245–53.
66. Herden J, Heidenreich A, Wittekind C, Weissbach L. Predictive value of the UICC and AJCC 8th edition tumor-nodes-metastasis (TNM) classification for patients treated with radical prostatectomy. Cancer Epidemiol. 2018;56:126–32.
67. Epstein JI, Walsh PC, Carmichael M, Brendler CB. Pathologic and clinical findings to predict tumor extent of nonpalpable (stage T1c) prostate cancer. JAMA. 1994;271:368–74.
68. Matoso A, Epstein JI. Defining clinically significant prostate cancer on the basis of pathological findings. Histopathology. 2019;74:135–45.
69. Van der Kwast TH, Roobol MJ. Defining the threshold for significant versus insignificant prostate cancer. Nat Rev Urol. 2013;10:473–82.
70. Chua MLK, Lo W, Pintilie M, Murgic J, Lalonde E, Bhandari V, et al. A prostate cancer "Nimbosus": genomic instability and SChLAP1 dysregulation underpin aggression of intraductal and cribriform subpathologies. Eur Urol. 2017;72:665–74.
71. Cuzick J, Swanson GP, Fisher G, Brothman AR, Berney DM, Reid JE, et al. Prognostic value of an RNA expression signature derived from cell cycle proliferation genes in patients with prostate cancer: a retrospective study. Lancet Oncol. 2011;12:245–55.
72. Klein EA, Cooperberg MR, Magi-Galluzzi C, Simko JP, Falzarano SM, Maddala T, et al. A 17-gene assay to predict prostate cancer aggressiveness in the context of Gleason grade heterogeneity, tumor multifocality, and biopsy undersampling. Eur Urol. 2014;66:550–60.
73. Nguyen JK, Magi-Galluzzi C. Unfavorable pathology, tissue biomarkers and genomic tests with clinical implications in prostate cancer management. Adv Anat Pathol. 2018;25:293–303.

74. Risbridger GP, Taylor RA, Clouston D, Sliwinski A, Thorne H, Hunter S, et al. Patient-derived Xenografts reveal that intraductal carcinoma of the prostate is a prominent pathology in BRCA2 mutation carriers with prostate cancer and correlates with poor prognosis. Eur Urol. 2015;67:496–503.
75. Shore ND, Kella N, Moran B, Boczko J, Bianco FJ, Crawford ED, et al. Impact of the cell cycle progression test on physician and patient treatment selection for localized prostate cancer. J Urol. 2016;195:612–8.
76. Trock BJ, Fedor H, Gurel B, Jenkins RB, Knudsen BS, Fine SW, et al. PTEN loss and chromosome 8 alterations in Gleason grade 3 prostate cancer cores predicts the presence of un-sampled grade 4 tumor: implications for active surveillance. Mod Pathol. 2016;29:764–71.
77. Carneiro A, Priante Kayano P, Gomes Barbosa ÁR, Langer Wroclawski M, Ko Chen C, Cavlini GC, et al. Are localized prostate cancer biomarkers useful in the clinical practice? Tumour Biol. 2018;40(9):1010428318799255.
78. Cucchiara V, Cooperberg MR, Dall'Era M, Lin DW, Montorsi F, Schalken JA, et al. Genomic markers in prostate cancer decision making. Eur Urol. 2018;73:572–82.
79. Kretschmer A, Tilki D. Biomarkers in prostate cancer – current clinical utility and future perspectives. Crit Rev Oncol Hematol. 2017;120:180–93.

What the Urologist Wants to Know from Prostate MRI

2

Ryan W. Speir, Adam C. Calaway, and Michael O. Koch

2.1 Introduction

The role of multi-parametric MRI (mpMRI) in the diagnosis and management of prostate cancer (PCa) has evolved rapidly over the previous decade. For many years, PCa was diagnosed after a suspicious PSA and/or digital rectal examination (DRE) prompted a transrectal ultrasound (TRUS)-guided template biopsy. The biopsies themselves were designed to sample the posterior prostate using a 6-core or 12-core template technique. The detection rate of PCa using this modality alone ranges from 13% to 63% based on PSA level and DRE suspicion [1–5]. Occurring along parallel pathways, two significant changes in the diagnosis and management of prostate cancer occurred. First, it became apparent that urologists were identifying and treating a significant portion of clinically insignificant cancers. Second, men were being biopsied based on an imperfect screening test. As MRI technology improved over the previous decade, its use in detection of PCa has expanded. At present, clinical indications include prior negative biopsies with ongoing clinical concern for underlying malignancy, presurgical planning, active surveillance, and local recurrence after prostatectomy. In this review, we will begin by discussing the role of mpMRI at time of initial diagnosis, both in the biopsy-naive and prior biopsy setting. We will discuss its use in active surveillance (AS), both in confirmatory biopsy and ongoing surveillance. Finally, we will review the role prior to local (or surgical) therapy of known PCa.

2.2 Initial Diagnosis

Most solid organ malignancies are identified using imaging, which may or may not prompt a biopsy for confirmation. Until recently, PCa was identified either by screening with PSA and/or DRE that would prompt a TRUS-guided biopsy or once the disease was already advanced and the patient was presenting with symptoms. An ideal screening test would be noninvasive and inexpensive and would identify men at risk for death or morbidity from disease and not identify men with clinically insignificant disease. This would minimize the rate of unnecessary biopsies and also the percentage of men found to have clinically insignificant disease.

The role of mpMRI in the screening or initial diagnosis began in the setting of a prior negative

R. W. Speir
Indiana University, Department of Urology, Indianapolis, IN, USA
e-mail: rwspeir@iu.edu

A. C. Calaway
Case Western University/University Hospitals, Department of Urology, Cleveland, OH, USA
e-mail: adam.calaway@uhhospitals.org

M. O. Koch (✉)
Indiana University Health, Department of Urology, Indianapolis, IN, USA
e-mail: miokoch@iupui.edu

T. Tirkes (ed.), *Prostate MRI Essentials*, https://doi.org/10.1007/978-3-030-45935-2_2

biopsy when there was still ongoing concern for malignancy. This represents a challenging group of patients, particularly when the PSA continues to rise. The fear is that clinically significant (CS) PCa still exists and many providers feel unprepared to offer their patients reassurance from the prior negative biopsy. The role of transperineal and extended or saturation biopsies has been previously evaluated, and while they do identify more cancers than the standard TRUS-guided biopsy, they are more invasive and associated with additional morbidity [6, 7]. There are also a number of blood and urine biomarkers designed to improve patient selection including Prostate Health Index (PHI), ConfirmMDx, SelectMDx, and the 4Kscore. While these tests have been validated to risk-stratify patients regarding their likelihood of having CS-PCa, they fail to improve the diagnostic yield of repeat biopsies. mpMRI has the potential advantage in this setting to not only improve patient selection for biopsy, but also to help guide the biopsy with the expectation the this will improve the diagnostic accuracy.

2.2.1 First Biopsy

As the mpMRI and TRUS/MRI fusion technology improved and the ability to identify CS PCa in the repeat biopsy setting became more accepted, interest shifted to the use of mpMRI prior to the initial biopsy. Tontilla et al. evaluated 130 biopsy naïve men referred for prostate biopsy based on PSA elevation alone. Patients were randomized to mpMRI/TRUS fusion targeted biopsies or standard TRUS-guided random biopsies. The overall cancer detection rate was 64% vs 57% ($p = 0.5$), while the CS PCa detection rate was 55% vs 45% ($p = 0.8$). They concluded that the use of mpMRI/TRUS fusion biopsies did not improve the cancer detection rates compared to TRUS random biopsies alone [8]. In contrast, Gaunay et al. evaluated 400 men, of which 231 patients had no prior biopsy. The overall prevalence of PCa in this subgroup was 55% with a CS PCa detection rate of 42%. The mpMRI sensitivity, specificity, positive predictive value (PPV), and negative predictive value (NPV) were 94%, 36%, 65%, and 82% for all PCa, while it was 95%, 30%, 50%, and 89% for CS PCa [9]. These results are in line with Siddiqui et al., who found an overall cancer detection rate of 56%, while the CS PCa detection rate was 32.7% in 196 biopsy naïve men who underwent mpMRI followed by targeted fusion biopsies and concurrent standard biopsies [10]. The PRECISION trial was a multicenter, randomized non-inferiority trial which assigned 500 biopsy naïve men to either MRI with/without biopsy or TRUS-guided biopsy. The men with a positive mpMRI underwent targeted biopsy alone without random biopsy while those with a negative mpMRI did not undergo biopsy. Of the men with a positive mpMRI, the CS PCa detection rate was 38% compared to 26% in the TRUS-guided biopsy group ($p = 0.005$). They concluded that using mpMRI to target lesions prior to initial biopsy was a better approach in regard to CS PCa detection when compared to standard TRUS-guided biopsy [11].

The utility of a negative mpMRI is also contested at the present time. Wysock et al. examined 75 patients with negative mpMRI prior to biopsy. In the biopsy naïve subset, the NPV was 81.3% for all cancer detection and 98.7% for CS PCa. These findings suggest that in patients with a negative mpMRI, the TRUS biopsy can be avoided [12]. Elkhoury et al. came to different conclusions when examining their subset of men with negative mpMRI. In this group without an identifiable lesion, the PCa detection rate was 15%. They concluded that the combined biopsy approach was superior to any biopsy approach in isolation. Additionally, given the 15% rate of CS PCa in men with normal mpMRI, a negative MRI should not obviate the need for systematic biopsy in men when it is otherwise indicated [13]. From the urologist's standpoint, taking 12 systematic cores samples in the at-risk patient with a negative mpMRI albeit with a small risk to the patient would be justified to miss the CS PCa present in 15% of patients.

2.2.2 Repeat Biopsy

There is increasing literature evaluating the patient population with a prior negative prostate biopsy with ongoing concern for malignancy. In the past, these patients have been subjected to multiple repeat systematic, non-targeted biopsies. The benefits of mpMRI in this clinical setting are twofold. It could potentially demonstrate a targetable area or could conversely be non-suspicious and may provide reassurance to continue to observe without necessitating a repeat biopsy.

Gaunay et al. evaluated 282 men who had a history of negative biopsy who underwent mpMRI guided prostate biopsy. Of these patients, the overall prevalence of prostate cancer was 42% with a CS PCa detection rate of 28%. The mpMRI sensitivity, specificity, PPV, and NPV were 94%, 37%, 52%, and 90% for all PCa, while it was 96%, 32%, 36%, and 96% for CS PCa [9]. This is in line with other studies which demonstrate a CS PCa detection rate of 16–40% when restricting to patients with Gleason ≥7 [14]. In 2016, Wysock reported that in the prior negative biopsy subset of men with negative prostate MRIs, the NPV was 86.2% for all cancer detection and 100% for CS PCa [12].

Several studies have also evaluated the mpMRI directed PCa detection rates stratified by the number of prior negative biopsies. While the rate of detection of CS PCa decreases with subsequent biopsies when not utilizing MRI, there appears to be consensus that the inclusion of MRI allows for similar rates of detection. Sonn et al. evaluated the diagnosis of CS PCa (as defined as Gleason ≥7) in patients with 1, 2, 3, or ≥ 4 prior biopsies and demonstrated no change in PCa detection between the groups (23–29%) [15].

2.3 Case 2.1

A 71-year-old gentleman who initially presented in 2004 for an elevated PSA as well as irritative voiding symptoms. He underwent a 12-core TRUS-guided biopsy at that time which was benign. He had a repeat biopsy in 2017 for a PSA of 4.4 which was also benign. He returned to the urology clinic in 2019 with a rise in his PSA from 4.4 to 6.9 over 10 months. Of note, he had had several febrile UTIs over the previous few years but had sterile urine at the time of his evaluation. A SelectMDX was sent showing a 36% chance of Gleason 7 prostate cancer or worse. Given this information, he was scheduled for an MRI fusion biopsy. The mpMRI completed prior to his biopsy showed no lesions (Fig. 2.1). As such no targeted biopsies were taken, but a standard 12-core biopsy was still obtained. This returned with chronic inflammation in a majority of the cores. This case represents the patient with the ongoing clinical suspicion for clinically significant prostate cancer to include both PSA and SelectMDX. While a standard 12-core prostate biopsy was again performed, the mpMRI demonstrated no targetable lesions. This represents a case where the patient who did not benefit from repeat biopsy. Given the previously reported NPV of

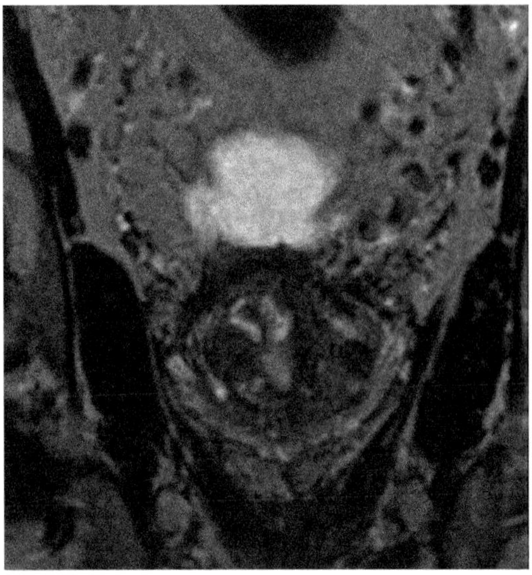

Fig. 2.1 (**Case 2.1**) No lesions within prostate as seen on coronal T2-weighted images. The prostate gland demonstrates areas of fibroglandular and stromal hyperplasia with well-circumscribed areas of benign appearing signal changes

90% for all cancer and 96% for CS PCa, we believe these patients could likely be observed without a biopsy at this time, particularly given the prior negative biopsies. Should there be ongoing increased suspicion in the future, the patient could undergo repeat imaging to assess for new lesions.

2.4 Case 2.2

A 52-year-old gentleman who was referred for persistently elevated PSA and concern for underlying prostate cancer in spite of three prior negative 12-core non-targeted biopsies. Over 1 year, his PSA had risen from 8.9 to 21.6. His previously measured prostate volume was 27.2 cc. mpMRI was obtained which revealed a highly suspicious PIRADS 4 lesion in the left anterior region of the prostate (Fig. 2.2).

He underwent a targeted fusion biopsy of the lesion, in addition to a standard 12-core biopsy. The pathology revealed Gleason 3 + 5 = 8 disease in the targeted region. Additionally, Gleason 3 + 4 was found in the left medial base and apex on the standard 12-core biopsy. After discussing the options with this patient, he elected to undergo a radical prostatectomy. The final pathology revealed Gleason 4 + 3 = 7 disease in the left anterior and left posterior prostate with extension into the bladder neck. This case demonstrates the situation of multiple prior negative non-targeted biopsies with ongoing clinical suspicion and the demonstration of a targetable lesion in the anterior gland. As reported earlier, misses of the non-targeted biopsies often occur in the anterior or apical regions of the gland, as in this patient. The dilemma in these patients is not whether to biopsy the target but what to do about the remainder of the gland. Our experience at the Indiana University, along with a review of the evidence, supports that using concurrent systematic biopsy along with the targeted fusion biopsy, 15% of cancers are discovered outside of the targeted region.

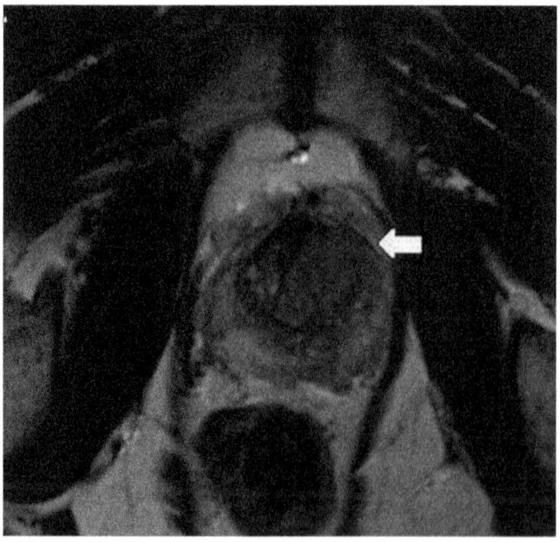

Fig. 2.2 **(Case 2.2)** Axial T2-weighted image showing a left anterior gland (PIRADS 4) lesion (arrow) in the peripheral zone

We extrapolate this to the initial biopsy patient without the need to present a further case. If we know that our standard biopsy template under US guidance missed a significant number of cancers and there is technology that will improve the accuracy of the biopsy, it naturally follows that this should be implemented earlier in the diagnostic process. Limiting the widespread use of mpMRI prior to initial biopsy is the hardware availability, the radiologist's expertise, and the cost of the exams. As these studies become more widespread, we would expect these issues to be resolved.

2.5 Active Surveillance

2.5.1 Confirmation

In men with clinically localized very low, low, and low-volume intermediate-risk PCa, active surveillance (AS) has emerged as an important management strategy. The benefit of AS over more definitive treatment strategies includes minimizing overtreatment with the potential side effects. There is still considerable anxiety related to this management paradigm, as both providers and patients alike fear underestimating the aggressiveness of the malignancy and the potential risk of missing the window of opportunity for curative intervention. Although it is accepted that TRUS-guided biopsies miss between 30% and 40% of clinically significant cancers and may underestimate the aggressiveness of cancer in

20–30% of cases, it remains the basis for patient selection into AS programs [16]. mpMRI aims to narrow this discrepancy and improve the diagnostic accuracy of the biopsy and thus better categorize the PCa patient. A meta-analysis reported that MRI was able to identify suspicious lesions suitable for AS in 2/3 of men [17].

Most patients that are entered on to an AS approach for PCa undergo a confirmatory biopsy prior to long-term management with an AS program. This represents an opportunity for improve risk assessment to better classify patients, serving to not only reassure providers and patients as to the extent of their disease but also to identify those patients with more aggressive appearing lesions potentially not sampled at the time of the initial biopsy [18]. If these targeted regions prove to be more aggressive disease, they would no longer be eligible for AS and would be offered definitive treatment instead.

Several studies have reported a NPV of MRI for CS PCa as high as 90% [19]. As such, a negative mpMRI at time of confirmatory biopsy has been shown to be a good predictor of appropriate enrollment in AS. Second, if the mpMRI findings are discordant with the initial biopsy findings, either with a high suspicion score lesion in the same region or a new lesion identified in a difficult to biopsy region, this should prompt targeted biopsies. While the PPV of the mpMRI in this setting when detecting high-risk disease is only 50–60%, it still upgrades patients in 40–60% of cases [20, 21]. Likewise, as the suspicion score to the lesion increases, so does the rate of upgrading [22].

2.6 Case 2.3

A 54-year-old gentleman with a BMI of 38 and a PSA of 4.1 who underwent a TRUS biopsy and was found to have low-volume Gleason 3 + 3 = 6 disease. He underwent a Prolaris score (examines cell cycle protein expression) which was 4.6, a low score predicting him to have a low mortality risk stratification. He underwent a repeat systematic non-guided TRUS biopsy demonstrating again Gleason 3 + 3 disease in the left apex and right mid gland. He was initiated on AS given the results of the repeat biopsy. Over the next few months, his PSA rose from 4.1 to 11.3, and he underwent a mpMRI prior to his confirmatory biopsy. There were two areas of concern: left posterior mid (PIRADS 3) and left anterior apex (PIRADS 4) lesions (Fig. 2.3). He underwent tar-

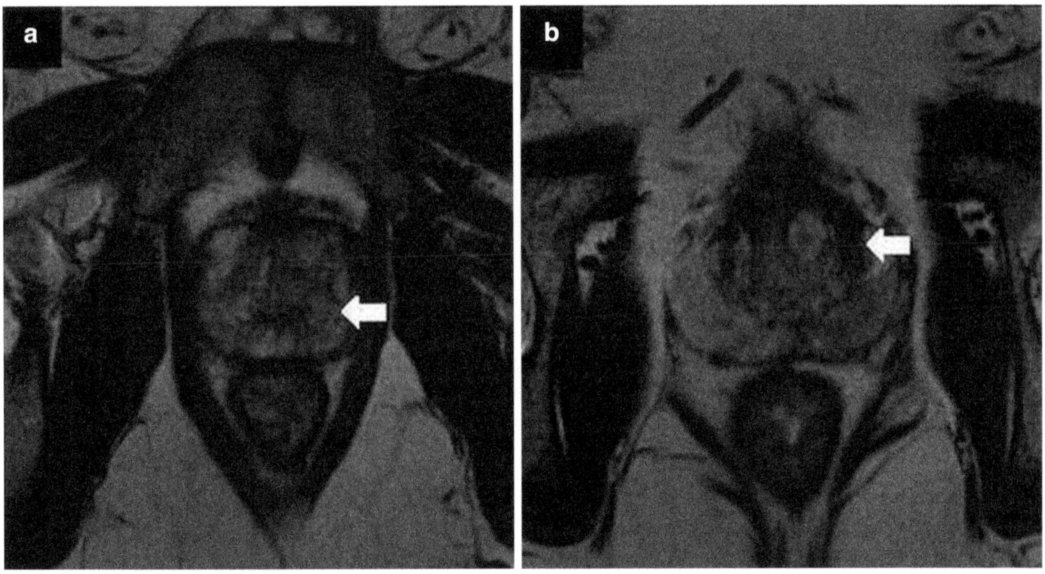

Fig. 2.3 (**Case 2.3**) Axial T2-weighted images of (**a**) left posterior mid (PIRADS 3) and (**b**) left anterior apex (PIRADS 4) lesions

geted biopsies of these two targets as well as a standard 12-core biopsy. Both the left posterior PIRADS 3 lesion and the left anterior apex lesion were Gleason 4 + 5 = 9 disease. Additionally, the 12-core standard biopsy returned with Gleason 4 + 4 = 8 and 4 + 5 = 9 along the left lateral biopsies.

After a thorough discussion regarding the patient's options, the patient elected to undergo a prostatectomy. Final pathology confirmed Gleason 4 + 4 = 8 with tertiary pattern 5. The cancer was located in the left anterior, left posterior, right anterior, and right posterior quadrants. He had one lymph node with a metastatic deposit.

This case highlights the 12-core systematic biopsy approach can clearly fail to detect very significant disease. The apical lesion was likely not sampled at the time of either TRUS biopsies due to not only the difficult location but also the patient's body habitus. The mpMRI allowed for identification of this and subsequent sampling. This case thus highlights the need to consider not only the PSA kinetics but also the synergistic use of both traditional and targeted biopsies.

2.6.1 Surveillance

Additionally, a potential role of mpMRI has emerged in patients already on AS during the surveillance phase. The goal of ongoing surveillance with the use of repeat biopsies is to catch disease progression and thus offer further treatment. Along the same line, a reassuring repeat biopsy without evidence of progression affords the patient further delay of the potential side effects from definitive treatment. While there is currently a lack of consensus as to what signifies progression while on AS, the following criteria are widely accepted: (a) detection of higher volume cancer and/or higher grade cancer on biopsy, (b) PSA doubling time of less than 3 years, or (c) unequivocal clinical progression [23]. Definition of progression relies heavily on the error-prone biopsy techniques and pathologic interpretation mentioned above. mpMRI has been suggested as an adjunctive diagnostic test to improve the classification of patient while on AS. The use of mpMRI appears to have a higher sensitivity than TRUS-guided biopsies for intermediate- and high-risk PCa [24]. Studies have evaluated whether or not it would be reasonable to observe, without repeat biopsy, the patient with a stable mpMRI, without the appearance of new suspicious lesions. mpMRI has been shown to have a high NPV for identification of men unlikely to be reclassified to higher-risk categories and thus change their management strategy [22]. This appears to be particularly promising when taking into account reassuring PSA kinetics, such as a stable absolute value, stable PSA density, and/or prolonged PSA doubling times. As the comfort level of urologists with negative mpMRI grows, this may become the preferred treatment approach.

Several challenges exist in reference to this particular use of MRI. Conceptually, those patients with highly suspicious mpMRI lesions more often than not have disease not suitable for AS in the first place. Those patients with PIRADS 4 or 5 lesions are likely selected out of this population prior to enrollment. As such, low-volume, lower-risk disease is often occult on imaging, and thus there is not a clear consensus as to what signifies the progression of an existing lesion radiographically. Some considerations include a change in size, changing characteristics as seen in DWI, or an increase in the PIRADS score. Some less controversial indicators of progression include the appearance of new highly suspicious lesions as well as evidence of disease progression locally (extraprostatic extension, seminal vesicle involvement, nodal involvement). When interpreting mpMRI imaging in this setting, we therefore use a multidisciplinary approach to the patient, taking into account the original biopsies, PSA kinetics, patient specific risk factors, as well as the most current imaging. In most cases, evidence of disease progression seen on MRI prompts a repeat biopsy prior to initiating active treatment.

2.7 Case 2.4

A 71-year-old gentleman who was diagnosed with Gleason 3 + 3 prostate cancer in 1/12 cores in 2015. He was enrolled in active surveillance at

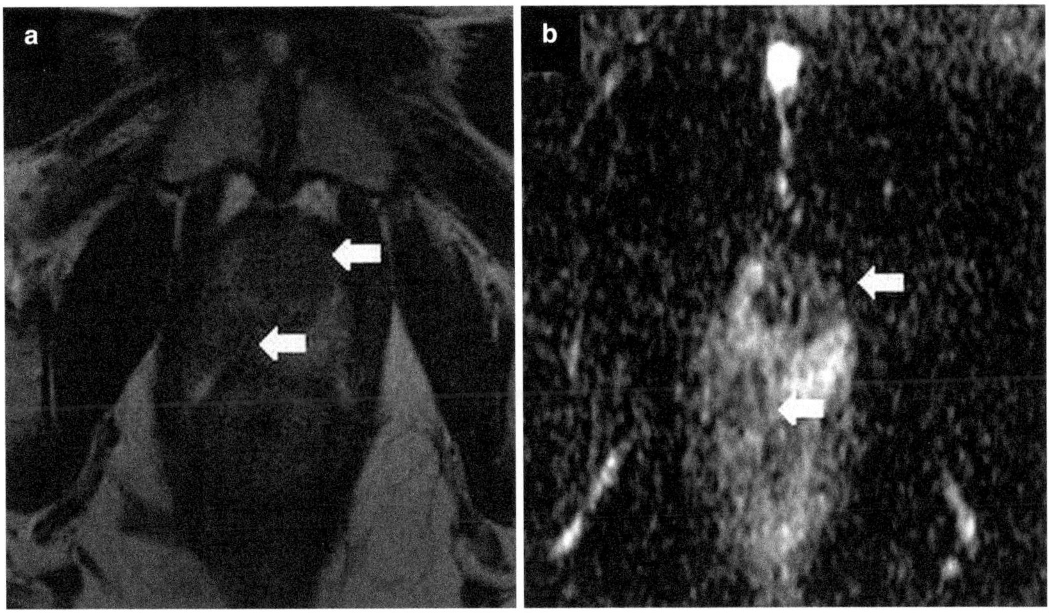

Fig. 2.4 **(Case 2.4)** Axial T2-weighted image (**a**) and DWI (**b**) of two lesions (arrows) in the prostate apex: left anterior (PIRADS 4) and right posterior (PIRADS 3)

that time and did not have a confirmatory biopsy or further imaging at that time. His PSA rose from 8.1 to 18.4 over 13 months, and he was seen for consultation. A mpMRI was obtained which revealed 2 lesions: left anterior (PIRADS 4) and right apex (PIRADS 3) (Fig. 2.4). He underwent a targeted fusion biopsy in addition to a standard 12-core biopsy. Pathology revealed Gleason 4 + 4 = 8 in the left anterior and Gleason 4 + 5 = 9 in the right apex. Additionally, the standard 12-core biopsy revealed Gleason 5 + 4 = 9 on all six 6 cores from the right side of the gland.

This case represents an example of a patient who was placed on AS without initial mpMRI or targeted biopsy. The first mpMRI showed clear evidence of disease. In this particular patient, the suspicions were confirmed and appropriate treatment was offered.

2.8 Staging Prior to Local (or Surgical) Therapy

Cancer staging is the most significant determinant of survival and often dictates the treatment strategies that should be considered. Clinical staging for prostate cancer has historically been determined by a combination of digital rectal exam (DRE), laboratory testing (PSA), and pathological assessment of biopsy tissue (Gleason Score, # cores positive, % of core involvement). Using these determinants, the NCCN, AUA, EAU, and ASCO have developed varying risk classification systems which stratify patients into very low-risk, low-risk, intermediate-risk, high-risk, or very high-risk disease [25–28]. Additional imaging studies to further help quantify the extent of disease may be warranted. In the past, staging for low-risk prostate cancer (cT1c, PSA < 10, and biopsy Gleason Score ≤ 6) with imaging (CT, bone scan, and/or MRI) was vastly overused [29–31]. The NCCN and the AUA has attempted to reduce the use of imaging studies in this population by including recommendations against imaging in their published guidelines and through the "Choosing Wisely" campaign [26, 32]. In men with more aggressive disease (or clinically significant prostate cancer), imaging studies may provide additional information to help physician and patients to decide the best treatment strategy in order to maximize oncological control while minimizing side effects of the treatment.

Radical prostatectomy is an accepted definitive treatment option for men with localized prostate cancer. Given the increased acceptance of active surveillance as an appropriate treatment option for men with very low, low and low-volume intermediate-risk disease, most men undergoing radical prostatectomy in the United States and Europe over the last decade have had intermediate or higher-risk disease [33–35]. More recently, the role of surgery in men with locally advanced or oligometastatic disease has garnered significant attention and is currently being assessed in SWOG-sponsored phase III randomized controlled trial (SWOG 1802). As such, the role of imaging for local staging has become increasingly more important in the group of men considering surgical therapy.

The goals of radical prostatectomy are to achieve oncologic control with negative surgical margins while maintaining urinary continence and erectile function when applicable. The technique of a nerve-sparing radical prostatectomy, popularized by Walsh in the 1980s, sought to maximize functional outcomes by sparing the neurovascular bundles that run on the posterolateral aspect of the prostate between the lateral prostatic fascia and the prostatic capsule [36]. A nerve-sparing procedure has been shown to improve erectile function and possibly urinary continence recovery [37–39]. Aggressive nerve sparing is associated with potential adverse events. The risk of positive surgical margins and subsequent potential for biochemical, local, and systemic recurrences may occur when nerve sparing is done in patients with extraprostatic extension (EPE) or when the capsule is violated in men with organ-confined disease [40–42].

There are two main differences between the concept of current prostate cancer treatment and the late 1980s when the nerve-sparing technique was described. First, in the previous era, the majority of patients had low-volume, low-risk prostate cancer. This cohort has very low risk of non-organ-confined disease; therefore, most positive margins incurred during nerve sparing were a result of surgical technique and not biology of the disease [43]. Currently, the majority of men being operated on have at least intermediate-risk prostate cancer which confers at least a 20% risk of pT3 disease which makes the decision to perform nerve sparing more complex [44]. Information obtained from local staging studies may be influential to aid in this decision. Moreover, in recent years, more physicians are aggressively treating men with high-risk prostate cancer with radical prostatectomy [33–35]. Although nerve sparing may still be feasible in certain instances in this population, more commonly surgeons are faced with the decision on whether or not to perform a wide resection or an extended pelvic lymph node dissection which may be aided by appropriate local staging [45, 46]. Second, imaging studies used for local staging have vastly improved since the 1980s. Spatial resolution for CT scans of the pelvis are poor making it hard to distinguish between the prostate and the surrounding soft tissue [47]. Prostate MRI has become a popular imaging technique in the 2000s due to its noninvasiveness, lack of ionizing radiation, and superior resolution. The use of MRI in the diagnosis, staging, and treatment of prostate cancer has exponentially increased in the last decade which was associated with significant improvements in MRI quality [48, 49]. In this section, we outline clinical cases in which prostate MRI prior to prostatectomy influenced operative approach and technique in order to achieve the oncological and functional goals of the operation.

2.9 Case 2.5

A 59-year-old man had been followed for 10 years due to an elevated PSA. His PSA has slowly risen to 4.86. A 4Kscore demonstrated a 10% risk of having aggressive prostate cancer. A standard 12-core TRUS biopsy was performed and showed 1 core positive for Gleason 3 + 4 disease and 1 core positive for Gleason 4 + 3 disease of the right side. He had an isolated core of low-volume Gleason 3 + 3 disease on the left. An Oncotype DX genomic test showed very low-risk prostate cancer. The patient had minimal nocturia at baseline and erections sufficient for intercourse without the use of medications.

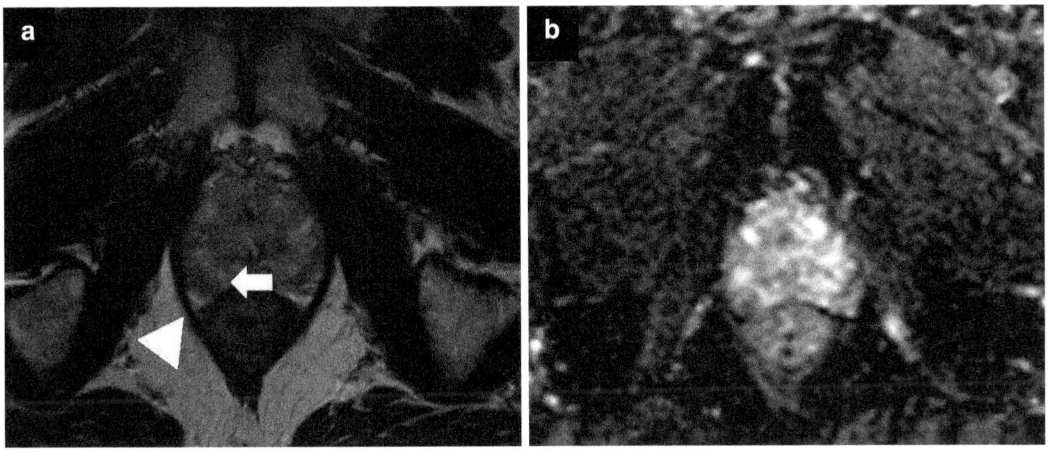

Fig. 2.5 **(Case 2.5)** Axial T2-weighted image (**a**) and ADC map (**b**) of a 1.4 cm right apical lesion (arrow). The lesion abuts but does not bulge or invade the prostatic capsule. A clear fat signal on the other side of the lesion and the prostatic capsule is clearly visualized on the T2 image (arrowhead). A successful bilateral nerve-sparing prostatectomy was completed as a result

An MRI was ordered to assess the extent of disease and evaluate the feasibility of nerve sparing. The study demonstrated one PIRADS 3 lesion in the right peripheral zone near the apex which corresponded to his TRUS biopsy pathology. The lesion measured 1.4 cm in diameter. The lesion was closely associated with prostatic capsule posteriorly but did not demonstrated definitive bulging or extraprostatic extension (Fig. 2.5). Given the reassuring MRI, he was taken to the operating room for a bilateral nerve-sparing prostatectomy and lymph node dissection. Final pathology demonstrated organ-confined Gleason 3 + 4 prostate cancer with negative margins.

It is important for the urologists to be familiar with the imaging sequences looking for signs of potential EPE and the vernacular that radiologists use when describing disease around the prostatic capsule. Extraprostatic disease has traditionally been evaluated using axial and coronal T2-weighted images. However, use of functional imaging sequences including diffusion-weighted imaging and dynamic contrast enhancement has been shown to aid in the detection of EPE [50, 51]. Criteria for detecting EPE have been suggested to include at least one of the following: irregular capsular bulge, disruption of the prostatic capsule, gross extension into the prostatic fat, broad capsular contact (>12 mm), obliteration of the rectoprostatic angle, or asymmetry of the neurovascular bundle [52]. At times, the radiology report may not specifically comment regarding the presence or absence of EPE but may include these other terms which may help the surgeon determine the risk of EPE and whether or not a nerve-sparing procedure is advisable. In this case, the MRI indicated that the lesion was abutting the capsule, but images did not meet any of the above outlined criteria for EPE.

One of the main concerns in using prostate MRI for local staging is the relatively poor sensitivity. A recently published meta-analysis of 75 studies and 9796 men indicated that the sensitivity of MRI in predicting pT3a disease was low (0.57) [53]. This is likely due to the inability of MRI to detect microscopic foci of EPE leading to high false-negative rates and thus low sensitivity. False-negative MRIs (negative MRI for EPE, positive pathology for EPE) may increase the patient's risk for a positive surgical margin and subsequent biochemical recurrence if nerve sparing is performed [40–42]. Surgeons must be cognizant of this limitation of MRI when planning operative approach. Some groups have suggested that combining MRI results with other readily available clinical and pathologic variables may improve the ability to accurately predict

EPE. Rayn et al. evaluated a cohort of 532 men who underwent 3 Tesla MRI and fusion biopsy prior to radical prostatectomy to determine if the results of the MRI improved the predictive ability of the Partin Tables and the MSKCC nomogram in determining pT3a disease. The predictive accuracy increased substantially when MRI results were added to the models (Partin Tables: AUC 0.66 vs 0.8, $p < 0.001$; MSKCC AUC 0.7 vs 0.8, $p = 0.003$) [54]. A similar study from the Mayo Clinic confirmed the beneficial predictive effects when combining MRI results to CAPRA-S and the Partin Tables [55]. Thus, it may be prudent to use these predictive models which incorporate clinical and pathological variables with radiographic findings rather than radiographic findings alone.

Nevertheless, numerous studies have evaluated the impact of MRI to effect a surgeon's operative plan. A single-center study of 438 men scheduled to undergo prostatectomy were randomized into MRI and no-MRI groups. The primary endpoint was positive surgical margin rates. Men in the MRI group had similar surgical margins rates (43, 19%) as men who did not have an MRI (49, 23%). Authors admitted numerous study limitations including the non-blinding of radiologists to clinical variables; therefore, the true impact of MRI on the primary outcome is unknown. More illuminating were the comments regarding suboptimal communication between radiologists and urologists which may have been the main reason a benefit was not seen in the MRI group [56]. Results of a single-institution cohort study emphasized this latter opinion. Authors demonstrated the importance of case presentation at an MRI conference prior to prostatectomy on surgical margin rates and degree of nerve sparing. Five-hundred fifty-seven men who underwent MRI and case discussion were compared with 410 men who did not. Positive surgical margin rates were lower in the MRI group (26.7% vs 33.3%) which may be due to the higher likelihood of men in the MRI group to have a non-nerve-sparing surgery [57]. We recommend that most centers, especially ones beginning an MRI prostate program, develop similar collaborative approaches in order to maximize benefit of imaging.

Other non-randomized studies have demonstrated potential benefits of using MRI prior to prostatectomy to guide operative approach. A multicenter European study evaluated 137 men who underwent MRI prior to prostatectomy over a 6-month period. The Tewari nerve-sparing classification system was used to grade the degree of nerve-sparing planned prior to and after the MRI was completed. In this grading system, nerve-sparing Grades 1–2 are more aggressive techniques which aim to preserve all (Grade 1) or most (Grade 2) of the neurovascular bundle, whereas Grade 3 is a partial nerve sparing and Grade 4 is a non-nerve-sparing procedure [58]. The results of the MRI forced a change in operative approach in 46.7% of patient-based and 56.2% of side-based cases. Remarkably, changes in approach were almost equally split between more aggressive resection of the neurovascular bundle and more aggressive nerve sparing. Appropriateness of change in operative approach was judged by presence of positive surgical margins or EPE and judged to be 75%. In comparing this cohort to a control group of 161 men without MRI prior to prostatectomy, the positive surgical margin rate was substantially lower in men who underwent MRI despite more aggressive clinical and pathological characteristics (13.4% vs 24.1%, $p < 0.01$) [59]. A second study similarly assessed if MRI could be better at selecting nerve-sparing candidates prior to surgery. In this prospective study of 105 men, all men were planned to undergo bilateral nerve sparing prior to MRI. After MRI, the operative plan changed in 30% of cases to either a unilateral or non-nerve-sparing approach. Appropriateness of decision was judged in a similar fashion as the previous study. The decision to undergo bilateral nerve sparing based on MRI results was appropriate in 70 of 73 cases. The decision to undergo unilateral nerve sparing based on MRI results was appropriate in 28/32 cases. One significant limitation of this cohort was that most men in the study had low-risk disease [60]. Finally, a larger cohort study of 353 men from who underwent MRI prior to prostatectomy at a single institution was designed similarly to the previous two studies. Authors concluded that MRI significantly improves decision-making during surgery [61]. A significant limitation of all of these studies is that it is unknown to what degree clinical factors or MRI data affected operative approach.

Finally, the above case underlines the increasingly complexity of managing patients with elevated PSA and prostate cancer. Numerous ancillary tests were completed to determine need for biopsy (4 K), need for treatment (Oncotype DX), and operative approach (MRI). Some of these studies had discordant results. It is important to recognize the limitations of these ancillary studies and discuss these challenging cases at multidisciplinary tumor boards.

2.10 Case 2.6

A 63-year-old retired physician was referred to clinic for a second opinion of recently diagnosed prostate cancer. His PSA acutely rose from 3.95 to 8.8. A standard 12-core TRUS biopsy was performed which showed all six cores taken from the left side of his prostate to be positive for high-risk Gleason 9 or 10 prostate cancer involving 5–90% of each core. The patient had minimal lower urinary tract symptoms at baseline and was able to achieve erections sufficient for intercourse without medication. On physical exam, he had a large firm nodule on the left side which corroborated with his biopsy results that seemed like it extended beyond the capsule of the prostate.

An MRI was ordered preoperatively to assess the extent of disease. There was a large 2.3 cm PIRADS 5 lesion on the left apex of the prostate. There was no evidence of EPE, seminal vesicle invasion (SVI), or adenopathy. Selected images from that study are depicted in Fig. 2.6. Prior to surgery and after consultation with our genitourinary radiologists, we believed that there was clear capsular invasion on the left side (arrowhead in Fig. 2.6a). There were no abnormalities on the right. Therefore, we planned to perform a wide resection on the left side and nerve sparing on the right. Intraoperatively, our suspicion for left-sided EPE was confirmed. His final pathology was Gleason 4 + 5 prostate cancer, pT3a with EPE on the left.

This case highlights a few important aspects for urologists to consider when using prostate MRI for operative planning. First, numerous studies have demonstrated high interobserver variability in interpreting prostate MRI images [62, 63]. Rosenkrantz et al. evaluated the interobserver variability of six experienced radiologists from six different institutions. While interobserver agreement was modest for detection of

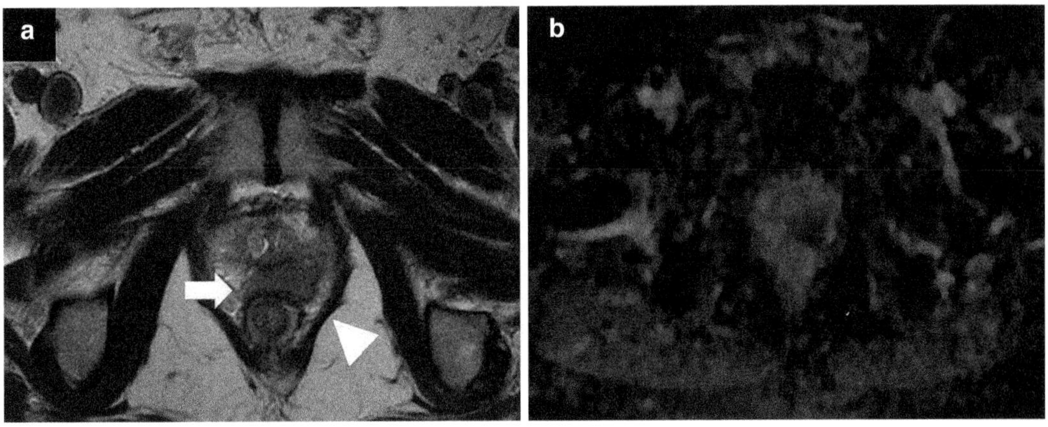

Fig. 2.6 (**Case 2.6**) T2-weighted image (**a**) and ADC map (**b**) of a large left apex lesion (arrow). Both images show abnormal MR signal beyond the prostatic capsule (arrowhead). A wide resection on the left was planned which allowed for negative surgical margins. Final pathology demonstrated pT3a disease on the left posterior-lateral aspect of the prostate

lesions with a PIRADS score of 4 or higher in the peripheral zone (kappa coefficient: 0.593) and the transition zone (kappa coefficient: 0.509), interobserver variability was high (kappa coefficient: 0.289) when evaluating for definitive EPE on T2-weighted imaging [62]. One proposed explanation for these findings is the presence of a radiologic learning curve when interpreting prostate MRI [64–68]. Most of these studies have suggested that learning curves are present for radiologists in the diagnosis of prostate cancer. In one initial study, Latchamsetty et al. evaluated a cohort of 80 men who underwent endorectal coil MRI prior to radical prostatectomy at an institution with little previous experience in prostate MRI. In this enriched cohort (all men included were at an elevated risk of having EPE based on clinical factors), MRI results were compared with pathologic specimens to determine the accuracy of MRI in predicting EPE. Learning curves were assessed by comparing the accuracy of the first 40 cases with the second 40 cases. Sensitivity (31.3% vs 64.7%), specificity (70.8% vs 78.3%), positive predictive value (41.7% vs 68.8%), and negative predictive value (60.7% vs 70.5%) increased with increasing experience [66]. Jansen and colleagues recently published a cohort of 430 patients which found different results. A cohort of 430 men who underwent MRI prior to prostatectomy were evaluated to assess staging accuracy and the effect of a radiologic learning curve. Sensitivity for EPE was low (0.45) and did not improve over time [68]. One potential way to improve the sensitivity of MRI interpretation and navigate a potential radiologic learning curve was proposed in a brief correspondence by Tay and colleagues. Authors suggested that combining a standard MRI report, a second specialized MRI provided by a genitourinary radiologist blinded to the standard report and clinical variables, and clinical variables could drastically improve the ability to predict pathologic pT3a disease [69]. These studies and the above case highlight the importance of discussing prostate MRI images prior to determining an operative plan. Prostate MRI has a poor sensitivity in detection pT3a disease likely due to the inability to visualize microscopic foci of disease beyond the capsule. Conversely and pertinent to this case, the specificity of MRI in detecting EPE is relatively high. The previously mentioned meta-analysis reported that the specificity of MRI for pT3a disease was 0.91 [53]. It seems most reasonable to adjust operative approach regarding nerve sparing based on MRI findings in situations where clear invasion on MRI is described. In instances where clear invasion is not described, decision to perform nerve sparing is best made by using predictive nomograms that incorporate clinical, pathological, and radiographic variables [54, 55].

A final salient point to consider is the size of the lesion found on the MRI. In the above case, the MRI described a relatively large (2.3 cm) primary lesion. Men with EPE had significantly larger tumor diameters on final pathology than men with organ-confined disease (2.49 vs 1.45 cm, $p < 0.0001$) [70]. Given that primary lesion size is a readily obtainable value on prostate MRI, this variable should be considered when determining operative plan. In fact, in the previously mentioned study by Rayn et al., the largest lesion diameter on MRI was the strongest predictor of EPE at the time of prostatectomy [54]. Thus, the index for suspicion for microscopic EPE should be higher in men with larger tumors even if the radiology report suggests organ-confined disease.

2.11 Case 2.7

A 69-year-old man has been followed for an elevated PSA for a number of years. He previously underwent a TRUS biopsy of his prostate in 2017 which showed low-volume low-risk disease and subsequently was placed on active surveillance. He was referred to our institution for a prostate MRI and fusion biopsy due to a rise in his PSA to 7.07. Selected images from the prostate MRI conducted prior to his consultation are shown in Fig. 2.7. There was a large T2 hypointense lesion incorporating the entirety of his left peripheral zone and extending into the transition zone and right side of the gland. There was clear evidence of EPE (Fig. 2.7b) and SVI (Fig. 2.7d). There

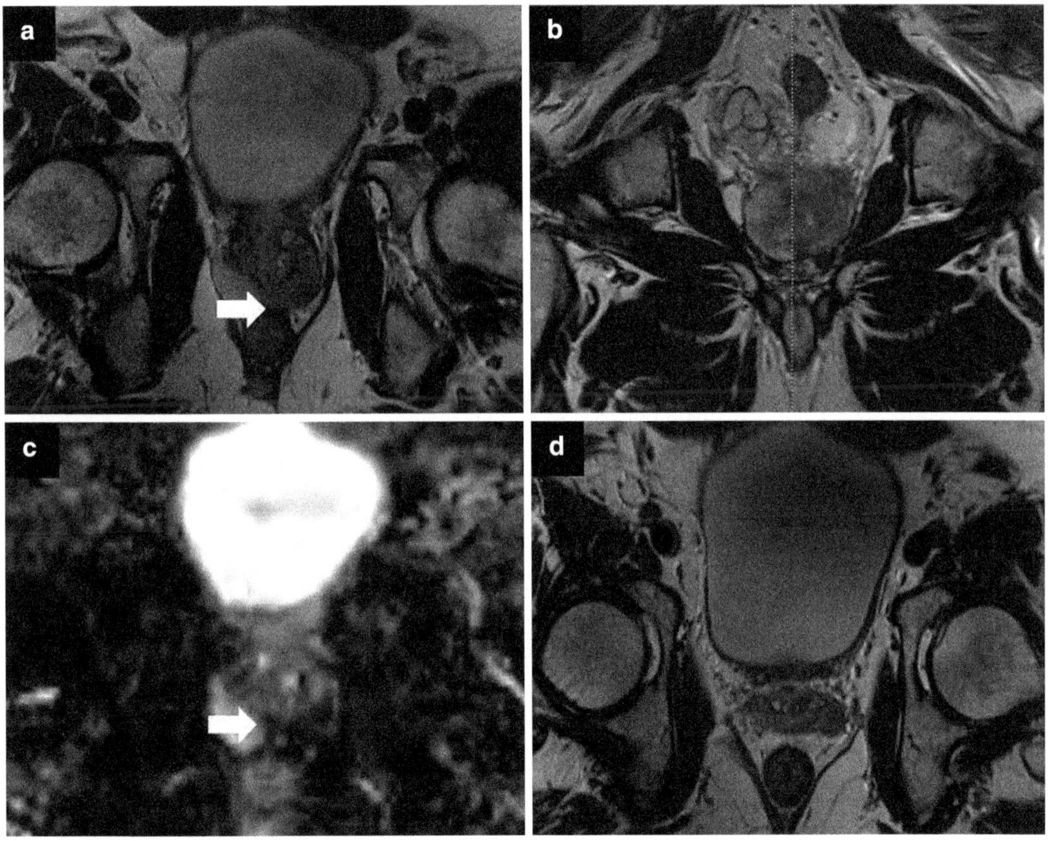

Fig. 2.7 (**Case 2.7**) Representative images of a large left-sided lesion (arrow) visible on (**a**). Axial T2-weighted (**b**). Coronal T2-weight and (**c**). ADC images. These images clearly demonstrate a large hypointense lesion originating on the left and extending past midline. Image (**d**) shows the left seminal vesicle invasion as an area of low signal intensity and abnormal gland architecture

appeared to be no evidence of disease on the right side of his gland. Pathology of his 2017 biopsy reported Gleason 3 + 4 disease and Gleason 3 + 3 disease all on the right side of his gland. This case is interesting due to disease demonstrated on MRI, and prostate biopsy was incongruent.

Given the findings of his MRI and previous prostate biopsy, a repeat biopsy was not conducted as the treatment was indicated. The patient elected for radical prostatectomy and bilateral pelvic lymph node dissection. A prostate exam was done prior to scheduling surgery to determine if the prostate was resectable. Exam demonstrated a large prostate nodule on the left with clear evidence of EPE. The prostate was not fixed to the pelvic sidewall. As a result, a robotic prostatectomy was schedule with the plan to perform a wide resection on the left and a nerve-sparing procedure on the right. Final pathology demonstrated a large 3.7 cm Gleason 4 + 3 primary tumor with EPE and SVI on the left. Surgical margins were negative.

High-risk prostate cancer is most commonly defined using D'Amico criteria as men with a PSA >20, Gleason Grade of ≥8, or ≥ cT3 disease [71]. More recently, NCCN guidelines have separated men in this group into high (cT3a, Gleason Grade Group 4 or 5, or PSA 20) and very high-risk disease (cT3b-T4, primary Gleason pattern 5, OR > 4 cores positive with Gleason Grade Group 4 or 5) [26]. Based on the physical exam findings, this man would be classified into the high-risk NCCN category. This patient's MRI result and physical examination gave a hint at the extent and significance of his disease and dictated the operative strategy. A wide resection operative approach is reserved for patients with high disease burden due to the potential lower rate of positive surgical margins which increases the likelihood of cancer control while potentially reducing the need for adjuvant therapy. This technique sacrifices the neurovascular bundle which allows for a generous margin on the posterior-lateral aspect of the prostate. This approach has been previously described in detail for open, laparoscopic, and robotic techniques [46, 72–75]. A retrospective cohort study evaluated oncologic and functional (urinary) outcomes in men undergoing wide resection (129 men) and non-wide resection (354 men) robotic prostatectomy for intermediate- or high-risk prostate cancer. As expected, men who underwent wide resection had more advanced clinical (clinical stage, biopsy Gleason Grade, CAPRA-9) and pathological disease (pathologic stage, prostatectomy Gleason Grade, CAPRA-S) than men who did not have a wide resection. However, the incidence of positive surgical margins was similar between the groups (20% wide resection vs 22% non-wide resection, $p = 0.505$), and a wide resection technique was responsible for a clinically meaningful reduction in odds of a positive posterolateral surgical margin on multivariate analysis (OR 0.73, 95%CI 0.38–1.41). Surgical technique in this series did not influence biochemical recurrence-free survival which is more likely driven by the biology of the disease than the surgical technique in men with high-risk disease. Finally, urinary control as assessed through two validated questionnaires was similar between the two groups with most of the improvement in urinary control occurring in the first 6 months [46]. In this particular case, a wide resection on the left allowed us to obtain negative surgical margins. A nerve-sparing approach on the right hopefully mitigated some of the potential urinary and erectile functional decline. Further follow-up regarding the association between surgical approach, recurrence, adjuvant therapy, and functional outcomes is certainly needed.

Finally, this case once again highlights some of the issues of using MRI solely to dictate operative plan. This particular case demonstrated macroscopic cT3a and cT3b disease which was appropriately reported by the radiologist. As mentioned, the specificity of MRI reported in a large meta-analysis in predicting pT3a disease (0.91) and pT3b (0.96) is exceptional which is due to low false-positive results [53]. High specificity of MRI makes intuitive sense; when lesions are large, they are easier to visualize and accurately predict. However, MRI has poor sensitivity in determining pT3a (0.57) and pT3b (0.58) disease preoperatively due to high false-negative rates given the inability of MRI to accurately visualize microscopic (or focal) disease outside of the prostate [53]. A recent study attempted to develop a model to predict pT3b disease preoperatively using clinical variables and MRI data (similar to the previously discussed studies developing models for prediction of pT3a disease). Results were limited as only 8% of the study cohort had pT3b disease. Nevertheless, MRI data (AUC 0.591) was inferior to clinical variables (AUC 0.85) in the ability to predict pT3b disease [76].

2.12 Case 2.8

A 65-year-old male was initially seen by his primary urologist for an elevated PSA to 12.9. A prostate MRI prior to any biopsy demonstrated two PIRADS 5 lesions. One was located in the right anterior lateral peripheral zone, and a smaller 6 mm lesion was located in the right posterior peripheral zone (Fig. 2.8a, b). The MRI also indicated that there were two lymph nodes visualized in the iliac chain that did not meet size criteria for metastasis but were suspicious (Fig. 2.8c). There was no formal comment on EPE or SVI.

A prostate biopsy was done which showed high-risk PCa. His disease was confined to the right side of his prostate. The patient had Gleason 4 + 3 and Gleason 4 + 4 disease in 5 cores with 10–70% core involvement. Staging CT of the abdomen and pelvis and bone scan was completed and demonstrated no obvious metastatic disease. Of note, the iliac chain lymph nodes

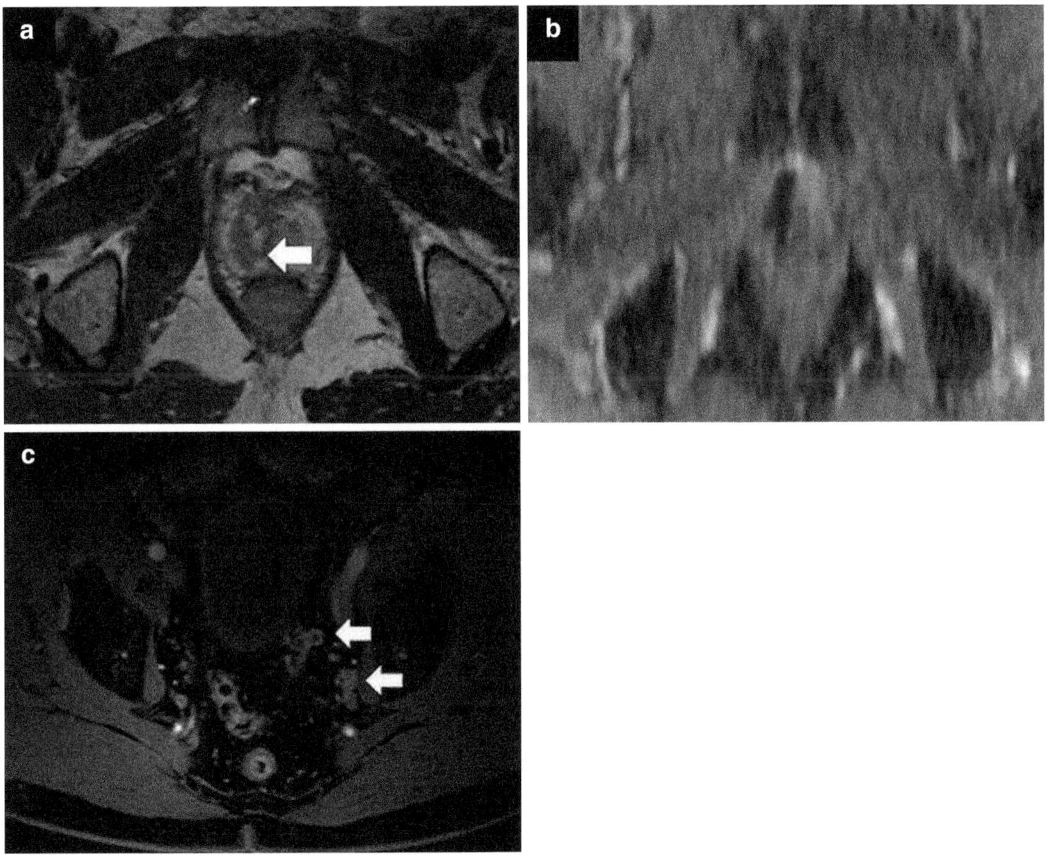

Fig. 2.8 **(Case 2.8)** Axial T2-weighted image (**a**) and ADC map (**b**) demonstrating one of the two large PIRADS 5 lesions (arrows) detected on the patients initial MRI. No obvious indication of EPE was noted. (**c**) Axial T2-weighted image with fat suppression demonstrates multiple suspicious lymph nodes in the left iliac chain (arrows)

demonstrated on the MRI were not mentioned in the CT report (images not shown). The patient underwent a PSMA-PET-MRI which confirmed the presence of two PIRADS 5 lesions on the right side of his prostate (Fig. 2.9a). There was no macroscopic EPE or visible SVI. Radiotracer uptake was visualized in the two left-sided iliac chain lymph nodes which corresponded to the enlarged lymph nodes reported by the MRI (Fig. 2.9b, c). There was no radiotracer uptake on the right-sided pelvic lymph nodes. The patient ultimately elected for surgical resection. The initial operative plan was for an extended pelvic lymph node dissection and a left unilateral nerve sparing due to the risk of having microscopic extracapsular extension on the right. Lymph node dissection included the external iliac, obturator, perirectal, and common iliac lymph nodes bilaterally. A frozen section of a lymph node at the bifurcation of the iliac vessels on the left was taken and came back consistent with metastasis. When dividing the prostatic pedicles, nerve sparing on the left was aborted due to grossly abnormal tissue resulting in poor surgical planes. Final pathology demonstrated a Gleason 4 + 3 prostate cancer with 30% ductal variant. The primary lesion was on the right side measured 3 cm in diameter and was associated with bilateral EPE and right SVI. Two of the 11 lymph nodes removed were positive for cancer. The positive nodes were all taken from the left-hand side. This and the next case highlight some of the emerging

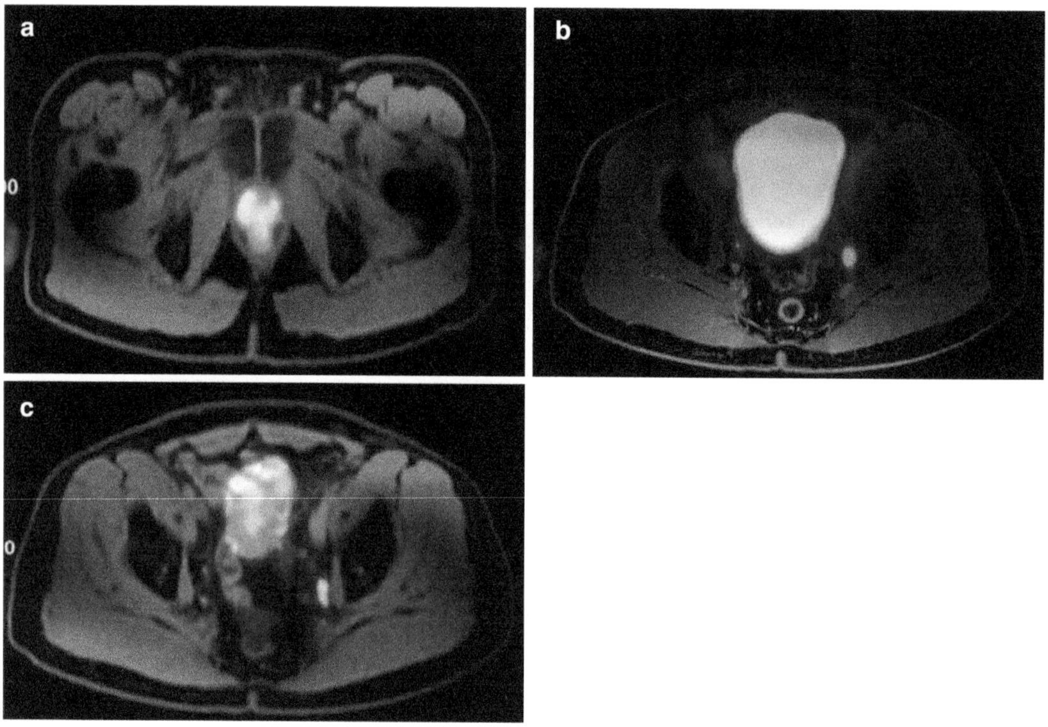

Fig. 2.9 (Case 2.8) PSMA-PET-MRI scans of the primary lesion (**a**) and pelvic lymph nodes (**b–c**) which correspond to the MRI findings. The prostate lesion and pelvic lymph nodes demonstrated PSMA avidity. Given these findings, a right-sided wide resection and extended pelvic lymph node dissection were planned which confirmed right sided extraprostatic disease and two positive lymph nodes on the left

imaging techniques which may have potential utility in the diagnosis, staging, management, and treatment of prostate cancer. PSMA, or prostate specific membrane antigen, is a transmembrane protein expressed in normal and prostate cancer cells which has been used as a target for functional imaging studies and may be a target for drug delivery and treatment in the future. The majority of data investigating functional imaging with PSMA in prostate cancer staging exists with PSMA-PET-CT scans. The largest study to date evaluating PSMA-PET-CT scans in staging was recently published by Yaxley et al. In a retrospective cohort study of 1253 men undergoing staging prior to primary treatment of prostate cancer, metastatic disease was suggested by PET avidity in 12.1% of men. Increasing PSA, International Society of Urological Pathology (ISUP) grade, and radiologic staging with MRI were all prognostic markers for PET avidity and suspected metastatic disease. Of note, this study did not confirm metastasis suspected on PSMA scans with pathology [77]. The same group addressed this issue partially in another recent study which the sensitivity, specificity, positive, and negative predictive values of PSMA-PET-CT on pelvic lymph node staging were calculated using surgical pathology as the reference standard. Only 21 of the 55 men with metastatic disease on surgical pathology had lymph nodes identified on presurgical staging (sensitivity 38.2%). One-hundred forty-three men did not have metastasis on imaging. Thirty-four of these men had metastasis on pathology for a negative predictive value of 80.8%. Authors concluded that while specificity was quite high (93.5%), sensitivity was low; therefore, pelvic lymph node dissection is still the gold standard way to stage the pelvic lymph nodes [78]. A big issue in our presented case, which is highlighted in the latter study by Yaxley et al., is the potential for controversy when using these functional tests in preoperative staging.

Traditionally, operative procedures have not been indicated in men with suspected or confirmed oligometastatic metastatic disease. With these newer imaging studies, there is potential to diagnose more men with lymph node or distant metastases prior to surgery when compared to standard staging imaging. Therefore, treatment dilemmas may arise. Results from a subgroup analysis of the randomized controlled trial STAMPEDE and several other population-based and prospective studies suggest potential benefit of treatment of the primary cancer in the setting of oligometastatic disease [79–83].

In this particular case, a PSMA-PET-MRI was completed. The benefits of performing a PET-MRI instead of a PET-CT scan are similar to the benefits of standard MRI compared to CT scans: better spatial resolution of soft tissues. A pilot study of eight patients evaluated the initial clinical feasibility and reproducibility of performing whole-body PSMA-PET-MRI in men with a new or recurrent diagnosis of high-risk prostate cancer. Scans were able to visualize the dominant intraprostatic lesion in all seven patients who previously did not have treatment. Local staging was also complimentary between PET and MRI images in the majority of patients. Authors suggested that their protocol was successful, yet further studies were needed [84]. A second larger cohort study of 122 men evaluated PSMA-PET-MRI for staging prior to a planned prostatectomy. Imaging was able to correctly identify prostate cancer lesions in 97% of cases and changed the therapeutic treatment plan in 28.7%. For those men who underwent surgery, PET-MRI were able to accurately predict T-stage in 82.5% and node positive disease in 93%, respectively [85]. In our study, the MRI and the PSMA-PET-MRI were both able to visualize the two PIRADS 5 lesions on the right side of his prostate. Additionally, the suspicious nodes in the left iliac chain initially visualized on MRI demonstrated PSMA avidity. These congruent findings dictated our initial operative plan. Resection of the neurovascular bundle on the right was planned due to the dominant PIRADS 5 lesions, Gleason Grade, and risk for EPE. A nerve-sparing procedure was planned on the left due to the reassuring images. Additionally, an extended pelvic lymph node dissection was planned due to the abnormal pelvic lymph nodes. Our case also highlights how visual cues and intraoperative assessment are a key component to performing oncologic efficacious surgery. During the operation, abnormal tissue was visualized outside of the prostate on the left which was presumed to represent extraprostatic disease. This was confirmed on final pathology. Surgeons should keep this in mind when using imaging to guide an operative approach: make a plan prior to the operation and be willing to change that plan intraoperatively if the surgery is not going well.

2.13 Case 2.9

A 52-year-old male initially presented to an outside institution for bloody ejaculate. His PSA was found to be elevated at 20.2. A PSA obtained 2 years previously was 2.7. He had no voiding issues or sexual dysfunction. A standard 12-core TRUS biopsy was done in early 2019 demonstrated high-volume Gleason 4 + 5 prostate cancer in all six cores taken from the right side of his prostate. Staging CT scan of the abdomen and pelvis and bone scan were negative except for some suspected post-biopsy artifact visualized on the right side of his prostate (not shown).

Given his young age, good health, and high-risk disease on biopsy, he was referred to our center for consideration of surgical therapy or possible enrollment in clinical trials investigating new imaging modalities. After informed consent, he was enrolled in a clinical trial designed to evaluate the utility of PSMA-PET-MRI in the pretreatment setting. Selected images from his PSMA-PET-MRI are shown in Fig. 2.10. The large primary lesion encompassing the entire right side of the prostate was visualized (Fig. 2.10a). Multiple lymph nodes demonstrated PET avidity predominantly in the right external iliac chain. After extensive discussion with the patient regarding the imaging study and potential treatment options, the patient elected for radical prostatectomy and bilateral pelvic lymph node dissection with the understanding that multi-

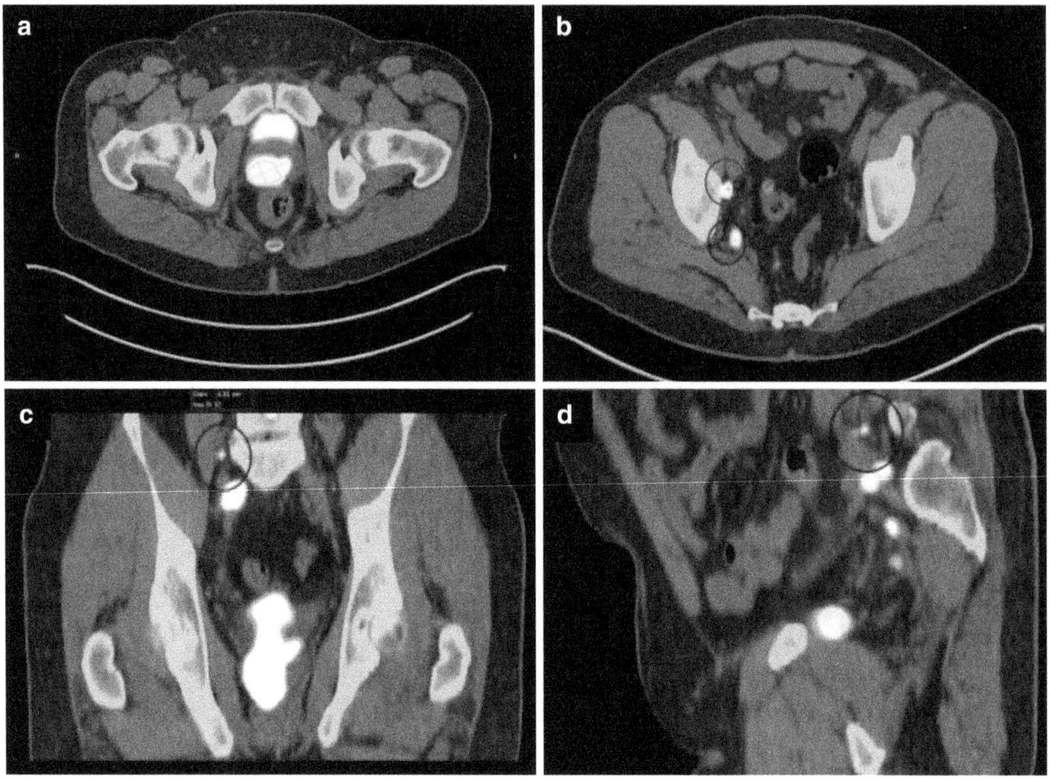

Fig. 2.10 (**Case 2.9**) Axial (**a** and **b**), coronal (**c**), and sagittal (**d**) PSMA-PET-CT images depict a large right-sided lesion which extends beyond midline. Evidence of PET avidity in the pelvic lymph nodes (circles) on axial (**b**), coronal (**c**), and sagittal images (**d**). Note on the coronal and sagittal images the cephalad extent of the suspicious lymph nodes

modal therapy for treatment was likely. Given the superior extent of the suspected positive lymph nodes, an open radical retropubic lymph node dissection was planned. A wide resection was planned on the right. A nerve-sparing procedure was planned on the left.

The prostatectomy and external iliac and obturator lymph nodes were removed prior to entering the peritoneum and performing an extended dissection on the right up to the mid paracaval region (Fig. 2.11). Final pathology demonstrated a large 3.8 cm right-sided Gleason 4 + 5 lesion with right-sided EPE and bilateral SVI. Six of 24 removed lymph nodes were positive for cancer including 2 lymph nodes in the left and right external iliac and obturator packets, 1 lymph node in the presacral packet, and 1 in the paracaval packet.

This case once demonstrates the utility of PSMA-PET in the ability to detect the primary lesion and accurately stage pelvic lymph nodes in the setting of high-risk disease. The abnormality in the prostate on the right side was thought to be post-biopsy hemorrhage artifact. However, on PSMA-PET-MRI, the primary lesion was easily visualized in MRI and PET sequences. CT scans, despite recent technology improvements and contrast enhancement, still lack the spatial resolution to distinguish between the prostate and adjacent structures to detect primary lesions and presence of periprostatic disease [86]. While MRI has been shown to be more effective in detecting primary tumors and periprostatic disease than CT imaging, both modalities perform poorly in staging the pelvic lymph nodes [87]. Hovels et al. performed a meta-analysis of 24

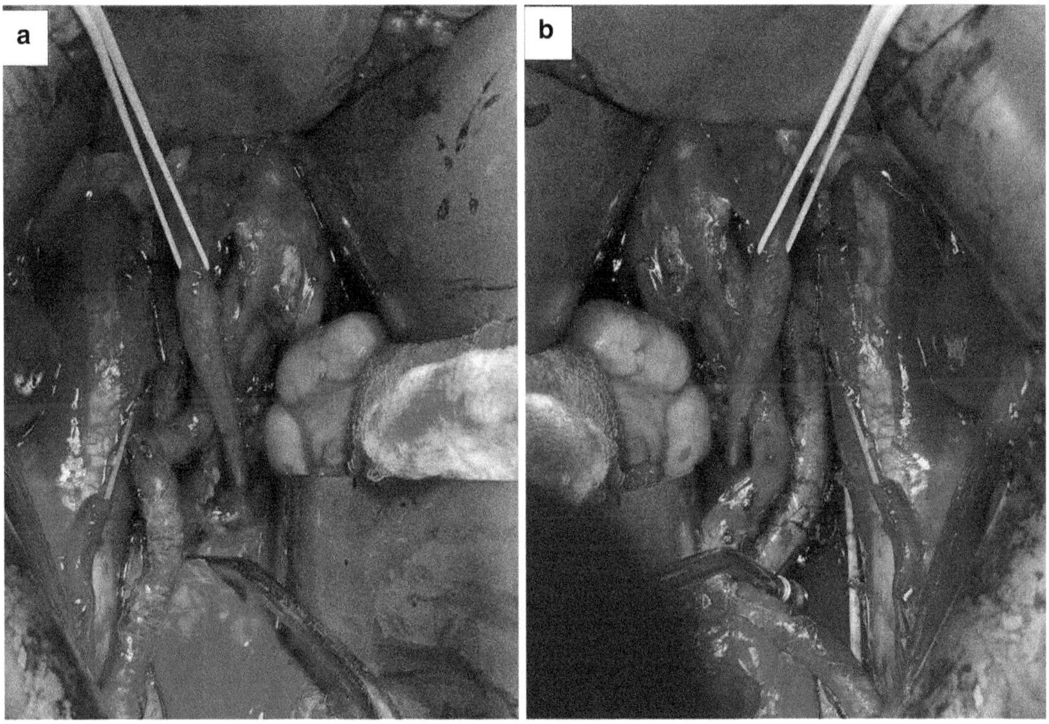

Fig. 2.11 (**Case 2.9**) Intraoperative images representing the extent of the lymph node dissection on the right (**a**) and left (**b**). The prostatectomy and lower pelvic lymph node dissection were done prior to opening the peritoneum. The superior extent of the node dissection was completed after opening the peritoneum and entrance into the retroperitoneum. The right ureter is encircled and retracted with a vessel loop. The lymph node packets medial and lateral to the iliac arteries and lateral the vena cava are clearly removed up to the level of the mid vena cava

studies to evaluate the diagnostic accuracy of CT and MRI in the diagnosis of lymph node metastases. Pooled sensitivity and specificity for CT and MRI were 0.42 and 0.82 and 0.39 and 0.82, respectively. There was no statistical difference between either modality. Therefore, CT and MRI performed equally poorly in detecting lymph node disease which is not surprising given that these studies rely on size criteria of ~1 cm to suggest metastatic disease [88]. These results suggest the need for better imaging studies, perhaps functional imaging, which may be able to more accurately stage the pelvic lymph nodes. As addressed in the previous case, numerous studies have investigated the efficacy of PSMA-PET imaging (either CT or MRI) in staging the pelvic lymph nodes with varying success. Further research in this area is ongoing and eagerly anticipated. At least in the two cases presented here, we found that PSMA-PET-MRI accurately predicted nodal disease.

References

1. Crawford ED, DeAntoni EP, Etzioni R, Schaefer VC, Olson RM, Ross CA. Serum prostate-specific antigen and digital rectal examination for early detection of prostate cancer in a national community-based program. The Prostate Cancer Education Council. Urology. 1996;47(6):863–9.
2. Catalona WJ, Partin AW, Slawin KM, Brawer MK, Flanigan RC, Patel A, et al. Use of the percentage of free prostate-specific antigen to enhance differentiation of prostate cancer from benign prostatic disease: a prospective multicenter clinical trial. JAMA. 1998;279:1542–7.
3. Schröder FH, van der Maas P, Beemsterboer P, Kruger AB, Hoedemaeker R, Rietbergen J, et al. Evaluation of the digital rectal examination as a screening test for prostate cancer. Rotterdam section of the European

randomized study of screening for prostate Cancer. J Natl Cancer Inst. 1998;90:1817–23.
4. Thompson IM, Pauler DK, Goodman PJ, Tangen CM, Lucia MS, Parnes HL, et al. Prevalence of prostate cancer among men with a prostate-specific antigen level < or =4.0 ng per milliliter. N Engl J Med. 2004;350:2239–46.
5. Andriole GL, Levin DL, Crawford ED, Gelmann EP, Pinsky PF, Chia D, et al. Prostate cancer screening in the Prostate, Lung, Colorectal and Ovarian (PLCO) Cancer Screening Trial: findings from the initial screening round of a randomized trial. J Natl Cancer Inst. 2005;97:433–8.
6. Shinohara K, Nguyen H, Masic S. Management of an increasing prostate-specific antigen level after negative prostate biopsy. Urol Clin North Am. 2014;41(2):327–38.
7. Crawford ED, Rove KO, Barqawi AB, Maroni PD, Werahera PN, Baer CA, et al. Clinical-pathologic correlation between transperineal mapping biopsies of the prostate and three-dimensional reconstruction of prostatectomy specimens. Prostate. 2013;73(7):778–87.
8. Tontilla PP, Lantto J, Paakko E, Piippo U, Kauppila S, Lammentausta E, et al. Prebiopsy multiparametric magnetic resonance imaging for prostate cancer diagnosis in biopsy-naïve men suspected prostate cancer based on elevated prostate-specific antigen values: results from a randomized prospective blinded controlled trial. Eur Urol. 2016;69(3):419–25.
9. Gaunay G, Patel V, Shah P, Moreira D, Hall SJ, Vira MA, et al. Role of multi-parametric MRI of the prostate for screening and staging: experience with over 1500 cases. Asian J Urol. 2017;4(1):68–74.
10. Siddiqui MM, Rais-Bahrami S, Turkbey B, George AK, Rothwax J, Shakir N, et al. Comparison of MR/ultrasound fusion-guided biopsy with ultrasound-guided biopsy for the diagnosis of prostate cancer. JAMA. 2015;313(4):390–7.
11. Kasivisvanathan V, Rannikko AS, Borghi M, Panebianco V, Mynderse LA, Vaarala MH, et al. MRI-targeted or standard biopsy for prostate-cancer diagnosis. N Engl J Med. 2018;378(19):1767–77.
12. Wysock JS, Mendhiratta N, Zattoni F, Meng X, Bjurlin M, Huang WC, et al. Predictive value of negative 3T multi-parametric prostate MRI on 12 core biopsy results. BJU Int. 2016;118(4):515–20.
13. Elkhoury FF, Felker ER, Kwan L, Sisk AE, Delfin M, Natarajan S, et al. Comparison of targeted vs systematic prostate biopsy in men who are biopsy naïve. JAMA Surg. 2019;1734:E1–8.
14. Mendhiratta N, Meng X, Rosenkrantz AB, Wysock JS, Fenstermaker M, Huang R, et al. Prebiopsy MRI and MRI-ultrasound fusion-targeted prostate biopsy in men with previous negative biopsies: impact on repeat biopsy strategies. Urology. 2015;86(6):1192–8.
15. Sonn GA, Chang E, Natarajan S, Margolis DJ, Macairan M, Lieu P, et al. Value of targeted prostate biopsy using magnetic resonance-ultrasound fusion in men with prior negative biopsy and elevated prostate-specific antigen. Eur Urol. 2014;65(4):809.
16. Ploussard G, Salomon L, Xylinas E, Allory Y, Vordos D, Hoznek A, et al. Pathological findings and prostate-specific antigen outcomes after radical prostatectomy in men eligible for active surveillance: does the risk of misclassification vary according to biopsy criteria? J Urol. 2010;183(2):539–44.
17. Schoots IG, Petrides N, Giganti F, Bokhorst LP, Rannikko A, Klotz L, et al. Magnetic resonance imaging in active surveillance of prostate cancer: a systematic review. Eur Urol. 2015;67:627–36.
18. Moore CM, Ridout A, Emberton M. The role of MRI in active surveillance of prostate cancer. Curr Opin Urol. 2013;23:261–7.
19. Abd-Alazeez M, Ahmed HU, Arya M, Allen C, Dikaios N, Freeman A, et al. Can multiparametric magnetic resonance imaging predict upgrading of transrectal ultrasound biopsy results at more definitive histology? Urol Oncol. 2014;32:741–7.
20. Vargas HA, Akin O, Afaq A, Goldman D, Zheng J, Moskowitz CS, et al. Magnetic resonance imaging for predicting prostate biopsy findings in patients considered for active surveillance of clinically low risk prostate cancer. J Urol. 2012;188:1732–8.
21. Marliere F, Puech P, Benkirane A, Villers A, Lemaitre L, Leroy X, et al. The role of MRI-targeted and confirmatory biopsies for cancer upstaging at selection in patients considered for active surveillance for clinically low-risk prostate cancer. World J Urol. 2014;32:951–8.
22. Hoeks CM, Somford DM, van Oort IM, Vergunst H, Oddens JR, Smits GA, et al. Value of 3-T multiparametric magnetic resonance imaging and magnetic resonance guided biopsy for early risk restratification in active surveillance of low-risk prostate cancer: a prospective multicenter cohort study. Investig Radiol. 2014;49:165–72.
23. Barrett T, Haider MA. The emerging role of MRI in prostate cancer active surveillance on ongoing challenges. Am J Roentgenol. 2017;208(1):131–9.
24. Hambrock T, Hoeks C, Hulsbergen-van de Kaa C, Scheenen T, Futterer J, Bouwense S, et al. Prospective assessment of prostate cancer aggressiveness using 3-T diffusion-weighted magnetic resonance imaging-guided biopsies versus a systematic 10-core transrectal ultrasound prostate biopsy cohort. Eur Urol. 2012;61:177–84.
25. Bekelman JE, Rumble RB, Chen RC, Pisansky TM, Finelli A, Feifer A, et al. Clinically localized prostate cancer: ASCO clinical practice guideline endorsement of an American Urological Association/American Society for Radiation Oncology/Society of Urologic Oncology Guideline. J Clin Oncol. 2018;36(32):3251–8.
26. Mohler JL, Antonarakis ES, Armstrong AJ, D'Amico AV, Davis BJ, Dorff T, et al. Prostate cancer, version 2.2019, NCCN clinical practice guidelines in oncology. J Natl Compr Cancer Netw. 2019;17(5):479–505.
27. Sanda MG, Dunn RL, Michalski J, Sandler HM, Northouse L, Hembroff L, et al. Quality of life and

satisfaction with outcome among prostate-cancer survivors. N Engl J Med. 2008;358(12):1250–61.
28. Mottet N, Bellmunt J, Bolla M, Briers E, Cumberbatch MG, De Santis M, et al. EAU-ESTRO-SIOG guidelines on prostate cancer. Part 1: screening, diagnosis, and local treatment with curative intent. Eur Urol. 2017;71(4):618–29.
29. Choi WW, Williams SB, Gu X, Lipsitz SR, Nguyen PL, Hu JC. Overuse of imaging for staging low risk prostate cancer. J Urol. 2011;185(5):1645–9.
30. Cooperberg MR, Lubeck DP, Grossfeld GD, Mehta SS, Carroll PR. Contemporary trends in imaging test utilization for prostate cancer staging: data from the cancer of the prostate strategic urologic research endeavor. J Urol. 2002;168(2):491–5.
31. Makarov DV, Desai RA, Yu JB, Sharma R, Abraham N, Albertsen PC, et al. The population level prevalence and correlates of appropriate and inappropriate imaging to stage incident prostate cancer in the medicare population. J Urol. 2012;187(1):97–102.
32. American Urological Association. Fifteen things physicians and patients should question. Available from: https://www.choosingwisely.org/wp-content/uploads/2015/02/AUA-Choosing-Wisely-List.pdf
33. van den Bergh R, Gandaglia G, Tilki D, Borgmann H, Ost P, Surcel C, et al. Trends in radical prostatectomy risk group distribution in a European multicenter analysis of 28 572 patients: towards tailored treatment. Eur Urol Focus. 2019;5(2):171–8.
34. Loft MD, Berg KD, Kjaer A, Iversen P, Ferrari M, Zhang CA, et al. Temporal trends in clinical and pathological characteristics for men undergoing radical prostatectomy between 1995 and 2013 at Rigshospitalet, Copenhagen, Denmark, and Stanford University Hospital, United States. Clin Genitourin Cancer. 2017;16(1):e181–92.
35. Onol FF, Palayapalayam Ganapathi H, Rogers T, Palmer K, Coughlin G, Samavedi S, et al. Changing clinical trends in 10,000 robot-assisted laparoscopic prostatectomy patients and impact of the 2012 USPSTF statement against PSA screening. BJU Int. 2019;124(6):1014–21.
36. Walsh PC, Mostwin JL. Radical prostatectomy and cystoprostatectomy with preservation of potency. Results using a new nerve-sparing technique. Br J Urol. 1984;56(6):694–7.
37. Ficarra V, Novara G, Rosen RC, Artibani W, Carroll PR, Costello A, et al. Systematic review and meta-analysis of studies reporting urinary continence recovery after robot-assisted radical prostatectomy. Eur Urol. 2012;62(3):405–17.
38. Catalona WJ, Basler JW. Return of erections and urinary continence following nerve sparing radical retropubic prostatectomy. J Urol. 1993;150(3):905–7.
39. Avulova S, Zhao Z, Lee D, Huang L-C, Koyama T, Hoffman KE, et al. The effect of nerve sparing status on sexual and urinary function: 3-year results from the CEASAR study. J Urol. 2018;199(5):1202–9.
40. Preston MA, Breau RH, Lantz AG, Morash C, Gerridzen RG, Doucette S, et al. The association between nerve sparing and a positive surgical margin during radical prostatectomy. Urol Oncol. 2015;33(1):18.e1–6.
41. Røder MA, Thomsen FB, Berg KD, Christensen IBJ, Brasso K, Vainer B, et al. Risk of biochemical recurrence and positive surgical margins in patients with pT2 prostate cancer undergoing radical prostatectomy. J Surg Oncol. 2014;109(2):132–8.
42. Godoy G, Tareen BU, Lepor H. Site of positive surgical margins influences biochemical recurrence after radical prostatectomy. BJU Int. 2009;104(11):1610–4.
43. Eggleston JC, Walsh PC. Radical prostatectomy with preservation of sexual function: pathological findings in the first 100 cases. J Urol. 1985;134(6):1146–8.
44. Hull GW, Rabbani F, Abbas F, Wheeler TM, Kattan MW, Scardino PT. Cancer control with radical prostatectomy alone in 1,000 consecutive patients. J Urol. 2002;167(2 Pt 1):528–34.
45. Abdollah F, Dalela D, Sood A, Sammon J, Cho R, Nocera L, et al. Functional outcomes of clinically high-risk prostate cancer patients treated with robot-assisted radical prostatectomy: a multi-institutional analysis. Prostate Cancer Prostatic Dis. 2017;20(4):395–400.
46. Yang DY, Monn MF, Kaimakliotis HZ, Cary KC, Cheng L, Koch MO. Oncologic and quality-of-life outcomes with wide resection in robot-assisted laparoscopic radical prostatectomy. Urol Oncol. 2015;33(2):70.e9–14.
47. Talab SS, Preston MA, Elmi A, Tabatabaei S. Prostate cancer imaging: what the urologist wants to know. Radiol Clin N Am. 2012;50(6):1015–41.
48. Kim SP, Karnes RJ, Mwangi R, Van Houten H, Gross CP, Gershman B, et al. Contemporary trends in magnetic resonance imaging at the time of prostate biopsy: results from a large private insurance database. Eur Urol Focus. 2019 Apr 29. pii: S2405-4569(19)30102-6. https://doi.org/10.1016/j.euf.2019.03.016. [Epub ahead of print]
49. Rosenkrantz AB, Hemingway J, Hughes DR, Duszak R, Allen B, Weinreb JC. Evolving use of prebiopsy prostate magnetic resonance imaging in the medicare population. J Urol. 2018;200(1):89–94.
50. Bloch BN, Genega EM, Costa DN, Pedrosa I, Smith MP, Kressel HY, et al. Prediction of prostate cancer extracapsular extension with high spatial resolution dynamic contrast-enhanced 3-T MRI. Eur Radiol. 2012;22(10):2201–10.
51. Hoeks CM, Barentsz JO, Hambrock T, Yakar D, Somford DM, Heijmink SWTPJ, et al. Prostate cancer: multiparametric MR imaging for detection, localization, and staging. Radiology. 2011;261(1):46–66.
52. Wang L, Mullerad M, Chen H-N, Eberhardt SC, Kattan MW, Scardino PT, et al. Prostate cancer: incremental value of endorectal MR imaging findings for prediction of extracapsular extension. Radiology. 2004;232(1):133–9.
53. de Rooij M, Hamoen EHJ, Witjes JA, Barentsz JO, Rovers MM. Accuracy of magnetic resonance imag-

ing for local staging of prostate cancer: a diagnostic meta-analysis. Eur Urol. 2016;70(2):233–45.
54. Rayn KN, Bloom JB, Gold SA, Hale GR, Baiocco JA, Mehralivand S, et al. Added value of multiparametric magnetic resonance imaging to clinical nomograms for predicting adverse pathology in prostate cancer. J Urol. 2018;200(5):1041–7.
55. Morlacco A, Sharma V, Viers BR, Rangel LJ, Carlson RE, Froemming AT, et al. The incremental role of magnetic resonance imaging for prostate cancer staging before radical prostatectomy. Eur Urol. 2017;71(5):701–4.
56. Rud E, Baco E, Klotz D, Rennesund K, Svindland A, Berge V, et al. Does preoperative magnetic resonance imaging reduce the rate of positive surgical margins at radical prostatectomy in a randomised clinical trial? Eur Urol. 2015;68(3):487–96.
57. Jäderling F, Akre O, Aly M, Björklund J, Olsson M, Adding C, et al. Preoperative staging using magnetic resonance imaging and risk of positive surgical margins after prostate-cancer surgery. Prostate Cancer Prostatic Dis. 2018;128:492.
58. Tewari AK, Srivastava A, Huang MW, Robinson BD, Shevchuk MM, Durand M, et al. Anatomical grades of nerve sparing: a risk-stratified approach to neural-hammock sparing during robot-assisted radical prostatectomy (RARP). BJU Int. 2011;108(6 Pt 2):984–92.
59. Schiavina R, Bianchi L, Borghesi M, Dababneh H, Chessa F, Pultrone CV, et al. MRI displays the prostatic cancer anatomy and improves the bundles management before robot-assisted radical prostatectomy. J Endourol. 2018;32(4):315–21.
60. Panebianco V, Salciccia S, Cattarino S, Minisola F, Gentilucci A, Alfarone A, et al. Use of multiparametric MR with neurovascular bundle evaluation to optimize the oncological and functional management of patients considered for nerve-sparing radical prostatectomy. J Sex Med. 2012;9(8):2157–66.
61. Park BH, Jeon HG, Jeong BC, Seo SI, Lee HM, Choi HY, et al. Influence of magnetic resonance imaging in the decision to preserve or resect neurovascular bundles at robotic assisted laparoscopic radical prostatectomy. J Urol. 2014;192(1):82–8.
62. Rosenkrantz AB, Ginocchio LA, Cornfeld D, Froemming AT, Gupta RT, Turkbey B, et al. Interobserver reproducibility of the PI-RADS version 2 lexicon: a multicenter study of six experienced prostate radiologists. Radiology. 2016;280(3):793–804.
63. Muller BG, Shih JH, Sankineni S, Marko J, Rais-Bahrami S, George AK, et al. Prostate cancer: interobserver agreement and accuracy with the revised prostate imaging reporting and data system at multiparametric MR imaging. Radiology. 2015;277(3):741–50.
64. Rosenkrantz AB, Ayoola A, Hoffman D, Khasgiwala A, Prabhu V, Smereka P, et al. The learning curve in prostate MRI interpretation: self-directed learning versus continual reader feedback. AJR Am J Roentgenol. 2017;208(3):W92–W100.
65. Gaziev G, Wadhwa K, Barrett T, Koo BC, Gallagher FA, Serrao E, et al. Defining the learning curve for multiparametric magnetic resonance imaging (MRI) of the prostate using MRI-transrectal ultrasonography (TRUS) fusion-guided transperineal prostate biopsies as a validation tool. BJU Int. 2016;117(1):80–6.
66. Latchamsetty KC, Borden LS, Porter CR, Lacrampe M, Vaughan M, Lin E, et al. Experience improves staging accuracy of endorectal magnetic resonance imaging in prostate cancer: what is the learning curve? Can J Urol. 2007;14(1):3429–34.
67. Akin O, Riedl CC, Ishill NM, Moskowitz CS, Zhang J, Hricak H. Interactive dedicated training curriculum improves accuracy in the interpretation of MR imaging of prostate cancer. Eur Radiol. 2010;20(4):995–1002.
68. Jansen BHE, Oudshoorn FHK, Tijans AM, Yska MJ, Lont AP, Collette ERP, et al. Local staging with multiparametric MRI in daily clinical practice: diagnostic accuracy and evaluation of a radiologic learning curve. World J Urol. 2018;36(9):1409–15.
69. Tay KJ, Gupta RT, Brown AF, Silverman RK, Polascik TJ. Defining the incremental utility of prostate multiparametric magnetic resonance imaging at standard and specialized read in predicting extracapsular extension of prostate cancer. Eur Urol. 2016;70(2):211–3.
70. Mizuno R, Nakashima J, Mukai M, Ookita H, Nakagawa K, Oya M, et al. Maximum tumor diameter is a simple and valuable index associated with the local extent of disease in clinically localized prostate cancer. Int J Urol. 2006;13(7):951–5.
71. D'Amico AV, Whittington R, Malkowicz SB, Schultz D, Blank K, Broderick GA, et al. Biochemical outcome after radical prostatectomy, external beam radiation therapy, or interstitial radiation therapy for clinically localized prostate cancer. JAMA. 1998;280(11):969–74.
72. Stephenson RA, Middleton RG, Abbott TM. Wide excision (nonnerve sparing) radical retropubic prostatectomy using an initial perirectal dissection. J Urol. 1997;157(1):251–5.
73. Dussinger AM, Beck SDW, Cheng L, Koch MO. Does wide primary perirectal dissection during radical retropubic prostatectomy alter pathologic and biochemical outcomes? Urology. 2005;66(5 Suppl):95–100.
74. Okajima E, Yoshikawa M, Masuda Y, Shimizu K, Tanaka N, Hirayama A, et al. Improvement of the surgical curability of locally confined prostate cancer including non-organ-confined high-risk disease through retropubic radical prostatectomy with intentional wide resection. World J Surg Oncol. 2012;10(1):249.
75. Miyake H, Fujimoto H, Komiyama M, Fujisawa M. Development of "extended radical retropubic prostatectomy": a surgical technique for improving margin positive rates in prostate cancer. Eur J Surg Oncol. 2010;36(3):281–6.
76. Martini A, Gupta A, Cumarasamy S, Lewis SC, Haines KG, Briganti A, et al. Novel nomogram for the prediction of seminal vesicle invasion including mul-

tiparametric magnetic resonance imaging. Int J Urol. 2019;26(4):458–64.
77. Yaxley JW, Raveenthiran S, Nouhaud F-X, Samaratunga H, Yaxley WJ, Coughlin G, et al. Risk of metastatic disease on 68 gallium-prostate-specific membrane antigen positron emission tomography/computed tomography scan for primary staging of 1253 men at the diagnosis of prostate cancer. BJU Int. 2019;44(Suppl. 3):1258.
78. Yaxley JW, Raveenthiran S, Nouhaud F-X, Samartunga H, Yaxley AJ, Coughlin G, et al. Outcomes of primary lymph node staging of intermediate and high risk prostate cancer with 68ga-PSMA positron emission tomography/computerized tomography compared to histological correlation of pelvic lymph node pathology. J Urol. 2019;201(4):815–20.
79. Parker CC, James ND, Brawley CD, Clarke NW, Hoyle AP, Ali A, et al. Radiotherapy to the primary tumour for newly diagnosed, metastatic prostate cancer (STAMPEDE): a randomised controlled phase 3 trial. Lancet. 2018;392(10162):2353–66.
80. Poelaert F, Verbaeys C, Rappe B, Kimpe B, Billiet I, Plancke H, et al. Cytoreductive prostatectomy for metastatic prostate cancer: first lessons learned from the multicentric prospective local treatment of metastatic prostate cancer (LoMP) trial. Urology. 2017;106:146–52.
81. Parikh RR, Byun J, Goyal S, Kim IY. Local therapy improves overall survival in patients with newly diagnosed metastatic prostate cancer. Prostate. 2017;77(6):559–72.
82. Löppenberg B, Dalela D, Karabon P, Sood A, Sammon JD, Meyer CP, et al. The impact of local treatment on overall survival in patients with metastatic prostate cancer on diagnosis: a national cancer data base analysis. Eur Urol. 2017;72(1):14–9.
83. Fossati N, Trinh Q-D, Sammon J, Sood A, Larcher A, Sun M, et al. Identifying optimal candidates for local treatment of the primary tumor among patients diagnosed with metastatic prostate cancer: a SEER-based study. Eur Urol. 2015;67(1):3–6.
84. Freitag MT, Kesch C, Cardinale J, Flechsig P, Floca R, Eiber M, et al. Simultaneous whole-body 18F-PSMA-1007-PET/MRI with integrated high-resolution multiparametric imaging of the prostatic fossa for comprehensive oncological staging of patients with prostate cancer: a pilot study. Eur J Nucl Med Mol Imaging. 2018;45(3):340–7.
85. Grubmüller B, Baltzer P, Hartenbach S, D'Andrea D, Helbich TH, Haug AR, et al. PSMA ligand PET/MRI for primary prostate cancer: staging performance and clinical impact. Clin Cancer Res. 2018;24(24):6300–7.
86. Ravizzini G, Turkbey B, Kurdziel K, Choyke PL. New horizons in prostate cancer imaging. Eur J Radiol. 2009;70(2):212–26.
87. Choi S. The role of magnetic resonance imaging in the detection of prostate cancer. J Urol. 2011;186(4):1181–2.
88. Hövels AM, Heesakkers RAM, Adang EM, Jager GJ, Strum S, Hoogeveen YL, et al. The diagnostic accuracy of CT and MRI in the staging of pelvic lymph nodes in patients with prostate cancer: a meta-analysis. Clin Radiol. 2008;63(4):387–95.

Zonal Anatomy of Prostate on MRI

3

Marcin B. Czarniecki and Joseph H. Yacoub

3.1 Introduction

The prostate is an accessory organ of the male reproductive system located within the midline of the pelvis and is contained within the subperitoneal space. The gland has the shape of an inverted pyramid, which encapsulates the prostatic urethra. The base of the gland is directly attached to the urinary bladder neck, while the apex of the gland is resting against the urogenital diaphragm. A normal gland is approximately the size of a walnut and weighs 15–20 g. Measurement on MRI or ultrasound is commonly performed using the approximation of an equation for a prolate ellipsoid, which is measured by multiplying Length × Width × Height × 0.52, where 0.52 approximates the constant of $\pi/6$. The prostate gland enlarges with age, with young males having an average volume of 11.5 cc (range 1.6–20.6), which is increased to 39.6 cc by 60 (range 38–83) [1, 2]. The prostate has a role of forming 15–20% of the excretion in the normal ejaculation, forming a liquid medium for the spermatozoa to swim in, as well as provide a concoction of proteolytic enzymes, increasing the likelihood of successful fertilization [3].

Human prostate anatomy was described as far back as 1543 by Andreas Vesalius, but a system of anatomical division of the prostate into lobes was not introduced until around 1912 [4]. Only in 1982, were the four distinct anatomical regions that are used today defined and histologically described by John McNeal [5]. The four regions are the peripheral (PZ), transition (TZ), and central zones (CZ), as well as the anterior fibromuscular stroma (AFS) (Fig. 3.1). In addition, non-anatomic carryover terms describing portions of the prostate are also in use, including "median lobe" or "central gland," which can be a source of confusion in understanding the prostatic anatomy. The practicing radiologist's role entails diagnosing prostate cancer, preparation and performing fusion biopsy, as well as staging and detection of recurrence. Each step requires an in-depth knowledge of prostate anatomy.

In this chapter, the authors aim to explain the currently accepted prostate anatomy, with an emphasis on its appearance on MRI. The relationships of the PZ, TZ, and CZ according to the division described by McNeal will be explained, as well as its importance for radiologists.

3.2 Vascularization

Vascular supply of the prostate arises from the prostatic arteries, which in turn typically arise from the anterior division of the internal iliac arteries. One should keep in mind that there is significant variability in origin of the prostatic arteries. It can arise from a common trunk with

M. B. Czarniecki · J. H. Yacoub (✉)
MedStar Georgetown University Hospital, Department of Radiology, Washington, DC, USA
e-mail: marcin.b.czarniecki@gunet.georgetown.edu; joseph.h.yacoub@medstar.net

T. Tirkes (ed.), *Prostate MRI Essentials*, https://doi.org/10.1007/978-3-030-45935-2_3

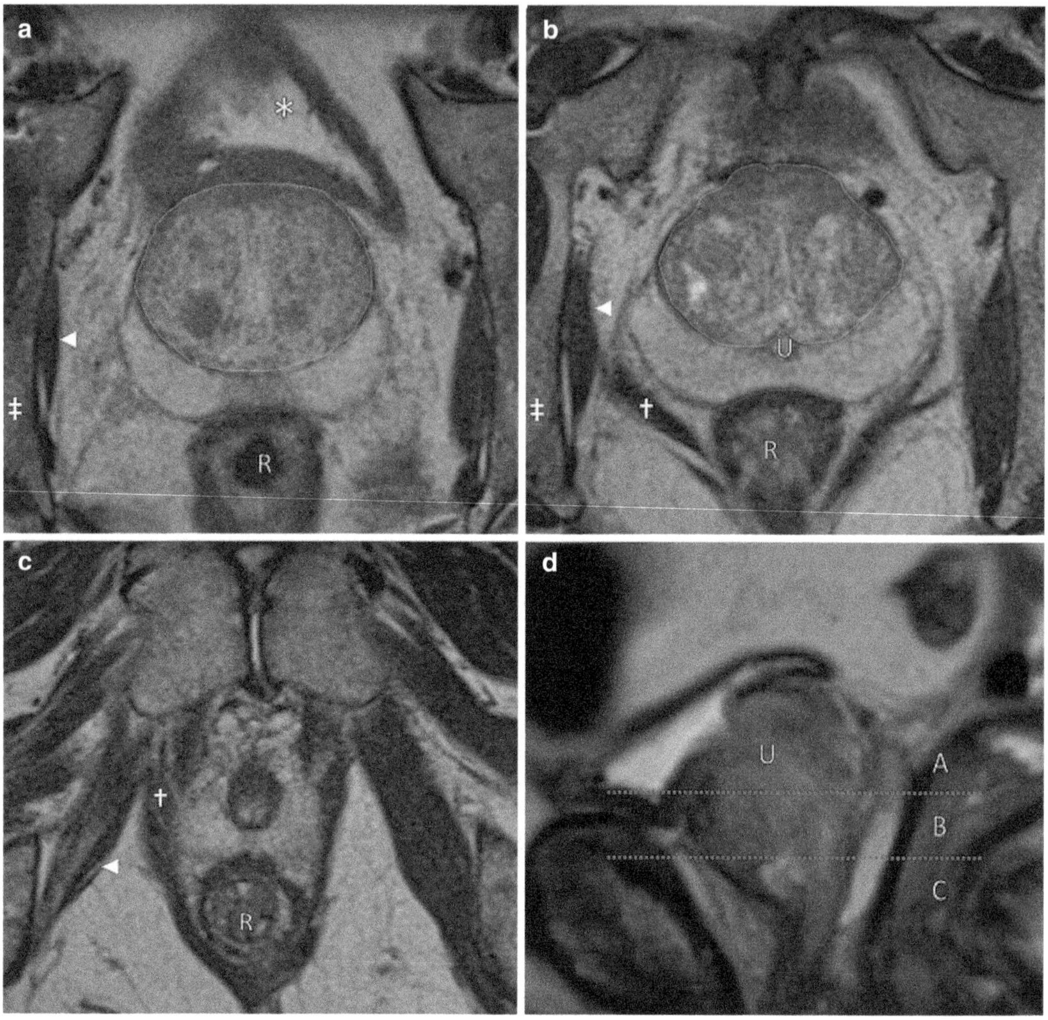

Fig. 3.1 Prostate zonal anatomy delineated at the base (**a**), midgland (**b**), and apex (**c**) showing the relationship of the peripheral (blue), transition (yellow), and central (orange) zones. The sagittal image shows the path of the prostatic urethra (U), which can help in dividing the prostate into three equal areas in the cariocaudal dimension (**d**). Posteriorly, the prostate is bounded by the rectum (R) from the base to the apex. The urinary bladder (*) is located cranial to the prostate base. The levator ani muscle is closely related to the lateral borders at the prostatic apex (†). Medial to the ischial bones (‡), the obturator internus muscles (arrowhead) forms the lateral border of the periprostatic tissues

the superior visceral artery, directly from the anterior division of the internal iliac artery just distal to the takeoff of the obturator artery, or from the obturator artery. Some variations in origin are of particular interest such as when arising from the pudendal and middle rectal arteries. This information is especially valuable in the setting of prostatic artery embolization (PAE) and could also be useful for urologists in surgical planning [6, 7]. Although arterial anatomy is variable to the extent that it may be supplied differently on each side, there are two main arterial branches that supply the gland itself on each side. The two branches can arise from a common trunk or from two independent prostatic arteries. The two branches are named according to the anatomical location where they enter the prostate as the anteromedial and posterolateral branch, with the former supplying the TZ, while the latter supply the PZ and apex. For the purpose of benign prostatic hyperplasia (BPH) treatment by PAE, selective embolization of the anteromedial branch is highly desired and is performed bilaterally [8]. There is, however, a high rate of prostatic revascularization, which most commonly happens from the posterolateral branch [8].

Venous drainage is from the prostatic venous plexus to the internal iliac veins. The venous plexus surrounds the prostate along its lateral and anterior margins [3, 9]. Age decreases the venous drainage within the lateral regions of the venous plexus, leaving the older men with a predominance of the anterior venous plexus [9]. Notably, the internal iliac veins are interconnected with the vertebral plexus, which is thought to be the route of osseous metastatic spread. The name "venous plexus" may be misleading. It was once thought that this vascular complex contains solely venous vessels, but newer studies found that small arterioles are also intertwined among the larger venous component. On imaging, the arterial and venous vasculature is not distinguishable from each other, but this finding has proven to be important for the surgeon as it may cause significant bleeding [10]. Recent literature also showed that there is a crucial role of the plexus in erectile dysfunction [11, 12]. Thus, current surgical and radiotherapy techniques aim to maximize the preservation of this complex in order to preserve sexual function by maintaining the perineurovascular network.

3.3 Lymphatic Drainage

Lymphatic drainage of the prostate follows the venous system and is important in the accurate staging of prostate cancer. Nodes that are located lateral to the prostate and medial to the obturator muscles are the sentinel obturator lymph nodes and may also be referred to as the medial chain of the external iliac nodal group [13]. Less commonly, there are lymph nodes which are directly adjacent to the prostate, seen in 4.4% of prostatectomy specimens [14]. Further drainage up the iliac chain follows along the external iliac nodes' medial and lateral chains. Alternatively, drainage may occur along the internal iliac nodes, although this is less common. In this case, the sentinel nodes are considered to be the junctional nodes at the confluence of the internal and external iliac vasculature. Some rarer routes of drainage include an anterior route following the perivesical nodes which then drain into the internal iliac chain and up along the aorta. Another rare route would be the presacral route, which drains along the paramedian margin of the sacrum to the sacral promontory and onto the common iliac chain [15].

Sensitivity of lymph node metastasis depends on the size and has a variable sensitivity ranging from 24% to 75%. Nodes measuring more than 10 mm in short axis on anatomical imaging are considered suspicious. However, there is increasing recognition that many smaller nodes can harbor the disease as well. Additional features such as shape, architecture, or functional imaging may add to the specificity and overall accuracy of detecting nodes.

3.4 Prostate Embryology and Anatomic Landmarks

3.4.1 Embryology

The primitive urogenital sinus extends from the embryonic hindgut as early as 8 weeks of gestation. Subsequently, the primitive urogenital sinus forms the rostral end (forming the urinary bladder), urogenital sinus (prostate), and penile urethra [16]. By 10 weeks, the prostate starts to form through the budding of epithelial cells through the urogenital sinus at the site of the Mullerian tubercle and is influenced by hormonal regulation [4]. The process is completed at full sexual maturation. Transition and peripheral zones have similar cell compositions, as both are derived from the urogenital sinus. The small differences in the cell ratios and patterns of glandular formation result in different signal intensities on MRI [17, 18]. The central zone is derived from the Wolffian duct, which has histological characteristics closely related to the lining of the ejaculatory ducts and seminal vesicles [18].

The McNeal's anatomical differentiation of zonal anatomy that is visible on MRI is distinctly related to the different embryological origins and its patterns of epithelial cells in each specific zone.

3.4.2 Prostatic Urethra and Verumontanum

The prostatic urethra is a key landmark in the prostate extending from the neck of the bladder to the external urethral sphincter. The verumontanum is a small section in the mid-prostatic urethra which drains the ejaculatory ducts and numerous small microscopic ducts from the CZ. It is an important anatomical landmark that divides the urethra into the proximal and distal parts (Fig. 3.2). It also demarcates the inferior extent of the transition zone, which is located superiorly [4]. Angulation of the prostatic urethra also occurs superior to the verumontanum and occurs at an angle of approximately 35 degrees [19]. With benign prostatic hyperplasia, the prostatic urethra elongates and becomes more angulated, causing obstructive symptoms in patients [9, 20, 21]. Numerous microscopic ducts drain from the PZ into the distal urethra. On MRI, the verumontanum may be identified as a focus of mid-prostatic urethral dilatation showing centrally increased T2 signal intensity surrounded by core of low T2 signal. These MR features correspond to increasing components of striated muscle fibers, which increase when moving caudally to the level of the external urethral sphincter [5, 7, 9].

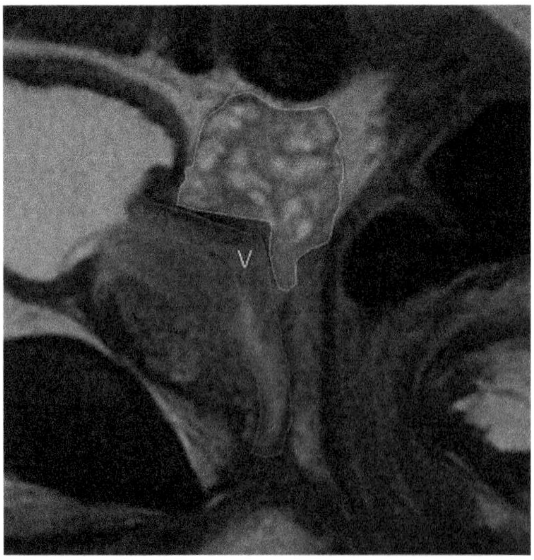

Fig. 3.2 Anatomy of the seminal vesicle in the sagittal plane. The seminal vesicle (yellow) joins at its caudal end with the vas deferens (not shown) to form the ejaculatory duct. The ejaculatory duct then runs caudally and medially to the verumontanum (V) and into the prostatic urethra (green)

3.4.3 Seminal Vesicles

The seminal vesicles are paired organs which comprise of convoluted and interconnected diverticula. This organ measures approximately 3 cm in length and has a diameter of 1.5 cm in a young, healthy male [22]. The seminal vesicles originate at the prostate base and extend superiorly toward the urinary bladder. At the base of the prostate, the seminal vesicles join with the ipsilateral vas deferens to form two symmetrical ejaculatory ducts. The conjoined ducts then course caudally and medially toward the midline of the prostate where both empty into the verumontanum [19, 23]. After ejaculation, the volume of the seminal vesicles decreases by approximately 40% [24].

On MRI, the fluid component of the seminal vesicles has an increased signal intensity on T2-weighted images. In older patients, the seminal vesicles are more likely to have a smaller volume due to extrinsic compression by BPH [25]. Assessment of the seminal vesicles is important in the staging of prostate cancer. For an optimal MR evaluation, the seminal vesicles are best evaluated when full. For this reason, abstinence from ejaculation for 3 days prior to imaging is recommended [26].

3.4.4 Sector Maps

Sector maps aide in anatomical localization of lesions; therefore it is important for the radiologist to know in order to help urologists and radiation oncologists in diagnosis and treatment planning. In PI-RADS v2.1, the revised sector map contains two additional sectors in the base PZ: right and left posterior PZ medial, as depicted in Fig. 3.3. With this revision, there are now 38 prostate sectors, plus 2 sectors for the seminal vesicles and 1 for the membranous urethra, amounting to a total 41 sectors [27]. The updated PI-RADS document continues to keep the general principles of dividing the prostate according to its histological makeup, as well as anatomical

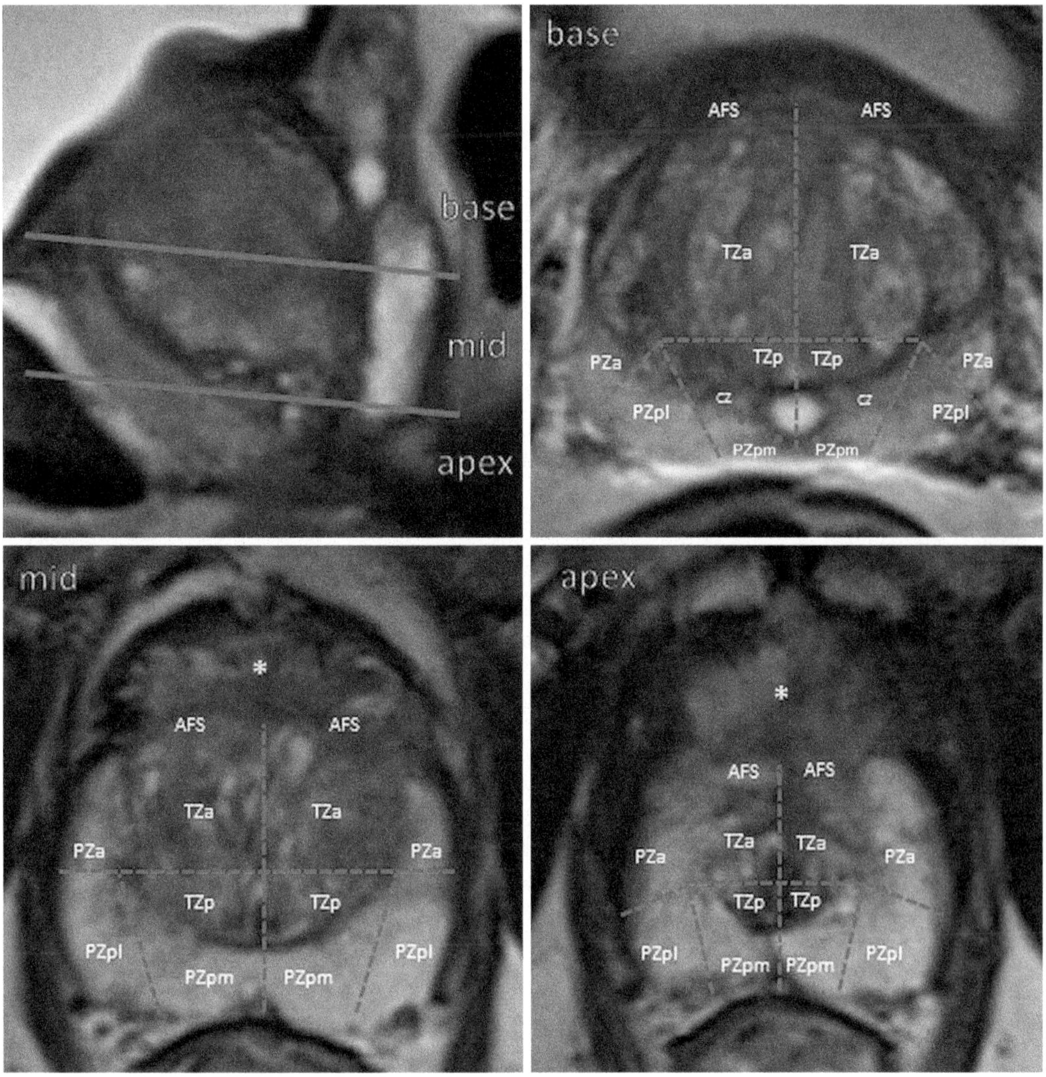

Fig. 3.3 Sector map according to PI-RADS v2.1. The segmentation model used in PI-RADS v2.1 employs 38 sectors for the prostate, 2 sectors for the seminal vesicles, and 1 for the membranous urethra (total 41). The prostate is divided into the base, midgland, and apex. The transition zone is divided into anterior (TZa) and posterior (TZp) portions at all three levels. The peripheral zone has an anterior (PZa), posterolateral (PZpl), and posteromedial (PZpm) portions at the base, midgland, and apex. The central zone (CZ) is seen only at the base. This figure is from a patient with mild BPH. Most patients have prostatic components that are enlarged or atrophied, and the PZ may be obscured by an enlarged TZ, and CZ may not be easily identifiable. In such instances, a diagram is used as an approximation of the gland, and a sector map can be marked to indicate the location of the findings in addition to the written report. Asterisk (∗) denotes the venous plexus seen anterior to the prostate

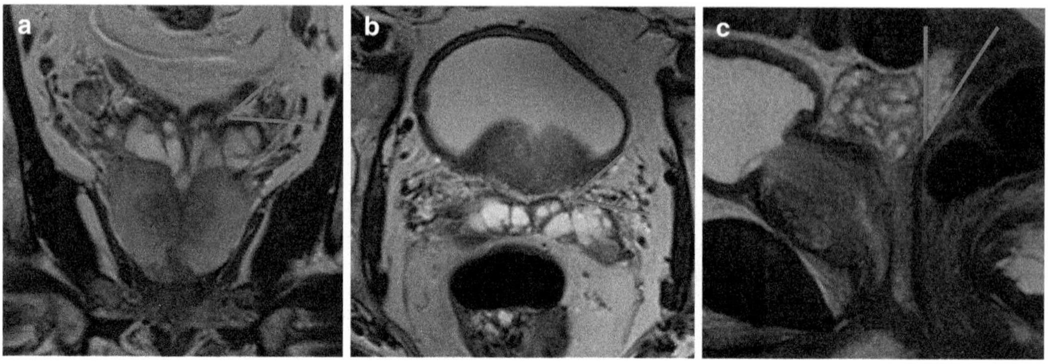

Fig. 3.4 Coronal (**a**), axial (**b**), and sagittal (**c**) T2-weighted images of a normal prostate demonstrating the prostate-seminal vesicle angle (**a, b**) and rectoprostatic angle (**c**)

locations to aid in the description of prostatic lesions. Thus, the TZ is divided into 12 sectors, with 4 sectors at each of the 3 levels: apex, mid, and base. At each of the three levels, the TZ is divided into an anterior (TZa) and posterior (TZp) sectors on both sides of the midline.

The PZ is divided into 18 sectors, anterior (PZa), posterolateral (PZpl), and posteromedial (PZpm) sectors at the base, midgland, and apex. The PZ occupies a larger proportion of the gland at the mid and apical levels and had increasing anterior component closer to the apex. The prostate base also contains two symmetrical areas in the medial portion of the gland, which represent the CZ.

The anterior fibromuscular stroma is divided into right and left sections at the prostate base, midgland, and apex. The seminal vesicles are likewise divided into right and left sections.

Other sectors maps exist, some of which are simpler with a smaller number of sectors. For example, one sector map is geared toward transperineal approach biopsies that sample the prostate from the apex longitudinally, which leads to a zonal sampling of prostate and is different from the more widely used transrectal approach [28].

3.4.5 Compartments and Angles

The prostate and its neighboring tissues can be separated into compartments [27]. The periprostatic compartment contains the tissues surrounding the prostate. Posteriorly, the rectoprostatic compartment contains the tissues posterior to the prostate and anterior to the rectum. The rectoprostatic angle is formed from the soft tissues between the rectum and prostate, with the angle measured between the anterior rectal wall and the posterior border of the seminal vesicles. Obliteration of this angle is considered as a sign of extraprostatic extension. Another angle is the prostate-seminal vesicle angle. This angle is measured best in the axial plane, and it can be obliterated with the extracapsular extension of the prostate cancer (Fig. 3.4).

3.5 Zonal Anatomy

Since the beginning of the MR imaging of the male pelvis in the 1980s, superior soft-tissue contrast of the MRI was found to be correlating with zones of the prostate [29]. The regions that were described by McNeal had a direct correlation on imaging. The central, transition, and peripheral zones are differentiated on T2-weighted imaging, which is currently used as the dominant sequence to evaluate its morphology.

3.6 Peripheral Zone (PZ)

The PZ forms up to 70% of the gland by volume [19]. It is composed of small glandular tubules lined by simple columnar epithelium which empty into larger ducts, surrounded by loosely bound muscle fibers [4]. The bilateral PZ form an incomplete ring encompassing the TZ in varying degrees along the gland. At the apex, almost all the tissue surrounding the urethra is PZ. Moving cranially, the PZ forms the outer border of the posterior, lateral, and anterolateral portions of the gland. At the base, the anterior horns are smaller and displaced by a larger fibromuscular stroma, which forms the anterior border of the gland at the level of the midgland and at the base [20]. The anterolateral portions of the PZ are often referred to as the "horns" and become less visible with development of benign prostatic hyperplasia (BPH).

On MRI, the PZ has a homogeneous high signal intensity on T2-weighted images that makes it easily distinguishable from the other zones; however, it is indistinguishable from the rest of the gland on T1-weighted images. Following the administration of intravenous contrast, the normal PZ demonstrates uniform enhancement. Uniform signal intensity of diffusion-weighted imaging is also expected in the normal PZ, without areas of diffusion restriction.

3.7 Transition Zone (TZ)

The TZ is composed of two symmetric lobes positioned on each side of the prostatic urethra above the level of the verumontanum. It is absent at the prostatic apex in a normal gland but is present on each side of the urethra at the midgland and base [20]. Histological features of the TZ vary somewhat from the PZ. First, the stromal component forms a dense layer and has a larger muscular component [30]. Ducts of the TZ are similar in number to PZ but are oriented laterally with substantially smaller, arborizing branches that curve anteriorly toward the bladder neck [19, 31].

The TZ comprises 5% of the gland in young adults and grows with age to nearly replacing the entire gland in patients with severe benign prostatic hyperplasia [19]. Progressive growth can result in lower urinary tract symptoms and chronic bladder outlet obstruction due to compression of the urethra.

On T1-weighted images, the TZ is usually indistinguishable from the rest of the gland but may contain blood products or proteinaceous material, which gives rise to foci of increased signal intensity. The TZ on T2-weighted images demonstrates signal heterogeneity, which progresses with age. In a young adult, it remains a minor component of the prostate with a uniform decreased signal intensity. With the progression of hyperplasia, TZ forms encapsulated nodules with variable signal intensities representing "glandular hyperplasia." Intervening area of low signal intensity is often seen between the nodules likely representing "stromal hyperplasia."

The TZ is variable in size and appearance on MRI, but its boundaries are well-demarcated. The outer border is well defined by the "surgical capsule," which is comprised of compressed stromal and fibromuscular tissue [32]. The term originates from the surgical field as the dissection field along which enucleation was performed for the treatment of BPH, currently considered an obsolete technique due to newer, less invasive methods of treating BPH. The surgical capsule is well delineated on MRI as a well-demarcated border between the TZ and PZ, with low signal intensity on T2-weighted images [33].

3.8 Central Zone (CZ)

The paired conical CZ extends along the ejaculatory ducts, with the apex directed toward the verumontanum (Fig. 3.5). The CZ is formed of small acini and ducts closely following the ejaculatory ducts. The cells are much larger and polyhedral compared to the peripheral zone [4]. The base of the CZ comprises the majority of the posteromedial sector of the prostatic base [33]. Histologically, it has a distinct structure, with a notably larger epithelial component compared to the PZ and TZ [33]. The glands are of larger caliber, with the formation of intraglandular lacunae formed by tall columnar cells and a prominent basal layer [18, 34]. Separate draining orifices along the ejaculatory duct develop, and thus the zone is thought to be remnant tissue related to the Wolffian ducts. Embryologically, it is more

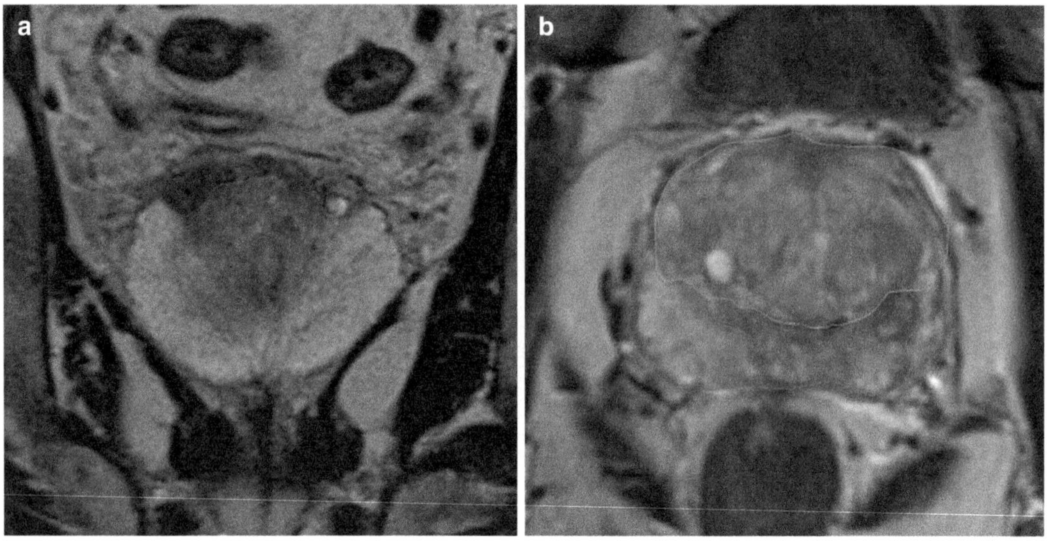

Fig. 3.5 The central zone (orange) in the coronal (**a**) and axial (**b**) plane. On the coronal plane, it may form a triangular shape of tissue which has a decreased signal intensity on T2-weighted images when compared to the peripheral zone (blue) and can be delinated from the transition zone (yellow) in most cases

closely related to the seminal vesicles than the remainder of the prostate [35]. Unlike the TZ, the volume of the CZ decreases with age [33]. The term "central gland" should not be confused with the central zone. The central gland was a term commonly used to refer to the combination of the TZ and CZ based on older literature that suggested that these two zones could not be distinguished on imaging. The use of this term is now discouraged.

3.8.1 Anterior Fibromuscular Stroma (AFS)

The anterior portion of the gland is histologically different from the rest of the prostate. Anatomically, the AFS forms the entire anterior surface of the prostate, extending like an apron from the bladder neck to the prostate apex. Superiorly it blends with the smooth and skeletal muscles of the bladder, and inferiorly, it blends into the muscle fibers forming the urethral sphincter at the apex [19]. Histologically, it is composed of smooth and skeletal muscle fibers, which in turn blend with the urogenital diaphragm along its caudal aspect [9, 33]. It is also inseparable from the glandular portions of the gland; therefore, it is removed together with the remainder of the prostate during prostatectomy.

The appearance of AFS on MRI is distinct from the rest of the gland. On T1- and T2-weighted imaging, it demonstrates a low signal intensity, much like skeletal muscle. It demonstrates no restricted diffusion with low signal intensity on all DWI sequences. The AFS is hypovascular relative to the glandular prostate on contrast-enhanced images [20, 33].

3.8.2 Prostate Capsule

The prostate capsule is comprised of concentrically oriented fibromuscular tissue surrounding the majority of the gland. It is an important anatomical landmark for the staging of prostate cancer. Some authors refer to it as pseudocapsule, because it is inseparable from the prostatic stroma and does not qualify as a true capsule in an anatomic or histologic sense [36]. At the base, there are small capsular defects at the origin of the ejaculatory ducts. Additionally, the prostatic apex has a poorly delineated capsule [5, 7]. Notably, there are innumerable areas of neurovascular

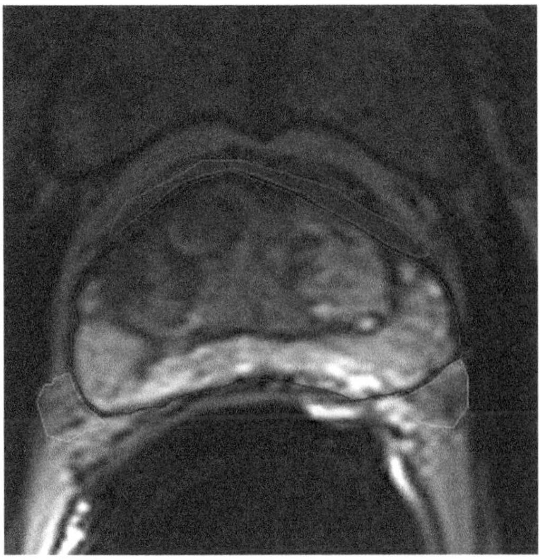

Fig. 3.6 Axial T2-weighted images of the prostate, showing the prostatic capsule (red) with a decreased signal intensity, anterior fibromuscular stroma (blue), and neurovascular bundles (yellow)

penetration through the capsule to supply the prostatic glandular structures, making the "capsule" porous.

The capsule is visible on MRI as a dark rind of a decreased signal on T2-weighted images surrounding the majority of the gland (Fig. 3.6). It has an important role in prostate cancer staging, as the extraprostatic extension has been associated with a higher risk of positive margins following prostatectomy hence increasing the risk for biochemical recurrence and metastatic disease [37–40].

3.8.3 Neurovascular Bundles

Combination of nerve fibers and small vessels seen along the posterolateral border of the prostate is named neurovascular bundles (NVBs). These are nestled between three periprostatic fascial planes creating a triangular structure (Fig. 3.6). Lateral fascia bounds the NVB laterally, Denonvilliers' fascia posteriorly, and the prostatic fascia along the medial border. The NVBs are classically described to be localized in a triangular-shaped area posterolateral to the gland at the 5 and 7 o'clock positions; however, the anatomy of the NVB is highly variable. Some studies show that more than half of the male population lack the expected triangular shape and are located anywhere along the prostatic lateral surface, with a significant portion positioned anteriorly [7, 41, 42]. The posterior part of the prostate at the 6 o'clock position has been shown to contain little to no nerve fibers [7, 43].

These paired structures contain nerve fibers originating from the pelvic plexus and ultimately innervate the bilateral corpora cavernosa and play an important role in erectile function [7]. Additional fibers arising from the pudendal nerve traverse along with the autonomic fibers and innervate the urethral sphincter and external urethral sphincter and help in maintaining urinary continence, which is another potential complication following prostatectomy [44]. Current surgical techniques aim to spare the excision of the neurovascular structures, which are needed to maintain these functions.

The triangular anatomy is best appreciated on MRI along the base where the fascial triangle is largest, and the NVBs are easiest to identify surrounded by a high signal from adipose tissue on T2-weighted images. They appear as small punctate and tubular structures, which correspond to vessels and fibers. As they travel caudally, they give off small branches innervating the prostatic capsule [45] and eventually partially supply the urethral sphincter. At the apex, these bundles become intimately adjacent to the prostatic capsule and are therefore less discernible on MRI.

3.8.4 Prostatic Cysts

Multiple different cystic entities have been described within and around the prostate, which is beyond the scope of this chapter. Having prostate anatomy in mind, most commonly seen intraprostatic cystic lesions are described below for the purpose of their identification on routine MR imaging. More in-depth reviews are available and may be of use for the practicing radiologist [46–49].

3.8.5 Utricle Cyst

As an embryological remnant of the Mullerian duct, utricle cyst is located at the midline and directly posterior to the prostatic urethra. It is the most common midline cyst, occurring in 1–5% of the population. On MR imaging, they are usually seen as pear-shaped cysts, which does not extend beyond the prostatic base but communicate with the prostatic urethra. Utricle cyst has shown to have an association with various genitourinary abnormalities and has rare reports of associated malignancies [48] (Fig. 3.7).

3.8.6 Mullerian Duct Cysts

Embryologically, these cysts result from failure of regression and cystic dilation of the mesonephric duct. Compared to the utricle cyst, they tend to be larger and extend cranially above the prostate base. Unlike utricle cysts, there is no communication with the urethra but have a similar appearance on MRI. These cysts show high signal intensity on T2-weighted images and can have variable intensity on T1-weighted images depended on hemorrhagic/proteinaceous content [48].

3.8.7 Aging Prostate

3.8.7.1 Benign Prostatic Hyperplasia

Benign prostatic hyperplasia (BPH) refers to changes occurring in the TZ and is a process of focal reorganization of cells related to aging (Fig. 3.8). In effect, two types of nodules develop, with either a predominantly "glandular" or "fibromuscular/stromal" proliferation [33]. McNeal first hypothesized that the nodules are invaded by epithelial cells and subsequently develop a more glandular histological architecture [4].

On MRI, benign prostatic hyperplasia has a heterogeneous signal pattern. On T1-weighted images, they usually appear isointense to the background prostate and can show foci of increased signal intensity from hemorrhage or proteinaceous material within a nodule. On T2-weighted images, the TZ is composed of well-demarcated or encapsulated nodules with intervening areas of low signal intensity. This

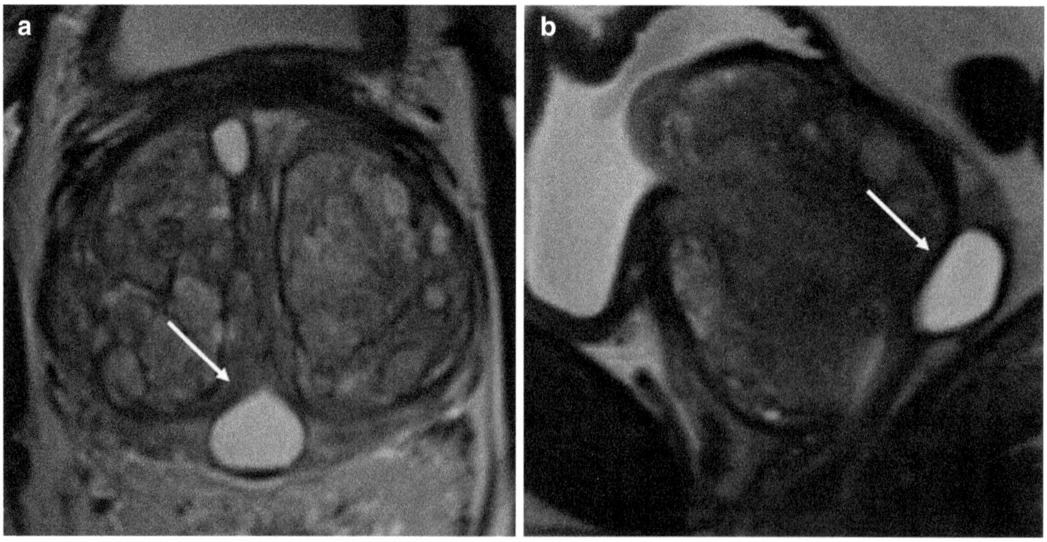

Fig. 3.7 Axial (**a**) and sagittal (**b**) T2-weighted images demonstrate a utricle cyst arising at the level of the verumontanum and extending cranially to the prostatic base (arrows). These are more common midline cysts and may be associated with certain congenital malformations. Mullerian duct cysts in comparison tend to be larger and extend beyond the level of the prostate base

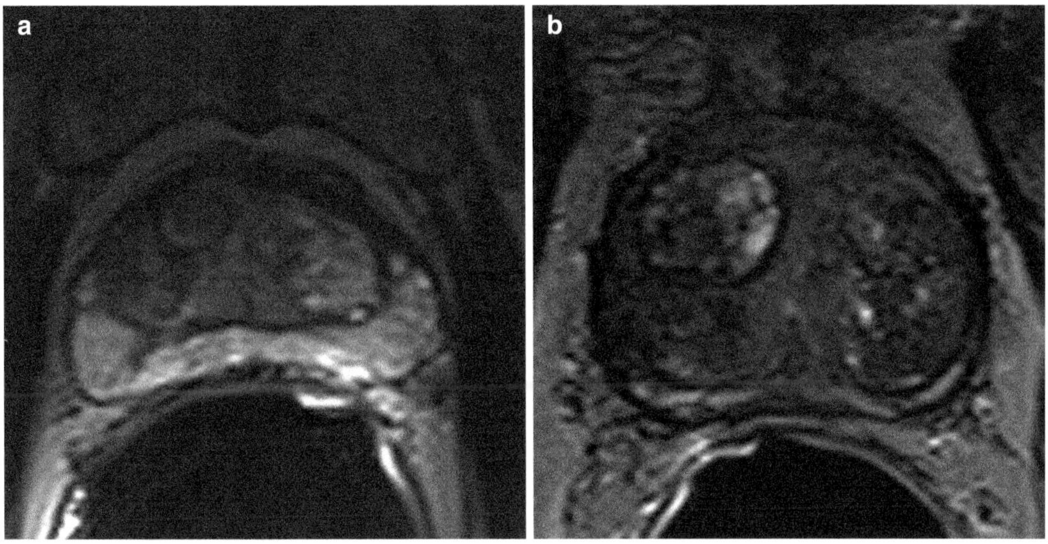

Fig. 3.8 T2-weighted axial images at baseline (**a**) and after 2 years (**b**) in the same patient. Over time, the transition zone has become heterogeneous with areas of stromal and glandular hyperplasia, while the peripheral zone decreased in volume by atrophy and compression by an enlarged transition zone

appearance has been described as "organized chaos." The nodules have variable T2 signal intensities, with some appearing predominantly hyperintense, while others show heterogeneous or low signal [33]. Nodules with diffuse low T2-weighted signal likely represent stromal hyperplasia, while other nodules likely represent glandular hyperplasia or a mix of stromal and glandular hyperplasia [50]. Nodules with stromal hyperplasia can be difficult to distinguish from prostate cancer and have also been shown to demonstrate restricted diffusion that makes them even more difficult to delineate from prostate cancer [51]. After the administration of contrast, nodules demonstrate variable enhancement with some demonstrating early hyperenhancement. One important variant that may be seen is the exophytic BPH nodule. This is a nodule within the PZ but is otherwise well encapsulated and follows the signal features of the TZ (Fig. 3.9).

Version 2.1 of the PI-RADS guidelines released in 2019 clarifies the distinctions between TZ prostate cancer and BPH. BPH nodules on T2-weighted images should be completely encapsulated with a well-defined border. Nodules that have an incomplete capsule in one of the planes on T2-weighted imaging or have a smudged appearance may be scored as suspicious TZ lesions [27].

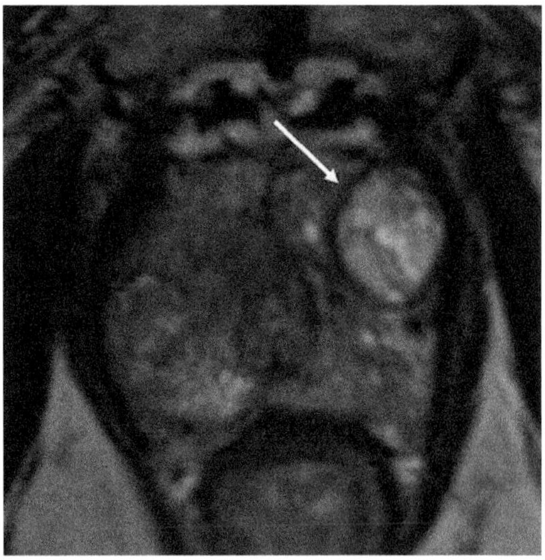

Fig. 3.9 Axial T2-weighted image at the level of the apex demonstrates an encapsulated lesion, which is well-defined in the left anterior peripheral zone (arrow). Signal features of the lesion are consistent with a glandular BPH nodule. Its location outside of the transition zone though suggests an exophytic BPH nodule

When the TZ is enlarged due to BPH, it may protrude into the base of the bladder, which is referred to as intravesical prostatic protrusion (IPP). This finding could be correlated with worse lower urinary tract symptoms [21] and is an important finding to recognize in surgical planning for prostatectomy [52]. This appearance is often referred to as "median lobe," which is carryover term from antiquated understanding of the prostate anatomy that divided the prostate into lobes instead of zones.

3.8.8 Atrophy

Atrophy, a phenomenon that primarily relates to the PZ, may be caused by inflammation, pharmacological treatment, ischemia, prior radiation, or compression by enlarging TZ. The nuclei decrease in size proportionally to the reduction of secretory cell volume and may lose the ability to stain for PSA and PAP [5]. The cells appear crowded with a decrease in the volume of the cytoplasm and nuclei. Most cases of atrophy present from diffuse whole-gland changes, whereas less typical focal atrophic changes are thought to be associated with prior inflammation than with aging [5] (Fig. 3.10). CZ can also demonstrate atrophy, which is primarily caused by its compression by the enlarging TZ (Fig. 3.9). On imaging, atrophy has nonspecific features but usually presents with volume loss and decreased signal intensity on T2-weighted images. The additional finding of mild restricted diffusion may lead to misdiagnosis with prostate cancer.

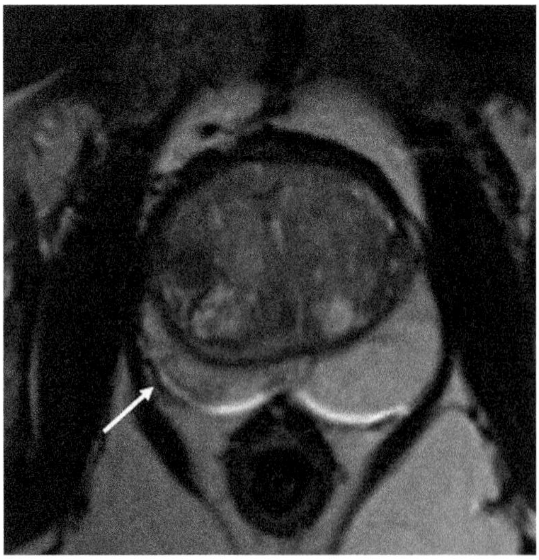

Fig. 3.10 Axial T2-weighted image at the level of the midgland demonstrates an asymmetry in the peripheral zones, with linear and wedge-shaped areas of decreased signal intensity and relative atrophy compared to the contralateral side. These changes, although nonspecific, may be seen in the setting of post-inflammatory fibrosis or atrophy

3.9 Conclusion

The prostate zonal anatomy is well delineated on MRI, with each zone having specific MRI characteristics. Benign prostatic hyperplasia of the transition zone and atrophy of the peripheral zone are associated with aging and result in variation of the proportions and signal characteristics of the zones. Understanding the normal appearance of the gland and the effects of aging is important in assessing prostate pathologies. Additionally, understanding the periprostatic anatomy is important for staging and directing the treatment plan.

References

1. Turkbey B, Huang R, Vourganti S, Trivedi H, Bernardo M, Yan P, et al. Age-related changes in prostate zonal volumes as measured by high-resolution magnetic resonance imaging (MRI): a cross-sectional study in over 500 patients. BJU Int. 2012;110(11):1642–7.
2. Ren J, Liu H, Wang H, Wen D, Huang X, Ren F, et al. MRI to predict prostate growth and development in children, adolescents and young adults. Eur Radiol. 2014;25:516–22.
3. Coakley FV, Hricak H. Radiologic anatomy of the prostate gland: a clinical approach. Radiol Clin N Am. 2000;38(1):15–30.
4. Aaron LT, Franco OE, Hayward SW. Review of prostate anatomy and embryology and the etiology of benign prostatic hyperplasia. Urol Clin North Am. 2016;43(3):279–88.
5. McNeal JE. Normal histology of the prostate. Am J Surg Pathol. 1988;12(8):619–33.
6. Carnevale FC, Soares GR, de Assis AM, Moreira AM, Harward SH, Cerri GG. Anatomical variants in prostate artery embolization: a pictorial essay. Cardiovasc Intervent Radiol. 2017;40(9):1321–37.
7. Walz J, Burnett AL, Costello AJ, Eastham JA, Graefen M, Guillonneau B, et al. A critical analysis of the current knowledge of surgical anatomy related to optimization of cancer control and preservation of continence and erection in candidates for radical pros-

tatectomy. Eur Urol. 2010;57(2):179–92. https://doi.org/10.1016/j.eururo.2009.11.009.
8. de Assis AM, Moreira AM, Carnevale FC. Angiographic findings during repeat prostatic artery embolization. J Vasc Interv Radiol. 2019;30(5):645–51. https://doi.org/10.1016/j.jvir.2018.12.734.
9. Hricak H, Dooms GC, McNeal JE, Mark AS, Marotti M, Avallone A, et al. MR imaging of the prostate gland: normal anatomy. Am J Roentgenol. 1987;148(1):51–8.
10. Power NE, Silberstein JL, Kulkarni GS, Laudone VP. The dorsal venous complex (DVC): dorsal venous or dorsal vasculature complex? Santorini's plexus revisited. BJU Int. 2011;108(6):930–2.
11. Spratt DE, Lee JY, Dess RT, Narayana V, Evans C, Liss A, et al. Vessel-sparing radiotherapy for localized prostate cancer to preserve erectile function: a single-arm phase 2 trial. Eur Urol. 2017;72(4):617–24.
12. Kaiho Y, Nakagawa H, Saito H, Ito A, Ishidoya S, Saito S, et al. Nerves at the ventral prostatic capsule contribute to erectile function: initial electrophysiological assessment in humans. Eur Urol. 2009;55(1):148–55.
13. Paño B, Sebastià C, Buñesch L, Mestres J, Salvador R, Macías NG, et al. Pathways of lymphatic spread in male urogenital pelvic malignancies. Radiographics. 2011;31(1):135–60.
14. Yacoub JH, Verma S, Moulton JS, Eggener S, Oto A. Imaging-guided prostate biopsy: conventional and. Radiographics. 2012;32(3):819–37.
15. Morisawa N, Koyama T, Togashi K. Metastatic lymph nodes in urogenital cancers: contribution of imaging findings. Abdom Imaging. 2006;31(5):620–9.
16. Toivanen R, Shen MM. Prostate organogenesis: tissue induction, hormonal regulation and cell type specification. Development. 2017;144(8):1382–98. https://doi.org/10.1242/dev.148270.
17. Gupta RT, Kauffman CR, Garcia-Reyes K, Palmeri ML, Madden JF, Polascik TJ, et al. Apparent diffusion coefficient values of the benign central zone of the prostate: comparison with low- and high-grade prostate cancer. Am J Roentgenol. 2015;205(2):331–6.
18. Vargas HA, Akin O, Franiel T, Goldman DA, Udo K, Touijer KA, et al. Normal central zone of the prostate and central zone involvement by prostate cancer: clinical and mr imaging implications. Radiology. 2012;262(3):894–902.
19. McNeal JE. The zonal anatomy of the prostate. Prostate. 1981;2(1):35–49.
20. Fine SW, Reuter VE. Anatomy of the prostate revisited: implications for prostate biopsy and zonal origins of prostate cancer. Histopathology. 2012;60(1):142–52.
21. Guneyli S, Ward E, Peng Y, Yousuf AN, Trilisky I, Westin C, et al. MRI evaluation of benign prostatic hyperplasia: correlation with international prostate symptom score. J Magn Reson Imaging. 2017;45(3):917–25.
22. Kim E, Lipshultz L, Howards S. Male infertility. In: Gillenwater J, Grayhack J, Howards S, Mitchell M, editors. Adult and pediatric urology. 4th ed. Philadelphia: Lippincott Williams & Wilkins; 2002. p. 1683–758.
23. Selman SH. The McNeal prostate: a review. Urology. 2011;78(6):1224–8.
24. Medved M, Sammet S, Yousuf A, Oto A. MR imaging of the prostate and adjacent anatomic structures before, during, and after ejaculation: qualitative and quantitative evaluation. Radiology. 2014;271(2):452–60.
25. Barrett T, Tanner J, Gill AB, Slough RA, Wason J, Gallagher FA. The longitudinal effect of ejaculation on seminal vesicle fluid volume and whole-prostate ADC as measured on prostate MRI. Eur Radiol. 2017;27(12):5236–43. https://doi.org/10.1007/s00330-017-4905-x.
26. Kabakus IM, Borofsky S, Mertan FV, Greer M, Daar D, Wood BJ, et al. Does abstinence from ejaculation before prostate MRI improve evaluation of the seminal vesicles? AJR Am J Roentgenol. 2016;207(6):1205–9.
27. Turkbey B, Rosenkrantz A, Haider M, Padhani A, Villeirs G, Macura K, et al. Prostate imaging reporting and data system version 2.1: 2019 update of prostate imaging reporting and data system version 2. Eur Urol. 2019;pii:S0302-2838(19)30180-0. https://doi.org/10.1016/j.eururo.2019.02.033. [Epub ahead of print]
28. Hansen N, Patruno G, Wadhwa K, Gaziev G, Miano R, Barrett T, et al. Magnetic resonance and ultrasound image fusion supported Transperineal prostate biopsy using the Ginsburg protocol: technique, learning points, and biopsy results. Eur Urol. 2016;70(2):332–40.
29. Sommer FG, McNeal JE, Carrol CL. MR depiction of zonal anatomy of the prostate at 1.5 T. J Comput Assist Tomogr. 1986;10(6):983–9.
30. Greene DR, Fitzpatrick JM, Scardino PT. Anatomy of the prostate and distribution of early prostate cancer. Semin Surg Oncol. 1995;11(1):9–22.
31. Villers A, Steg A, Boccon-Gibod L. Anatomy of the prostate: review of the different models. Eur Urol. 1991;20(4):261–8.
32. Semple JE. Surgical capsule of the benign enlargement of the prostate. BMJ. 2009;1(5346):1640–3.
33. Kitzing YX, Prando A, Varol C, Karczmar GS, Maclean F, Oto A. Benign conditions that mimic prostate carcinoma: MR imaging features with histopathologic correlation. Radiographics. 2016;36(1):162–75.
34. Hansford BG, Peng Y, Jiang Y, Al-Ahmadie H, Eggener S, Yousuf A, et al. Revisiting the central gland anatomy via MRI: does the central gland extend below the level of verumontanum? J Magn Reson Imaging. 2014;39(1):167–71.
35. Cheng L, Jones TD, Pan C-X, Barbarin A, Eble JN, Koch MO. Anatomic distribution and pathologic characterization of small-volume prostate cancer (<0.5 ml) in whole-mount prostatectomy specimens. Mod Pathol. 2005;18(8):1022–6.
36. Lee CH, Akin-Olugbade O, Kirschenbaum A. Overview of prostate anatomy, histology, and pathology. Endocrinol Metab Clin N Am. 2011;40(3):565–75.

37. Mikel Hubanks J, Boorjian SA, Frank I, Gettman MT, Houston Thompson R, Rangel LJ, et al. The presence of extracapsular extension is associated with an increased risk of death from prostate cancer after radical prostatectomy for patients with seminal vesicle invasion and negative lymph nodes. Urol Oncol. 2014;32(1):26.e1-7. https://doi.org/10.1016/j.urolonc.2012.09.002.
38. Wheeler TM, Dillioglugil Ö, Kattan MW, Arakawa A, Soh S, Suyama K, et al. Clinical and pathological significance of the level and extent of capsular invasion in clinical stage T1-2 prostate cancer. Hum Pathol. 1998;29(8):856–62.
39. Feng TS, Sharif-Afshar AR, Wu J, Li Q, Luthringer D, Saouaf R, et al. Multiparametric MRI improves accuracy of clinical nomograms for predicting extracapsular extension of prostate cancer. Urology. 2015;86(2):332–7. https://doi.org/10.1016/j.urology.2015.06.003.
40. Augustin H, Fritz GA, Ehammer T, Auprich M, Pummer K. Accuracy of 3-tesla magnetic resonance imaging for the staging of prostate cancer in comparison to the partin tables. Acta Radiol. 2009;50(5):562–9. https://doi.org/10.1080/02841850902889846.
41. Kiyoshima K, Yokomizo A, Yoshida T, Tomita K, Yonemasu H, Nakamura M, et al. Anatomical features of periprostatic tissue and its surroundings: a histological analysis of 79 radical retropubic prostatectomy specimens. Jpn J Clin Oncol. 2004;34(8):463–8.
42. Lee SB, Hong SK, Choe G, Lee SE. Periprostatic distribution of nerves in specimens from non–nerve-sparing radical retropubic prostatectomy. Urology. 2008;72(4):878–81.
43. Sievert KD, Hennenlotter J, Laible IA, Amend B, Nagele U, Stenzl A. The commonly performed nerve sparing total prostatectomy does not acknowledge the actual nerve courses. J Urol. 2009;181(3):1076–81. https://doi.org/10.1016/j.juro.2008.10.154.
44. Kasabwala K, Patel NA, Hu JC. Review of optimal techniques for robotic-assisted radical prostatectomy. Curr Opin Urol. 2018;28(2):102–7. https://doi.org/10.1097/MOU.0000000000000473.
45. Tewari A, Peabody JO, Fischer M, Sarle R, Vallancien G, Delmas V, et al. An operative and anatomic study to help in nerve sparing during laparoscopic and robotic radical prostatectomy. Eur Urol. 2003;43(5):444–54.
46. McDermott VG, Meakem TJ, Stolpen AH, Schnall MD. Prostatic and periprostatic cysts: findings on MR imaging. AJR Am J Roentgenol. 1995;164(1):123–7.
47. Priyadarshi V, Singh JP, Mishra S, Vijay MK, Pal DK, Kundu AK. Prostatic utricle cyst: a clinical dilemma. APSP J Case Rep. 2013;4(2):16. eCollection 2013
48. Shebel HM, Farg HM, Kolokythas O, El-Diasty T. Cysts of the lower male genitourinary tract: embryologic and anatomic considerations. Radiographics. 2013;33(4):1125–43. https://doi.org/10.1148/rg.334125129.
49. Curran S, Akin O, Agildere AM, Zhang J, Hricak H, Rademaker J. Endorectal MRI of prostatic and periprostatic cystic lesions and their mimics. AJR Am J Roentgenol. 2007;188(5):1373–9.
50. McNeal JE. Pathology of benign prostatic hyperplasia. Insight into etiology. Urol Clin North Am. 1990;17(3):477–86.
51. Oto A, Kayhan A, Jiang Y, Tretiakova M, Yang C, Antic T, et al. Prostate cancer: differentiation of central gland cancer from benign prostatic hyperplasia by using purpose: methods: results. Radiology. 2010;257(3):715–23.
52. Jeong CW, Lee S, Oh JJ, Lee BK, Lee JK, Jeong SJ, et al. Quantification of median lobe protrusion and its impact on the base surgical margin status during robot-assisted laparoscopic prostatectomy. World J Urol. 2014;32(2):419–23.

T2-Weighted Imaging

4

Ryan D. Ward and Andrei S. Purysko

4.1 Introduction

Though prostate MRI has been performed for over three decades, only in recent years has it become more widely adopted, largely driven by improved standardization and increasing clinical validation [1, 2]. Despite technical advances in MRI leading to the development of functional sequences capable of assessing tissue properties such as tissue cellularity, microvascularity, and metabolites, T2-weighted imaging (T2WI) remains a critical component of the prostate evaluation. T2WI has the following key roles in a state-of-the-art multiparametric MRI examination of the prostate:

- Localization of normal anatomical structures and pathologic conditions
- Assessment of the transition zone (TZ) and, to a lesser extent, the peripheral zone (PZ), according to the prostate imaging reporting and data system (PI-RADS) scoring system
- Staging of prostate cancer
- Segmentation (i.e., contouring) of the prostate gland to calculate gland volume
- Planning and real-time guidance of prostate biopsies and focal therapies

R. D. Ward
Massachusetts General Hospital, Division of Abdominal Imaging, Boston, MA, USA
e-mail: rward4@mgh.harvard.edu

A. S. Purysko (✉)
Cleveland Clinic, Section of Abdominal Imaging and Nuclear Radiology Department, Cleveland, OH, USA
e-mail: puryska@ccf.org

The interpretation of prostate MRI using T2WI and other sequences will be discussed in depth in Chap. 7 of this book. In this chapter, we will (1) compare and contrast the different types of T2 acquisitions, (2) discuss the hardware considerations and technical parameters to optimize image quality based on PI-RADS recommendations [3], (3) provide insights on patient preparation and other patient-specific parameters that may affect the quality of T2WI, and (4) address some of the inherent limitations of T2WI.

4.2 T2 Imaging Techniques

Over the decades, different T2WI techniques have been developed and validated, each with distinct advantages and disadvantages (Table 4.1). These types of acquisitions can be broadly divided into 2D and 3D techniques.

4.2.1 Two-Dimensional (2D) T2-Weighted Imaging

Historically the prostate was imaged with conventional 2D spin echo (SE) technique, whereby a 90-degree pulse was followed with a 180-degree pulse and an echo. Modern imaging of the prostate relies on 2D rapid acquisition with refocused echo (RARE) techniques, also known as fast spin echo (FSE) or turbo spin echo (TSE) depending

T. Tirkes (ed.), *Prostate MRI Essentials*, https://doi.org/10.1007/978-3-030-45935-2_4

on vendor (Table 4.2). In contrast to SE, FSE/TSE techniques permit multiple 180-degree pulses and echoes for each 90-degree pulse, permitting substantial reduction of imaging time, up to an order of magnitude faster than conventional spin echo techniques [4]. These time savings can be applied toward increasing the echo time (TE) and repetition time (TR) for increased signal intensity and contrast, to acquire greater signal averages, or to increase the matrix size for better spatial resolution and greater contrast resolution (Fig. 4.1).

Studies have found that compared with conventional spin echo, these modern techniques have improved overall image quality, pelvic organ differentiation, conspicuity of fluid, and identification of pathologic conditions [5]. FSE/TSE techniques have also demonstrated improved diagnostic accuracy in staging (seminal vesicle invasion and identifying T3 disease) compared with conventional spin echo [6].

2D T2 motion reduction sequences such as periodically rotated overlapping parallel lines with enhanced reconstruction (PROPELLER or BLADE, depending on the vendor) continuously acquire low-resolution images with radial filling of k-space and oversampling at its center. The result is less motion sensitivity at the expense of reduced T2 contrast (Fig. 4.2). This sequence does not routinely replace TSE/FSE sequences; however in some cases, it can be employed to salvage an otherwise limited exam (Fig. 4.3). 2D T2 PROPELLER/BLADE is often used in a single axial plane when motion-related artifacts are identified. One study found that it had comparable tumor localization when utilized in combination with diffusion-weighted images (DWI) and dynamic contrast-enhanced (DCE) images but not while utilized alone [7].

Table 4.1 Comparison of various T2WI techniques

Technique	Advantages	Disadvantages
2D RARE/FSE/TSE	Fast Highest SNR	Sensitive to motion
2D radial k-space sampling	Less motion sensitive	Lower resolution
Isotropic 3D	High resolution Potential for multiplanar reformats Lessened partial volume effects	Sensitive to motion Altered T2 contrast resolution

Abbreviations: *RARE* rapid acquisition with refocused echoes, *FSE* fast spin echo, *TSE* turbo spin echo, *SNR* signal-to-noise ratio

4.2.2 Three-Dimensional (3D) T2-Weighted Imaging

Isotropic volumetric 3D T2WI can be performed as an adjunct to 2D T2WI. These sequences use long echo train lengths combined with ultrashort echo spacing and nonspatially selective refocusing pulses. The major advantages include higher-resolution imaging and decreased partial volume effects. The high-resolution submillimeter slice thickness can help troubleshoot areas where volume averaging may affect interpretation. For example, in some cases, it can help examine the integrity of the T2-hypointense signal of the prostate capsule in the evaluation of extraprostatic extension (EPE) (Fig. 4.4). The hypointense capsule around benign prostatic hyperplasia (BPH) nodules, an important feature that distinguishes BPH from prostate cancer in the transition zone, can also potentially be demonstrated on the thin slice images when they are not well

Table 4.2 Vendor-specific T2WI sequence nomenclature cross-reference

	Vendor				
Technique	Siemens	GE	Phillips	Hitachi	Toshiba
2D RARE	TSE	FSE	TSE	FSE	FSE
Radial k-space sampling	BLADE	PROPELLER	MULTIVANE	RADAR	JET
Isotropic 3D	SPACE	CUBE	VISTA	ISOFSE	–

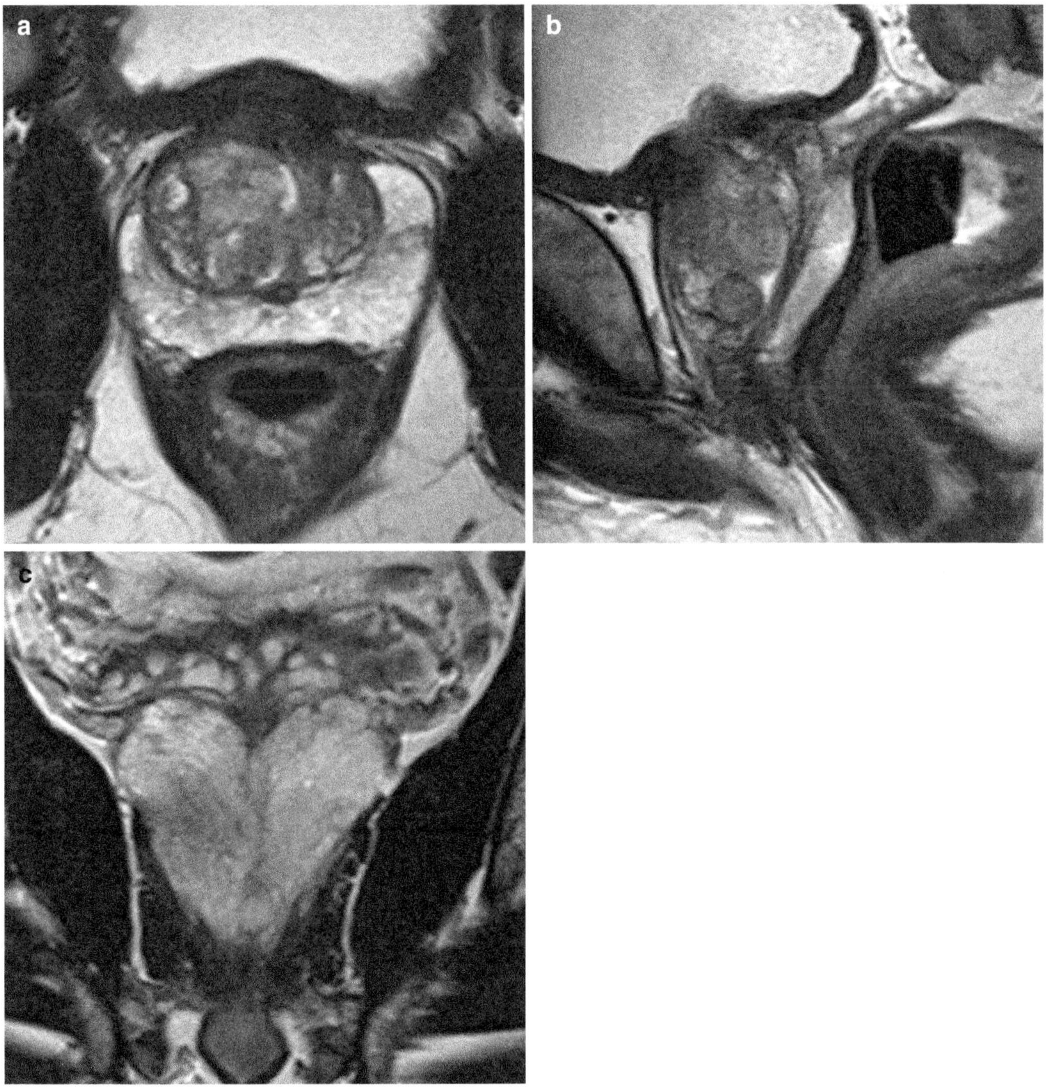

Fig. 4.1 Axial (**a**), sagittal (**b**), and coronal (**c**) T2WI FSE/TSE images of the prostate obtained in a 3T scanner with a pelvic phased-array surface coil

defined on 2D images. Finally, the data set acquired with isotropic voxels can be used for multiplanar reconstructions (Fig. 4.5). For this reason, some manufacturers of MR/ultrasound (US) fusion-guided biopsy devices recommend the use of 3D T2WI for the segmentation of the gland, although 2D acquisitions are also acceptable (Fig. 4.6).

A 3D acquisition has a longer scan time compared with a 2D acquisition in a single plane. However, if reconstructions are created from the 3D slab in lieu of acquiring multiple 2D sequences in individual planes, the overall acquisition time would be significantly less with a 3D sequence. One caveat of 3D imaging is that in order to obtain the 3D volume in reasonable scan time, the TR may need to be shortened which can influence T1 weighting and cause subsequent alteration of image contrast [8]. An additional challenge is that 3D acquisitions are more sensitive to motion, and furthermore, the images are not available for review until the slab is completely imaged, so if motion is present, the entire scan time may be lost.

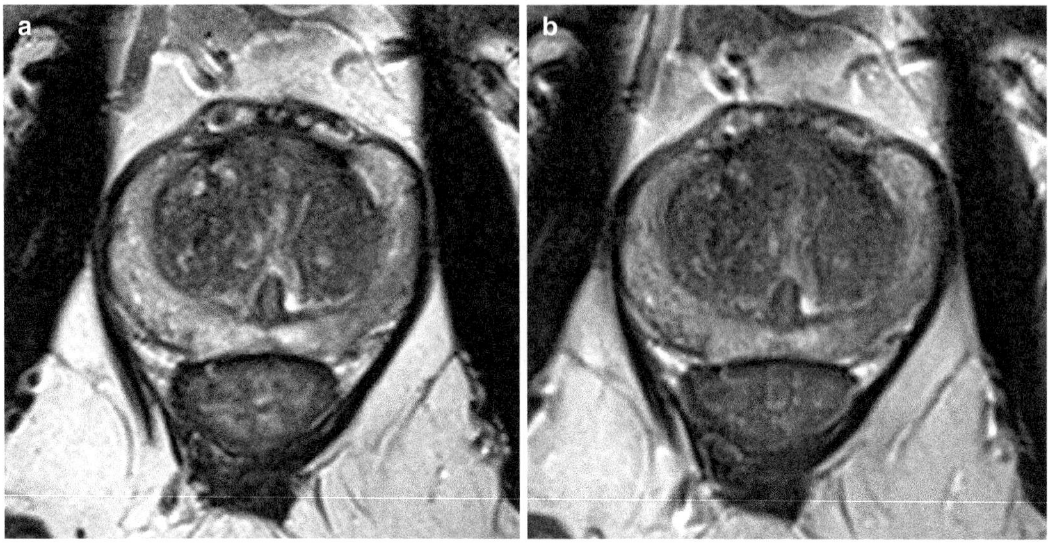

Fig. 4.2 Comparison between axial 2D TSE (**a**) and BLADE (**b**) T2W images of the prostate obtained in a 3T scanner with a pelvic phased-array surface coil

In a comparison of 3D to conventional 2D TSE sequences, one study using a 1.5T magnet without endorectal coil (ERC) found no significant difference in sensitivity, specificity, PPV, NPV, or accuracy between the two in terms of prostate cancer detection and presence of extracapsular extension [9]. Furthermore, while the 2D TSE sequences had a higher signal-to-noise ratio (SNR), the 3D T2 sequence had better tumor contrast and was equivalent in terms of subjective image quality. In terms of time savings, the authors found that the use of a single 3D volumetric slab saved approximately 8 min of acquisition time compared with 2D TSE sequences acquired in the individual planes. Using a 3.0T magnet and ERC, another study found that the two sequences were not different in their ability to delineate the prostatic zonal anatomy and capsule or to depict cancerous lesions based on the comparison of reader's confidence in tumor identification and tumor conspicuity. In addition, no differences were noted in regard to image distortion and motion artifact [8]. Similarly, the authors also note a 44% reduction in scan time to acquire a 3D slab compared with acquiring the individual planes (4:30 vs. 8–9 mins). In a more recent study using a 3.0T magnet without an endorectal coil, the authors found that 3D T2WI significantly increased the sensitivity and reader's confidence for detection of EPE [10].

4.2.3 Anatomic Planes

According to the PI-RADS recommendations, 2D T2WI should always be obtained in the axial plane, either as straight axial to the patient or in an oblique axial plane matching the long axis of the prostate (Fig. 4.7). A minimum of one additional orthogonal plane (i.e., sagittal and/or coronal) is recommended. It is also important to emphasize that DWI, DCE, and T1-weighted images (T1WI) should be obtained in the exact same plane as axial T2WI to facilitate the precise correlation of findings observed on other pulse sequences.

The axial T2WI optimally depicts the prostate zonal anatomy and its relationship to the urethra and is useful in the evaluation of extra-prostatic extension. Most initial anatomic and prostate cancer diagnostic assessments are based on the axial images, with further corroboration and localization using the other planes.

The coronal T2WI depicts the peripheral and central zones well. The urethra and verumonta-

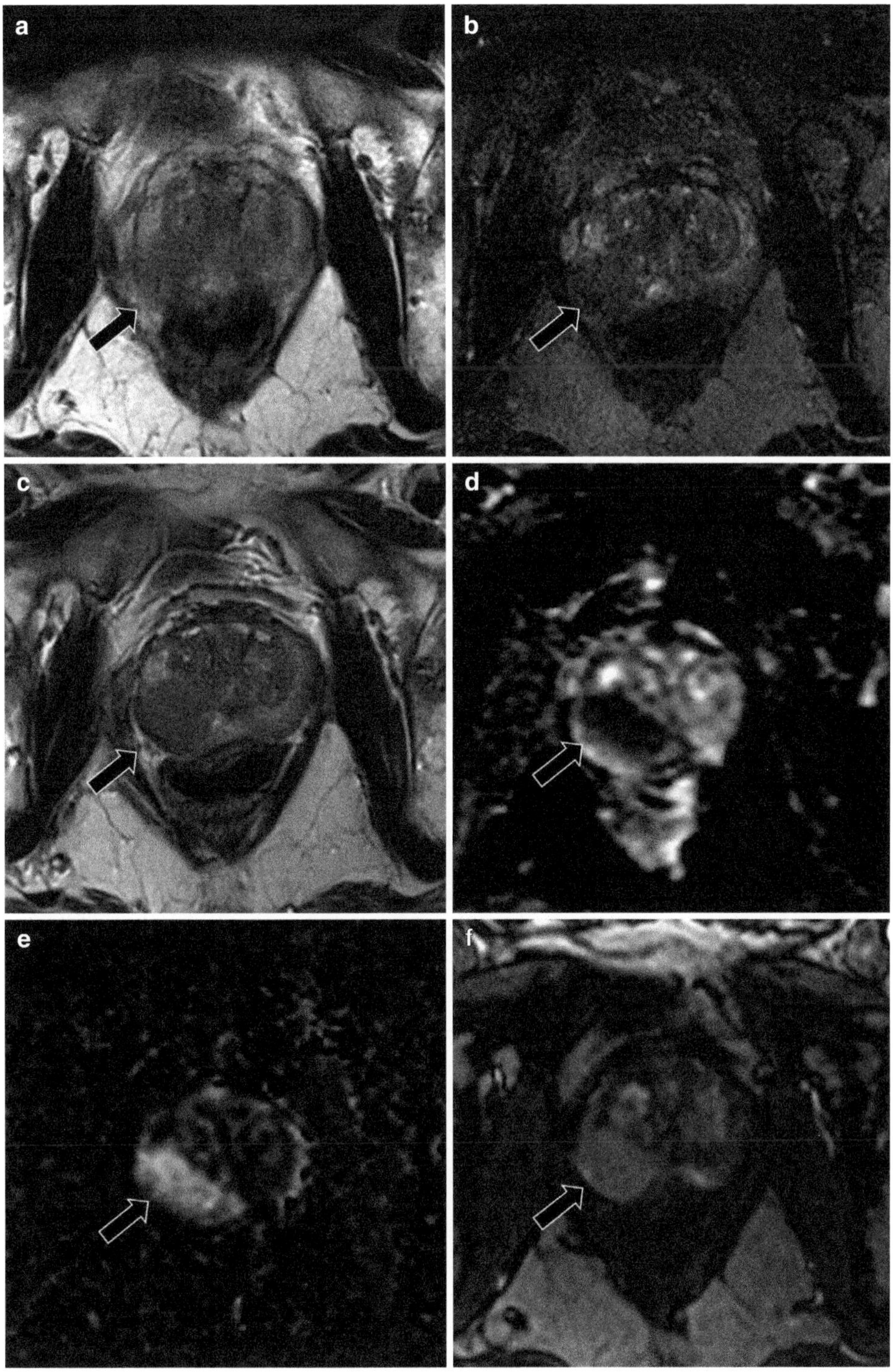

Fig. 4.3 Axial 2D TSE (**a**) and 3D (**b**) T2WI of the prostate have motion-related artifacts with blurring of the prostate capsule and poor conspicuity of a focal lesion with low signal intensity in the right posterolateral peripheral zone (arrow, **a** and **b**). Axial 2D T2WI BLADE (**c**) shows no motion artifact, with improved lesion conspicuity and better definition of capsular bulge that suggests the presence of extra-prostatic extension (arrow, **c**). The lesion had markedly restricted diffusion (i.e., markedly low signal intensity on ADC map [**d**] and markedly high signal intensity on DWI [**e**]) and early arterial enhancement on DCE (arrow, **d**-**f**). The lesion was biopsied and found to be a prostate adenocarcinoma ISUP grade group 4

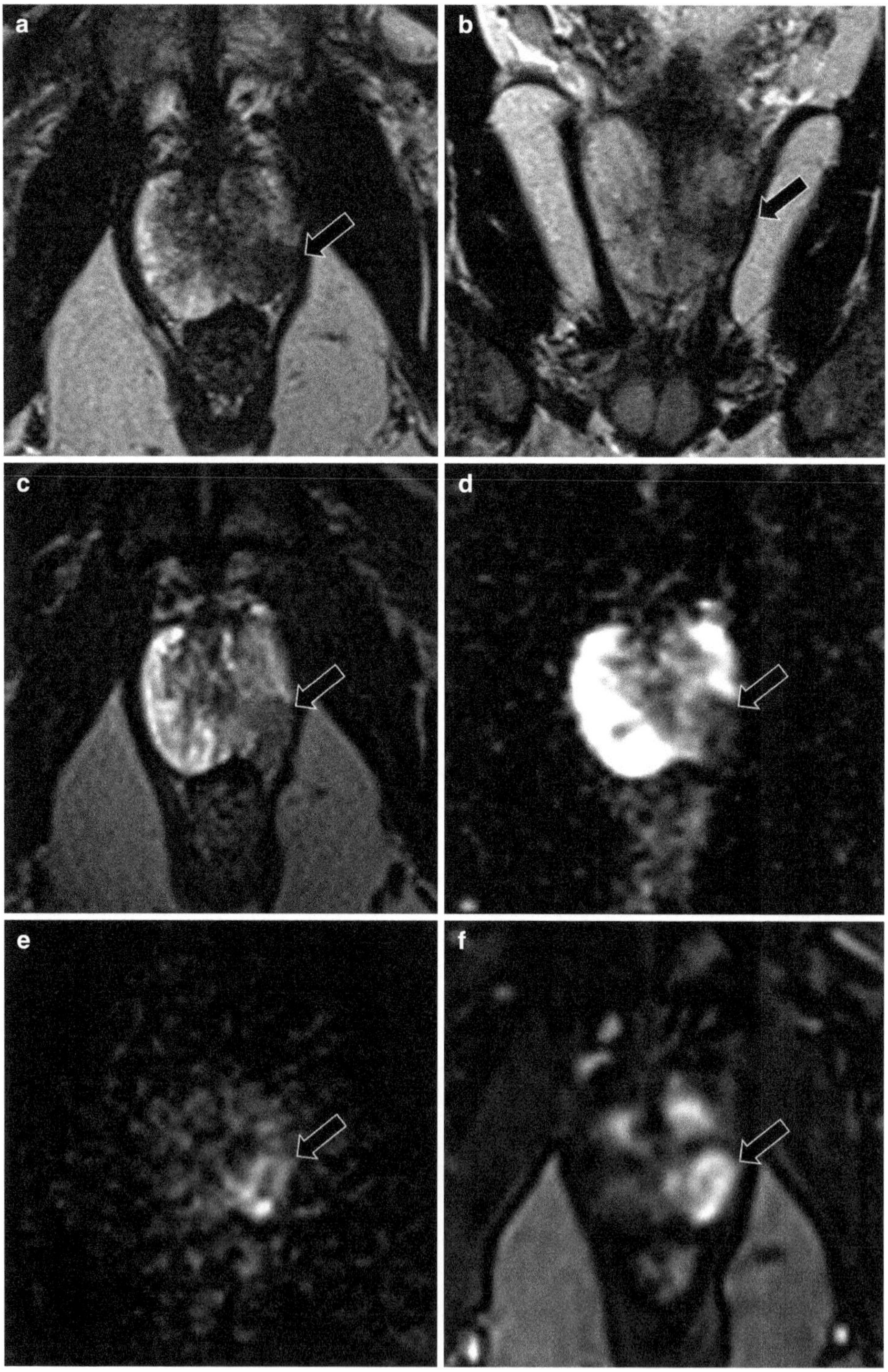

Fig. 4.4 Axial (**a**) and coronal (**b**) 2D T2WI demonstrates a left mid-posterior lateral peripheral zone lesion that abuts the capsule (arrow). There are corresponding restricted diffusion (**d**, ADC map; **e**, DWI, arrows) and enhancement on the post-contrast images (**f**, arrow). The high-resolution, thin-slice axial 3D T2 (**c**) demonstrates a definite extracapsular extension, which was not apparent on the 2D sequences (arrow). The lesion was biopsied and found to be an ISUP grade group 3 adenocarcinoma with cribriform glands

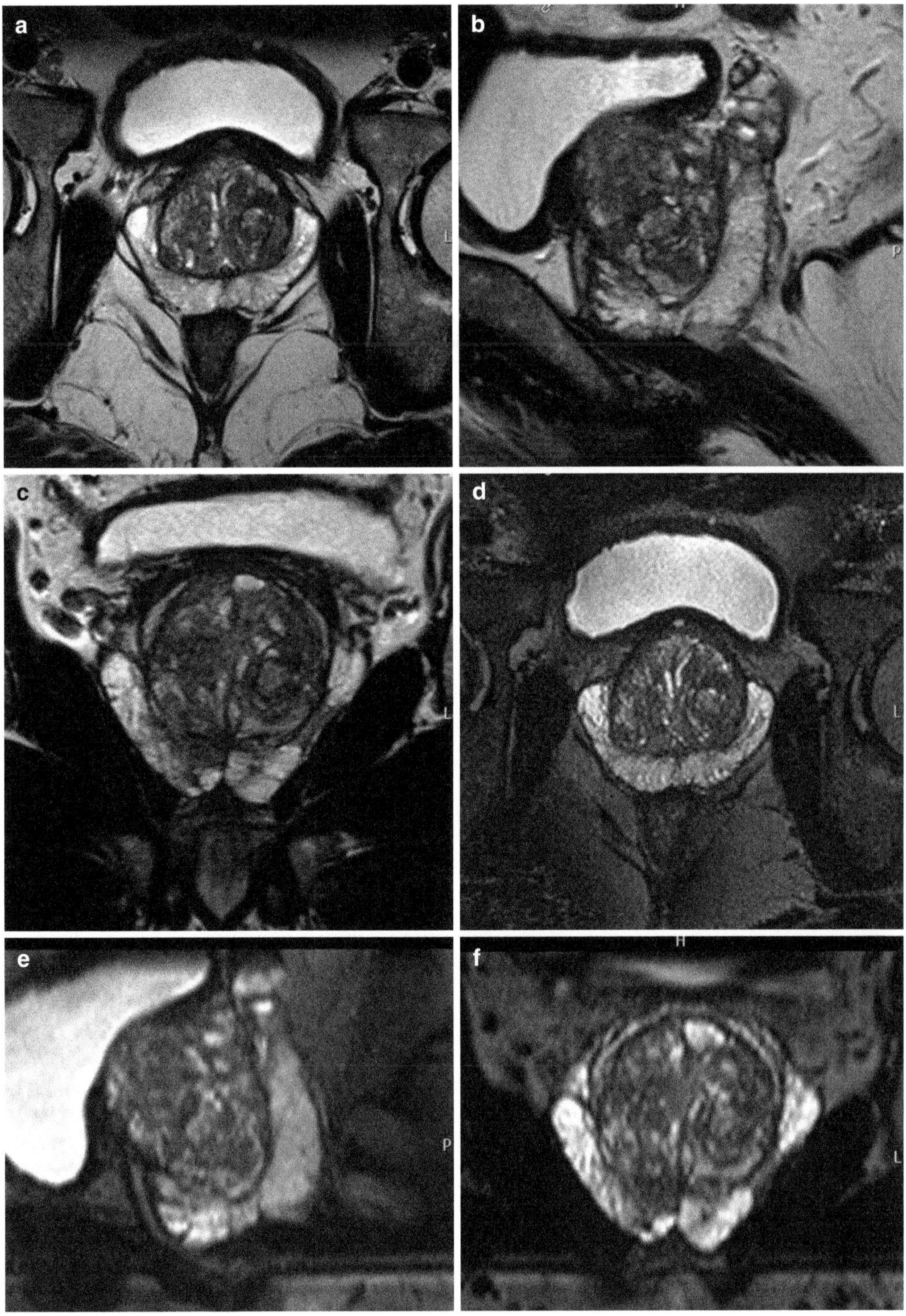

Fig. 4.5 2D TSE T2W images acquired in the oblique axial (**a**), sagittal (**b**), and coronal (**c**) planes with 3 mm-slice thickness. 3D T2W image acquired in the oblique axial plane (**d**) with 0.75 mm-slice thickness and reformatted in the sagittal (**e**) and coronal (**f**) planes with 2.5 mm-slice thickness. Overall, 2D and 3D T2WI show comparable image quality

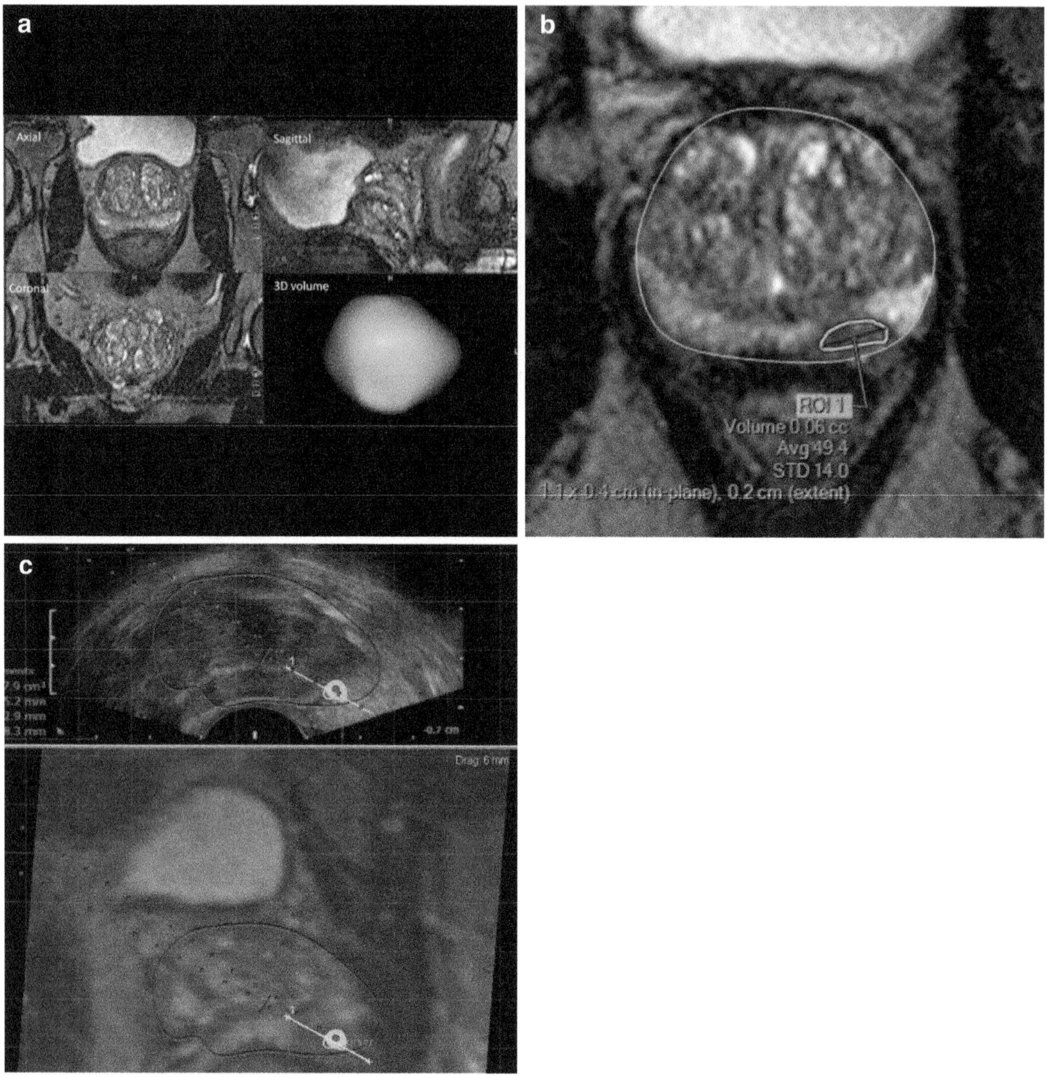

Fig. 4.6 MRI-targeted biopsy using MR/TRUS fusion system. Axial T2WI is used for segmentation of the gland, which provides the 3D measurement of the gland volume and the contour (green line) that will be overlaid on the TRUS images (**a**). Once the segmentation is performed, lesions of interest will be marked on the same T2WI (blue line [**b**]). Image obtained during the MR/US fusion-guided biopsy shows the US image with overlaying MR contour (purple line) and target (green and red circle) while the biopsy needle (yellow line) hits the target. The bottom part of the image shows the T2WI for reference (**c**)

num can be seen in their long axes. The coronal T2WI also depicts the prostate's relationship to the levator musculature, and it may also better evaluate the convergence of structures at the prostate base where partial volume averaging can impact evaluation [11]. The sagittal plane can be used to establish the relationship between the bladder, prostate, and rectum, and one can also see the full course of the prostatic urethra and bladder neck in a single image.

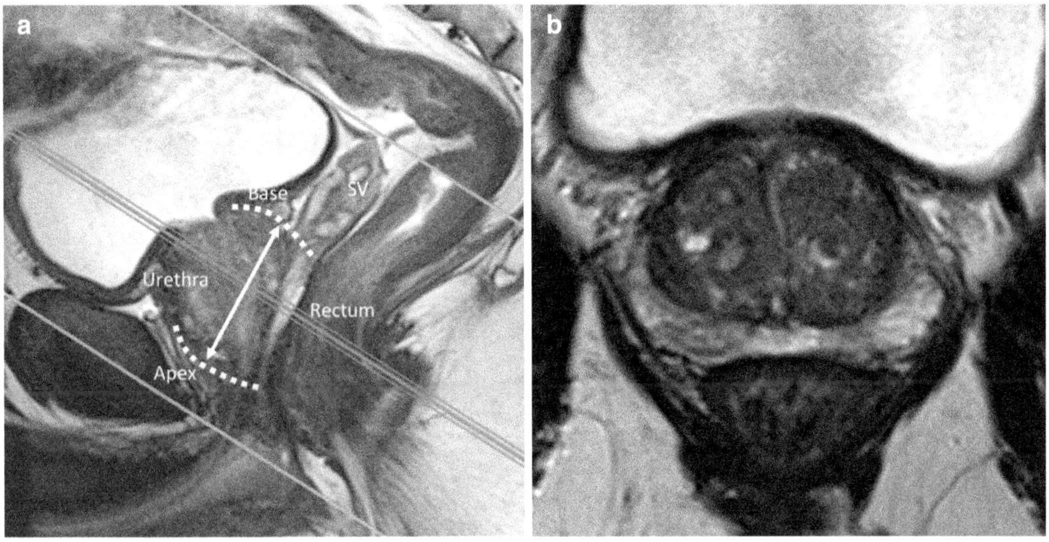

Fig. 4.7 Plane orientation and scan range. (**a**) Orange lines demarcate the range of acquisition of oblique axial T2WI, which extends from apex to the most superior aspect of the seminal vesicles. Green line represents the reference line for the oblique axial images (**b**), which are obtained perpendicular to the long axis of the prostate that extends from apex to base (white arrow). The urethra and anterior rectal wall can serve as a reference for the long axis of the prostate although these structures can be altered by benign prostatic hyperplasia and gaseous distension of the rectum

4.2.4 Field of View and Other Technical Parameters

The field of view should be set at 12–20 cm, which is large enough to image the entire prostate and seminal vesicles but small enough to not adversely impact resolution [3]. For 2D acquisitions, slice thickness should be set to 3 mm and obtained without gaps. The in-plane dimensions should be set at ≤0.7 mm in the phase-encoding direction and ≤0.4 mm in the frequency-encoding direction. A TE 90–120 ms has been suggested to provide optimal soft tissue contrast needed to identify prostate cancer [12], though adjustments will need to be made based on available equipment due to differences in relaxation times between 1.5 and 3.0T scanners [13]. An example T2WI protocol, including these technical parameters, is included in Table 4.3.

4.3 Hardware Considerations

4.3.1 Magnet Strength

While 1.5T magnets are acceptable for imaging of the prostate, 3.0T magnets are generally preferred [14]. For patients with pelvic/hip prostheses, brachytherapy seeds, or other metallic implants in the pelvis, it may be preferred to image on a 1.5T scanner to mitigate susceptibility artifacts. While the theoretical gain in signal between 1.5 and 3.0T should be 2×, the actual incremental gain is 1.6–1.8× increase in SNR depending on the type of sequence due to a number of technical factors [15]. The gain in SNR can be leveraged to reduce acquisition time or to obtain higher-resolution images [16]. The improvements in SNR using a higher-strength magnet are not without trade-offs though, as susceptibility, chemical shift, and other artifacts

Table 4.3 Sample T2WI protocol for a prostate MRI performed in a 3T system with pelvic phased-array surface coil

Multiparametric MR imaging sequence parameters at 3T					
Parameter	SAG 2D T2	COR 2D T2	AX 2D T2	T2 BLADE	3D T2 weighted (SPACE)
Field of view (mm)	210	210	180	210	240
Acquisition matrix	269 × 384	269 × 384	256 × 320	256 × 320	228 × 320
Repetition time (msec)	3340	3260	3730	2500	2500
Echo time (msec)	116	126	121	115	225
Flip angle (degrees)	120	120	138	135	Variable
Section thickness (mm), no gaps	3	3	3	3	1
Voxel size (mm)	0.5 × 0.5 × 3	0.5 × 0.5 × 3	0.6 × 0.6 × 3	0.7 × 0.7 × 3	0.8 × 0.8 × 1
Time for acquisition (min/sec)	1:55	2:31	2:53	2:54	6:04

increase proportionally with increasing magnetic field strength.

4.3.2 Receiver Coil Selection

There is variable utilization of endorectal coils across imaging centers. Studies have shown that 3.0T scanners with pelvic phased-array coil are comparable to 1.5T scanners with ERC in terms of prostate image quality [17]. However, patient discomfort, potential to distort pelvic anatomy, cost, and time requirement have caused routine ERC use to fall out of favor at many institutions, particularly when 3.0T imaging is available. When used, a pelvic phased-array with at least 16 channels should be employed, as the use of dedicated multichannel pelvic phased-array coils allows for improved SNR which permits smaller FOV and higher-resolution images [18].

4.4 Patient Preparation

Many patient-related factors can influence the quality of prostate MRI. Several different patient preparation measures have been described, in some cases with mixed results. No consensus exists regarding recommendations for patient preparation, and practice patterns are largely driven by personal preferences.

4.4.1 Time Interval Between Prostate Biopsy and MRI

A prostate biopsy can cause alterations in the normal signal characteristics and morphology of the gland that can last from weeks to months. Post-biopsy hemorrhage can have low signal on T2WI that can be difficult to distinguish from cancer (Fig. 4.8) [19]. On T1WI, hemorrhage appears as hyperintense signal owing to the presence of methemoglobin. Therefore, T2WI should always be interpreted in correlation with T1WI in the setting of a recent biopsy. Prostate contour changes can also occur after biopsy, which can mimic extracapsular extension [20]. In light of these effects, patients should ideally wait at least 6-weeks post-biopsy before receiving MRI [3, 21].

4.4.2 Abstinence from Ejaculation

Ejaculation has been shown to decrease the peripheral zone signal on T2WI [22]. Additionally, after ejaculation, the seminal vesicles may become collapsed, which can limit their evaluation in men aged more than 60 years [23]. Some institutions request that their patients abstain from ejaculation for up to 3 days before a prostate MRI. However, because of the lack of robust evidence confirming the benefit of this measure for prostate cancer detection and staging, PI-RADS guidelines do not routinely recommend it.

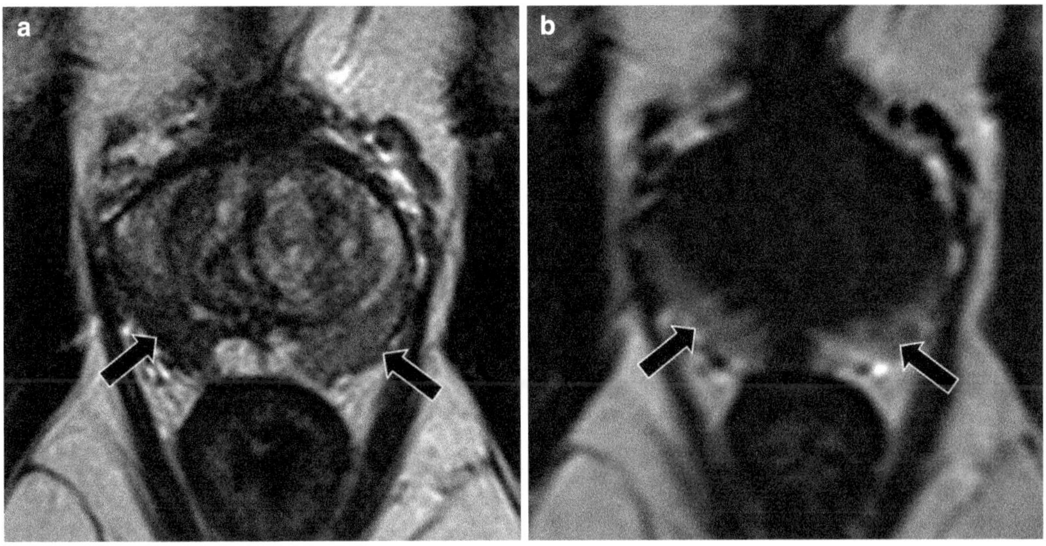

Fig. 4.8 MRI performed 3 weeks after the transrectal ultrasound-guided biopsy. Focal areas of low T2 signal intensity in the peripheral zone (arrows, **a**). The same areas demonstrate high signal intensity on T1WI (**b**), which represents residual post-biopsy changes

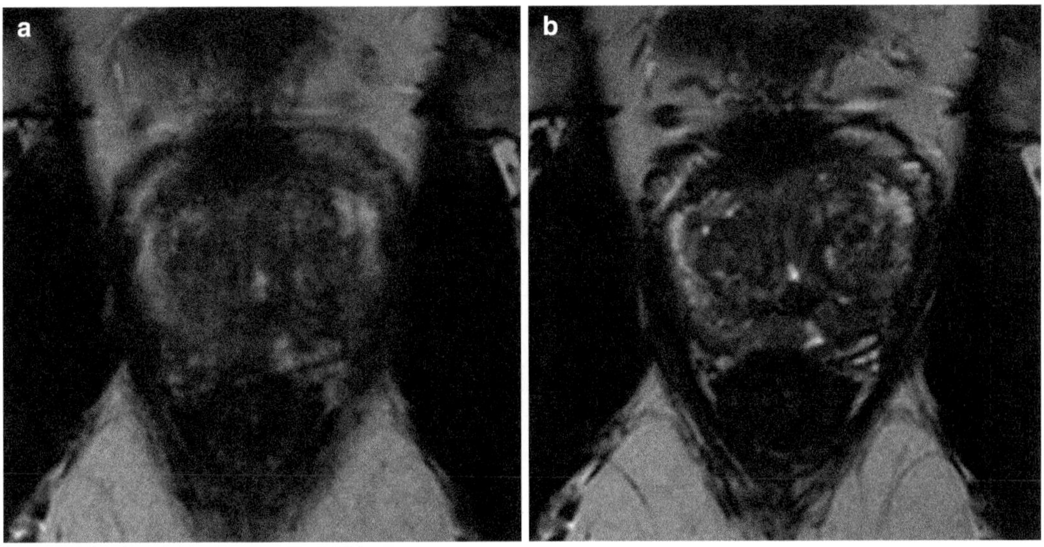

Fig. 4.9 2D TSE T2WI performed on 3T magnet with pelvic phased-array surface coil obtained before (**a**) and after (**b**) administration of antiperistaltic agent shows a significant reduction in motion-related artifacts

4.4.3 Bowel Preparation and Antiperistaltic Agents

Rectal distension with gas and stool can increase motion artifact on T2WI by inducing rectal contractions (Fig. 4.9) [24]. It can also cause susceptibility artifacts that can distort DWI. Patients should try to evacuate their rectum prior to the exam. Self-administration of a fleet enema is frequently used and can help reduce the rectal load. Some institutions also use antiperistaltic agents such as glucagon or hyoscine butylbromide

(HBB, also known as scopolamine butylbromide under the trade name Buscopan) to reduce motion, but the evidence is mixed. For example, Wagner et al. using a 1.5T scanner with ERC found no significant difference in image quality or in the assessment of the prostate, neurovascular bundle, or lymph nodes using HBB [25]. However, the lack of benefit in that study could be due to the use of ERC, which can immobilize the rectum. Two more recent studies using 3.0T scanners without ERC demonstrated improved visualization of anatomical structures on T2WI due to less motion and blur with the use of HBB [26, 27]. Fasting and use of glucagon have also been shown to improve MRI imaging of the pelvis, though there are limited studies specifically for prostate imaging [28]. The possibility of adverse reactions as well as the additional cost of administering these medications should be factored when assessing the potential risks and benefits of including these agents in routine clinical practice.

4.5 Conclusion

T2WI play important roles in the MRI evaluation of the prostate. Different types of T2WI pulse sequences are available, each with distinct advantages and disadvantages. Each sequence included in a protocol must be carefully weighed for incremental clinical utility over additional exam time. A meticulous selection of imaging parameters, appropriate hardware, and adequate patient preparation can contribute to optimal image quality.

References

1. Steyn JH, Smith FW. Nuclear magnetic resonance (NMR) imaging of the prostate. Br J Urol. 1984;56(6):679–81. https://doi.org/10.1111/j.1464-410X.1984.tb06145.x.
2. Hricak H, Williams RD, Spring DB, Moon KL Jr, Hedgcock MW, Watson RA, Crooks LE. Anatomy and pathology of the male pelvis by magnetic resonance imaging. AJR Am J Roentgenol. 1983;141(6):1101–10. https://doi.org/10.2214/ajr.141.6.1101.
3. Turkbey B, Rosenkrantz AB, Haider MA, Padhani AR, Villeirs G, Macura KJ, et al. Prostate imaging reporting and data system version 2.1: 2019 update of prostate imaging reporting and data system version 2. Eur Urol. 2019;76(3):340–51. https://doi.org/10.1016/j.eururo.2019.02.033.
4. Kier R, Wain S, Troiano R. Fast spin-echo MR images of the pelvis obtained with a phased-array coil: value in localizing and staging prostatic carcinoma. AJR Am J Roentgenol. 1993;161(3):601–6. https://doi.org/10.2214/ajr.161.3.8352116.
5. Nghiem HV, Herfkens RJ, Francis IR, Sommer FG, Jeffrey RB Jr, Li KC, et al. The pelvis: T2-weighted fast spin-echo MR imaging. Radiology. 1992;185(1):213–7. https://doi.org/10.1148/radiology.185.1.1523311.
6. Engelbrecht MR, Jager GJ, Laheij RJ, Verbeek AL, van Lier HJ, Barentsz JO. Local staging of prostate cancer using magnetic resonance imaging: a meta-analysis. Eur Radiol. 2002;12(9):2294–302. https://doi.org/10.1007/s00330-002-1389-z.
7. Rosenkrantz AB, Bennett GL, Doshi A, Deng FM, Babb JS, Taneja SS. T2-weighted imaging of the prostate: impact of the BLADE technique on image quality and tumor assessment. Abdom Imaging. 2015;40:552–9. https://doi.org/10.1007/s00261-014-0225-7.
8. Westphalen AC, Noworolski SM, Harisinghani M, Jhaveri KS, Raman SS, Rosenkrantz AB, Wang ZJ, Zagoria RJ, Kurhanewicz J. High-resolution 3-T endorectal prostate MRI: a multireader study of radiologist preference and perceived interpretive quality of 2D and 3D T2-weighted fast spin-echo MR images. AJR Am J Roentgenol. 2016;206(1):86–91. https://doi.org/10.2214/AJR.14.14065.
9. Rosenkrantz AB, Neil J, Kong X, Melamed J, Babb JS, Taneja SS, Taouli B. Prostate cancer: comparison of 3D T2-weighted with conventional 2D T2-weighted imaging for image quality and tumor detection. AJR Am J Roentgenol. 2010;194(2):446–52. https://doi.org/10.2214/AJR.09.3217.
10. Caglic I, Povalej Brzan P, Warren AY, Bratt O, Shah N, Barrett T. Defining the incremental value of 3D T2-weighted imaging in the assessment of prostate cancer extracapsular extension. Eur Radiol. 2019;29(10):5488–97. https://doi.org/10.1007/s00330-019-06070-6.
11. Gupta RT, Spilseth B, Patel N, Brown AF, Yu J. Multiparametric prostate MRI: focus on T2-weighted imaging and role in staging of prostate cancer. Abdom Radiol (NY). 2016;41(5):831–43. https://doi.org/10.1007/s00261-015-0579-5.
12. Diaz de Leon A, Costa D, Pedrosa I. Role of multiparametric MR imaging in malignancies of the urogenital tract. Magn Reson Imaging Clin N Am. 2016;24(1):187–204. https://doi.org/10.1016/j.mric.2015.08.009.
13. de Bazelaire CM, Duhamel GD, Rofsky NM, Alsop DC. MR imaging relaxation times of abdominal and pelvic tissues measured in Vivo at 3.0 T: preliminary results. Radiology. 2004;230(3):652–9. https://doi.org/10.1148/radiol.2303021331.

14. Barentsz JO, Richenberg J, Clements R, Choyke P, Verma S, Villeirs G, et al. European society of urogenital radiology. ESUR prostate MR guidelines 2012. Eur Radiol. 2012;22(4):746–57. https://doi.org/10.1007/s00330-011-2377-y.
15. Soher BJ, Dale BM, Merkle EM. A review of MR physics: 3T versus 1.5T. Magn Reson Imaging Clin N Am. 2007;15(3):277–90. https://doi.org/10.1016/j.mric.2007.06.002.
16. Jambor I. Optimization of prostate MRI acquisition and post-processing protocol: a pictorial review with access to acquisition protocols. Acta Radiol Open. 2017;6(12):2058460117745574. https://doi.org/10.1177/2058460117745574.
17. Sosna J, Pedrosa I, Dewolf WC, Mahallati H, Lenkinski RE, Rofsky NM. MR imaging of the prostate at 3 tesla. Acad Radiol. 2004;11(8):857–62. https://doi.org/10.1016/j.acra.2004.04.013.
18. Hayes CE, Hattes N, Roemer PB. Volume imaging with MR phased arrays. Magn Reson Med. 1991;18(2):309–19. https://doi.org/10.1002/mrm.1910180206.
19. Hoeks CM, Barentsz JO, Hambrock T, Yakar D, Somford DM, Heijmink SW, et al. Prostate cancer: multiparametric MR imaging for detection, localization, and staging. Radiology. 2011;261(1):46–66. https://doi.org/10.1148/radiol.11091822.
20. Qayyum A, Coakley FV, Lu Y, Olpin JD, Wu L, Yeh BM, et al. Organ-confined prostate cancer: effect of prior transrectal biopsy on endorectal MRI and MR spectroscopic imaging. Am J Roentgenol. 2004;183:1079–83. https://doi.org/10.2214/ajr.183.4.1831079.
21. White S, Hricak H, Forstner R, Kurhanewicz J, Vigneron DB, Zaloudek CJ, et al. Prostate cancer: effect of postbiopsy hemorrhage on interpretation of MR images. Radiology. 1995;195:385–90. https://doi.org/10.1148/radiology.195.2.7724756.
22. Medved M, Sammet S, Yousuf A, Oto A. MR imaging of the prostate and adjacent anatomic structures before, during, and after ejaculation: qualitative and quantitative evaluation. Radiology. 2014;271:452–60. https://doi.org/10.1148/radiol.14131374.
23. Kabakus IM, Borofsky S, Mertan FV, Greer M, Daar D, Wood BJ, et al. Does abstinence from ejaculation before prostate MRI improve evaluation of the seminal vesicles? Am J Roentgenol. 2016;207:1205–9. https://doi.org/10.2214/AJR.16.16278.
24. Caglic I, Hansen NL, Slough RA, Patterson AJ, Barrett T. Evaluating the effect of rectal distension on prostate multiparametric MRI image quality. Eur J Radiol. 2017;90:174–80. https://doi.org/10.1016/j.ejrad.2017.02.029.
25. Wagner M, Rief M, Busch J, Scheurig C, Taupitz M, Hamm B, Franiel T. Effect of butylscopolamine on image quality in MRI of the prostate. Clin Radiol. 2010;65:460–4. https://doi.org/10.1016/j.crad.2010.02.007.
26. Slough RA, Caglic I, Hansen NL, Patterson AJ, Barrett T. Effect of hyoscine butylbromide on prostate multiparametric MRI anatomical and functional image quality. Clin Radiol. 2018;73:216.e9–216.e14. https://doi.org/10.1016/j.crad.2017.07.013.
27. Ullrich T, Quentin M, Schmaltz AK, Arsov C, Rubbert C, Blondin D, et al. Hyoscine butylbromide significantly decreases motion artefacts and allows better delineation of anatomic structures in mp-MRI of the prostate. Eur Radiol. 2018;28:17–23. https://doi.org/10.1007/s00330-017-4940-7.
28. Winkler ML, Hricak H. Pelvis imaging with MR: technique for improvement. Radiology. 1986;158:848–9. https://doi.org/10.1148/radiology.158.3.3945763.

5 Diffusion-Weighted Imaging

Oguz Akin and Yousef Mazaheri

5.1 Introduction

Prostate cancer (PCa) is a major public health problem in the USA. An estimated 174,650 men will be diagnosed with prostate cancer in 2019 and an estimated 31,620 men will die, making it the second leading cause of cancer-related death in the USA [1]. On T2-weighted MR images, the zonal anatomy of the prostate is clearly depicted [2]. Prostate cancer usually appears as T2-hypointense signal within the peripheral zone (PZ) which is T2 hyperintense. T2-hypointense signal of the PCa may be less conspicuous in the transition zone (TZ) which has mixed T2 signal intensity [3].

Diffusion-weighted MR imaging (DW-MRI) has become an increasingly important component of clinical evaluation of the prostate for detection and characterization of PCa. In many areas of oncology, DW-MRI has proven to be a clinically useful, noninvasive functional imaging technique used in tumor detection and staging and for monitoring response to treatment in a variety of tumor types. The advantages of this technique include short acquisition times, no need for intravenous administration of contrast agent, and the ability to indirectly study tissue cellularity through noninvasive probing of the diffusion of water molecules in tissue.

In this review, we evaluate and summarize the published literature pertaining to DW-MRI and prostate cancer. We highlight recent modes of acquisition and analysis available for DW-MRI and suggest how these may be further improved. Finally, we review the literature and make recommendations for future research.

5.2 Technical Overview

In biological tissues, microscopic motion detected by DW-MRI includes both diffusion of water molecules, influenced by the structural components of the tissue, and microcirculation of blood in the capillary network. DW-MRI derives its image contrast from differences in the motion of water molecules between tissues. The degree of water diffusion in biologic tissue is inversely correlated to tissue cellularity and the integrity of cell membranes. The motion of water molecules is more restricted in tissues with high cellular density associated with numerous intact cell membranes (e.g., tumor tissue).

O. Akin
Memorial Sloan Kettering Cancer Center, Department of Radiology, New York, NY, USA
e-mail: akino@mskcc.org

Y. Mazaheri (✉)
Memorial Sloan Kettering Cancer Center, Department of Medical Physics and Radiology, New York, NY, USA
e-mail: mazahery@mskcc.org

T. Tirkes (ed.), *Prostate MRI Essentials*, https://doi.org/10.1007/978-3-030-45935-2_5

5.2.1 Hardware: Field Strength and Coils

MR prostate imaging was originally obtained on 1.5-Tesla (1.5T) scanners. A body coil was used for excitation, and a pelvic phased-array coil combined with an expandable endorectal coil was used for signal acquisition to ensure images with sufficient SNR [4]. As comparted to images obtained with pelvic phased-array coils alone, endorectal coil images have a ~10-fold improved SNR and spatial resolution [5, 6]. An endorectal coil consists of a coil inside an inflatable balloon which can be filled with 40–80 ml of either air, water, or an inert fluid that matches the susceptibility of the prostatic tissues, such as perfluorocarbon (PFC) or barium sulfate [6, 7]. The advantages of using an inert fluid are the reduced susceptibility artifacts between the rectum and the prostate due to the improved homogeneity of the magnetic field [7]. The reception signal providers of endorectal coils are highly inhomogeneous although post-processing methods have been suggested to reduce the signal inhomogeneities [8].

With the availability of 3-Tesla (3T) clinical scanners, improved SNR was achieved using the benefit of higher field strength. The theoretical SNR gain of 3T vs. 1.5T is in the range of 1.5–1.8 [9]. This in turn provided opportunities to increase spatial resolution and temporal resolutions as the doubling of field strength results in a twofold SNR improvement due to field strength alone. Additional factors effecting SNR include acquisition time, voxel volume, receiver bandwidth, longitudinal relaxation time (T1), and sequence-specific factors.

Additional improvements were achieved with the use of more advanced pulse sequence designs and the use of surface phased-array coils including 6–32 channels. A number of studies have reported comparisons of images obtained with 1.5T scanners with an endorectal coil to phased-array surface coils at 3T [10–14]. Bloch et al. demonstrated the clinical utility of endorectal 3T for the evaluation of the prostate with imaging features and quality not achievable at 1.5T [10]. Sosna et al. compared image quality at of the prostate at 3T with a phased-array coil to imaging with an endorectal coil at 1.5T and found that the image quality can be comparable [11]. For the local staging of prostate cancer, Park et al. demonstrated that 3T phased-array MRI is equivalent to the 1.5T endorectal MRI in evaluating local staging accuracy for prostate cancer without significant loss of imaging quality [12]. Turkbey et al. compared T2-weighted (T2W) MRI and DWI-MRI obtained without endorectal coil (surface coil alone) with a dual coil (combination of surface and endorectal coils) at 3T for localizing prostate cancer and found that by using endorectal MR coil, more cancer foci can be detected [14]. At 3T, imaging with surface coil had a sensitivity of 0.45 and positive predictive value (PPV) of 0.64. In comparison with dual coil, the sensitivity was 0.75 and the PPV was 0.80. However, additional considerations that need to be considered include patient comfort, patient preparation, costs, coil placement time, and anatomical distortions due to placement of the endorectal coil [15].

5.2.1.1 Imaging Strategies

DW-MRI is performed without breath-holding, due to long acquisition times. Most commonly, a single-shot echo-planar (ssEPI) sequence is used for acquisition (Fig. 5.1). The sequence provides a rapid and reliable method to acquire DW data, although it suffers from severe image distortion due to the presence of susceptibility-related field inhomogeneity.

The standard ssEPI commonly available suffers from image distortion due to the presence of susceptibility-related field inhomogeneity. The air in the rectum located directly behind the prostate could result in severe field inhomogeneities. Several pulse sequences have been presented in the literature to reduce image distortions [16–19]. A common strategy to reduce image distortions is to reduce the readout time. A promising approach is the segmented readout method [17] where segments of k-space are acquired along the readout direction. The decrease in readout time results in a reduction of geometric distortions. Another approach is the single excitation imaging based on multiple spin echo sequence [20].

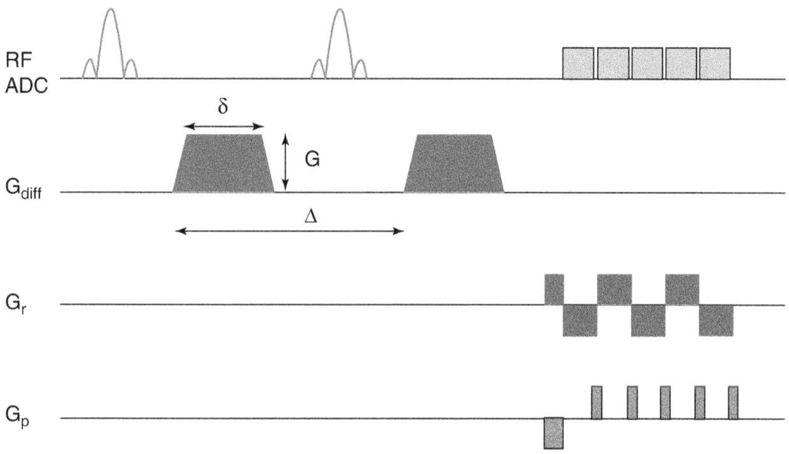

Fig. 5.1 The pulsed gradient spin echo (PGSE) for measuring diffusivity in MRI. The bipolar gradient recalled echo (GRE) dephases the spins in the first monopolar lobe and then refocuses the spins in the second monopolar lobe. A diffusion time Δ is introduced between dephasing and rephrasing diffusion-sensitizing gradient pulses, G is the diffusion gradient amplitude, and δ is the diffusion gradient duration

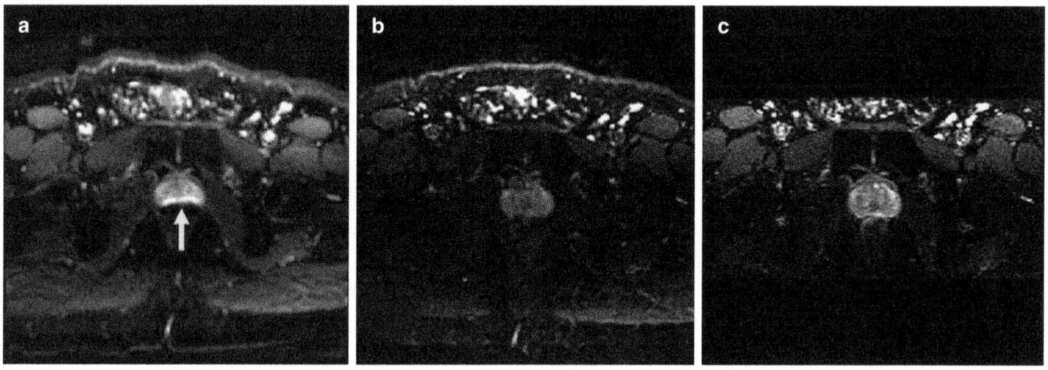

Fig. 5.2 Comparison of DW images of prostate obtained using (**a**) the standard ssEPI diffusion sequence, (**b**) the MUSE sequence with three shots, and (**c**) a rFOV diffusion-weighted sequence where the FOV in the phase-encoding direction has been reduced by 50%

Although these sequences are much less sensitive to chemical shift artifacts and geometric distortions as compared to EPI, they suffer from a theoretical loss of 50% in signal compared with EPI. Alternative strategies include radial readout such as periodically rotated overlapping parallel lines (PROPELLER) [21] or spiral readout [22]. Another approach is to reduce the field of view (FOV) [16] using a 2D spatially selective echo-planar RF excitation pulse and 180-degree refocusing pulse. Images can be generated with a reduced FOV (rFOV) in the phase-encode (PE) direction without the need for a longer readout. Finally, a promising approach is to use multi-shot EPI (msEPI) acquisitions which enable shorted readout times resulting in image distortions to be reduced. Importantly, msEPI methods are typically susceptible to motion-induced phase errors among excitations. Recently, a novel technique termed multiplexed sensitivity-encoding (MUSE) was developed to reliably correct nonlinear shot-to-shot phase variations without the use of navigator echoes [19] (Fig. 5.2). A recent study by Zhang et al. evaluated the reproducibility of quantitative diffusion measurements obtained with rFOV and msEPI acquisitions for prostate DW-MRI. The results demonstrate both msEPI and rFOV can generate reproducible high image quality quantitative diffusion measurements relative to ssEPI [23].

5.2.1.2 Quantification of DW-MRI Data

Numerous diffusion models have been evaluated in the literature for prostate cancer imaging. The actual choice of model depends on any of the three tissue properties measurable by DW-MRI: cellularity, vascularity, and microstructure (Fig. 5.3). In this section, we will review models that are commonly discussed for each of the three tissue properties and provide a brief comparison of their related trade-offs.

Standard Monoexponential Diffusion-Weighted Model of the Prostate

In the simplest case, the diffusion coefficient is described by a single exponential function:

$$S(b) = S(0) \cdot \exp(-b \cdot \mathrm{ADC}) \tag{5.1}$$

where $S(b)$ and $S(0)$ are signal intensities of each voxel with and without diffusion weighting and the quantity b is the diffusion-sensitizing factor (commonly referred to as the b-value). The gradient properties including amplitude, duration, and temporal spatial of the two motion-probing gradients determine the b-value commonly expressed in seconds per millimeter squared (s/mm^2):

$$b = \gamma^2 G^2 \delta^2 \left(\Delta - \frac{\delta}{3} \right) \tag{5.2}$$

where γ denotes the gyromagnetic ratio, G is the diffusion gradient amplitude, δ the diffusion gradient duration, and Δ the time between the leading edges of the diffusion gradient pulses.

The apparent diffusion coefficient, ADC, is a single diffusion coefficient, which describes a multitude of diffusion properties of tissue, including both diffusion and perfusion, and is assumed to be independent of b-value, that is, ADC is constant (Fig. 5.4). Commonly, two or more DW images are acquired, with one low b-value (often 0 s/mm^2) and the remaining b-values extending up to 1000 s/mm^2; these images are fitted to a monoexponential model to calculate ADC values, which can then be displayed as ADC parametric maps.

Changes in ADC due to tumor are typically attributed to tissue "cellularity." Although correlation between ADC and tissue cellularity is well established in neural tissue, there is insuf-

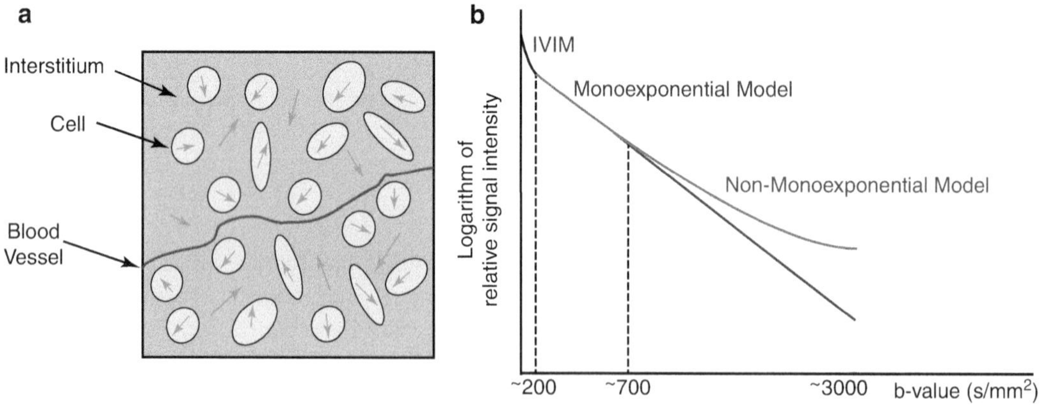

Fig. 5.3 (**a**) Individual water models diffuse through a random process in the cellular and interstitial compartment. The displacement due to blood flow in randomly oriented capillary segments can be modeled as a pseudo-diffusion process which forms the basis of the IVIM model. (**b**) Attenuation of diffusion MR signal (shown as the logarithm of the relative signal intensity) as a function of b-value. Three regions are noted. The rapid signal decay due to blood displacement in the capillaries at low b-values (less than 200 s/mm^2), the monoexponential signal attenuation resulting in a Gaussian distribution of molecular displacement (free diffusion) at intermediate b-values, and at higher b-values, there is deviation from the free diffusion due to hindrance effects which results in non-monoexponential (or non-Gaussian) diffusion behavior

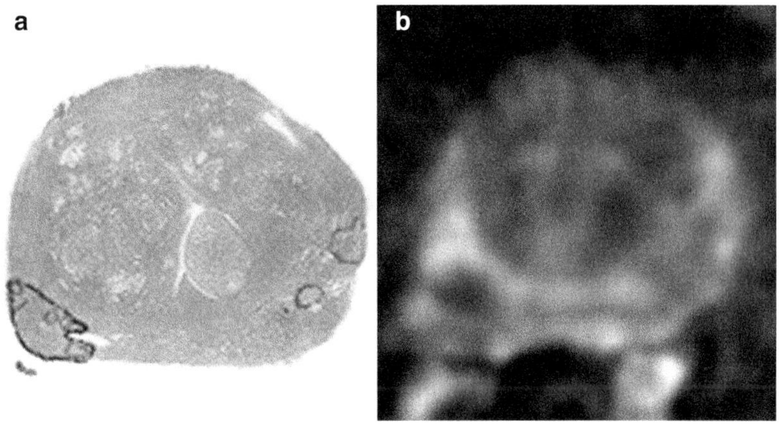

Fig. 5.4 Representative data from a 64-year-old patient with surgical Gleason score 7 (4 + 3) prostate cancer, pre-surgical PSA level of 9.43 ng/mL, and clinical stage T1c. (**a**) Whole-mount step-section histopathologic map with tumor outlined. (**b**) Axial ADC map corresponding to the lesion location

ficient biological evidence for this correlation in other tumors. Several factors could contribute to prostate cancer ADC in addition to cell density, including cell type, membrane permeability, and multiple intra- and extracellular structural features. A study found that both ADC and Gleason pattern changes correlate more strongly with relative proportion of the gland components, i.e., epithelium, stroma, and lumen than with cellularity metrics [24].

Low *b*-Value Diffusion-Weighted Model of the Prostate

Intravoxel Incoherent Motion (IVIM)

Le Bihan et al. [25, 26] proposed the intravoxel incoherent motion (IVIM) biexponential model. In this model, diffusion signal was measured from many *b*-values to estimate diffusion parameters, ranging from very low to high. Although it is more detailed than the monoexponential model, the biexponential model makes assumptions regarding the microcirculation and provides estimates of perfusion that are not sufficiently reproducible to be reliable [27].

The effect of perfusion on the total signal was modeled by incorporating the volume fraction f of the water flowing through the microvessels [28]. Accordingly, the signal attenuation is given by

$$S(b) = S(0)\cdot\left[(1-f)\cdot\exp(-b\cdot D) + f\cdot F\right] \tag{5.3}$$

where D is the diffusion coefficient, f is the volume fraction of water in perfused capillaries, and F is due to microcirculation and has a value of 1 or less that depends on capillary geometry and blood velocity.

According to a model presented by Le Bihan et al. [28], perfusion can also be considered an incoherent motion, and the signal component due to microcirculation of blood is given by $F = \exp(-b \cdot D^*)$. Hence the IVIM model of diffusion is given by

$$S(b) = S(0)\cdot\begin{bmatrix}(1-f)\cdot\exp(-b\cdot D)\\ +f\cdot\exp\left(-b\cdot D^*\right)\end{bmatrix} \tag{5.4}$$

where the pseudo-diffusion coefficient, $D*$, is dependent on the mean path length and blood velocity within the capillary network (Fig. 5.5).

A major limitation of the biexponential model is that it makes assumptions regarding the microcirculation and provides estimates of perfusion that are not sufficiently reproducible to be reliable [29–33]. Riches et al. [29] compared biexponential and monoexponential models of diffusion and associated perfusion coefficients of the prostate and rectal wall using 11 *b*-values in the range 0–800 s/mm^2. They found that when the minimum *b*-values are greater than 20 s/mm^2, the monoexponential model describes the data better than the biexponential model. However, when low *b*-values were included, the biexponential model better describes the low *b*-value signal in PCa, normal PZ, and rectal wall. Like Pang et al. [34], they highlighted the importance of selecting *b*-values in the measurement of diffusion- and perfusion-related parameters. Overall, the variability of very large variation in the perfusion coefficients

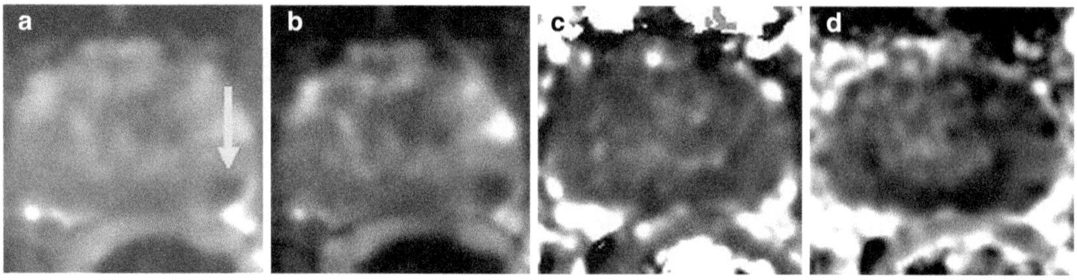

Fig. 5.5 Parametric maps of the prostate generated using 8 *b*-values in the range of 0–1000 s/mm^2 (0, 50, 100, 200, 400, 600, 800, and 1000 s/mm^2). (**a**) ADC map generated using the monoexponential model and parameters generated based on the IVIM model, (**b**) the diffusion coefficient *D*, (**c**) the pseudo-diffusion coefficient $D*$, and (**d**) the volume fraction of water in perfused capillaries, *f*. The area suspicious for cancer is shown with the arrow

limits its ability to reliably estimate perfusion effects. Kuru et al. found that IVIM parameters were not significantly different between PCa and areas of normal areas [30]. Dopfert et al. found that although ADC, *D*, and *f* were significantly lower in PCa compared to benign tissue, ADC maps provided better diagnostic performance than IVIM maps [32]. Shinmoto et al. reported that in 81% of patients with histologically proven prostate cancer, biexponential fit of multi-*b*-value images provided statistically improved fit over monoexponential fit [33].

High *b*-Value Diffusion-Weighted Model of the Prostate

Several studies investigated deviations of diffusion signal from monoexponential (ME) behavior using high-*b*-value DW-MRI (typically considered to be DW-MRI with a *b*-value range up to or beyond 2000 s/mm^2) [35–38]. Models considered for the analysis of high-*b*-value prostate data include the biexponential (BE) model, in which the relative contributions from "fast" and "slow" components of the signal decay are quantified; diffusion kurtosis (DK) imaging [37, 39], which estimates the diffusion coefficient as well as the kurtosis, a metric for the degree of non-Gaussian behavior [40]; and the stretched exponential (SE) formalism, which, similarly to DK imaging, makes no assumption as to the tissue compartmentalization but, rather, uses a stretching parameter to measure heterogeneity of the environment [38, 41] (Fig. 5.6).

Biexponential (BE) Model of Diffusion

The BE signal decay equation provides a four-parameter model of signal as follows [35, 36]:

$$S(b) = S(0) \cdot \begin{bmatrix} f_{\text{fast}} \cdot \exp(-b \cdot D_{\text{fast}}) \\ +(1 - f_{\text{fast}}) \cdot \exp(-b \cdot D_{\text{slow}}) \end{bmatrix} \quad (5.5)$$

In this model, the signal decay is assumed to be due to two components: the fast component with diffusion coefficient D_{fast} and fraction of f_{fast} and the slow component with diffusion coefficient D_{slow} and fraction ($1\text{-}f_{\text{fast}}$). Shinmoto et al. found that both D_{fast} and D_{slow} of PCa were significantly lower than those of TZ and PZ. Furthermore, f_{fast} was significantly smaller in cancer than in PZ [36].

Diffusion Kurtosis (DK) Model of the Prostate

The DK model provides a three-parameter signal decay equation given by [40]:

$$S(b) = S(0) \cdot \left[\exp\left(-b \cdot D + b^2 \cdot K \cdot D^2 / 6\right)\right] \quad (5.6)$$

where *D* is the diffusion coefficient adjusted for non-Gaussian behavior and *K* is the diffusion kurtosis, which quantifies non-Gaussian diffusion. *K* is a dimensionless statistical metric that quantifies the non-Gaussian behavior of an arbitrary probability distribution. When $K = 0$, the standard ME model is recovered. Due to the complex histology of cancer cells in PCa, it has been suggested that the DK model could provide better

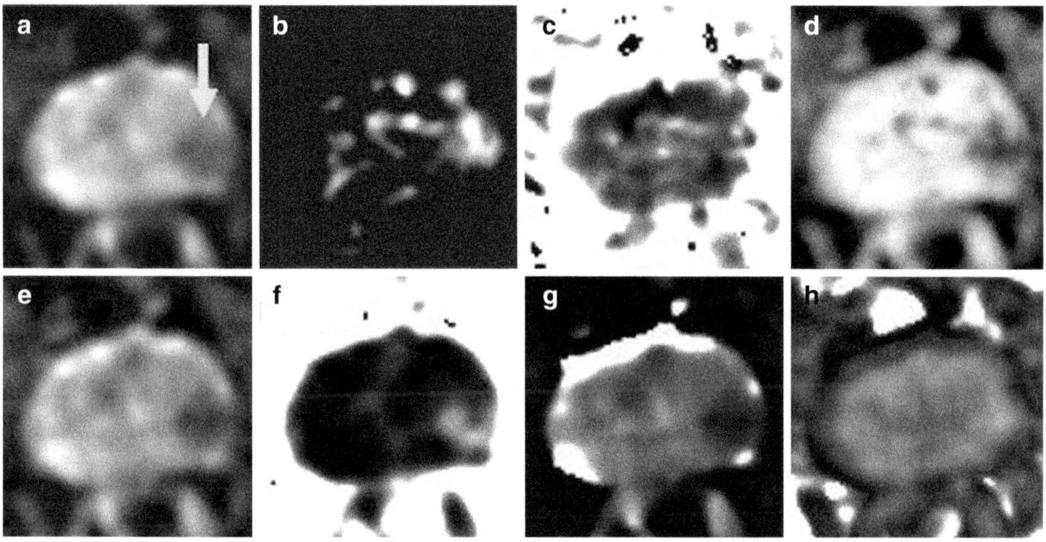

Fig. 5.6 Transverse parametric maps of the prostate obtained at high b-values using 10 b-values ($b_{max} = 2000$ s/mm^2). (**a**) For the ME model, the ADC map is shown. From the BE model, diffusion coefficients for the (**b**) slow diffusion (D_{slow}), (**c**) fast diffusion (D_{fast}) component, and (**d**) fraction of fast component, f_{fast}, are shown. From the DK model, (**e**) diffusion coefficient D and (**f**) kurtosis K are shown. From the SE model, (**g**) distributed diffusion coefficient DDC and (**h**) α are shown. The area suspicious for cancer is shown with the arrow

characterization of prostate cancer than the standard ME model [37, 39]. A study by Rosenkrantz et al. evaluating the feasibility of DK imaging to distinguish benign form malignant regions in PZ, found that K was significantly greater in cancerous sextants than in benign PZ. They also found that K showed significantly greater sensitivity for differentiating cancerous sextants from benign PZ than ADC or D. The same study evaluated the ability of DK imaging to distinguish low- from high-grade malignant regions and found K had significantly greater area under the curve for differentiating sextants with low- and high-grade cancer than ADC.

Stretched Exponential (SE) Model of the Prostate

The SE model allows gauging in a simple way the deviations from the monoexponential model through a three-parameter SE signal decay equation [41]:

$$S(b) = S(0) \cdot \exp\left\{-(b \cdot \mathrm{DDC})^{\alpha}\right\} \quad (5.7)$$

where DDC is the distributed diffusion coefficient. Alpha (α) is a dimensionless parameter with a value between 0 and 1; it characterizes deviation of the signal attenuation from monoexponential form and is used to measure heterogeneity of the environment. The stretched exponential model assumes a continuous distribution of diffusion coefficients where α represents deviation from monoexponential decay. A study comparing stretched-exponential and monoexponential model of DW-MRI (DWI) in PCa and normal tissues found that ADC was significantly higher than DDC in PCa but lower than DDC in the PZ and normal central gland [38].

Several investigators have evaluated the performance of DW-MRI at various b-values. In a study by Kim et al. detection of prostate at b = 1000 s/mm^2 was compared to 2000 s/mm^2 at 3T, and this study reported that b-value of 1000 s/mm^2 was more sensitive and more accurate in predicting localized prostate cancer than DW-MRI performed using b-value of 2000 s/mm^2 [42]. Another study reported significantly higher contrast ratios (defined as the ratio of ADC values of tumors to reference) at b = 1500 and 2000 s/mm^2 as compared to b-values of 800 and 1000 s/mm^2 [43].

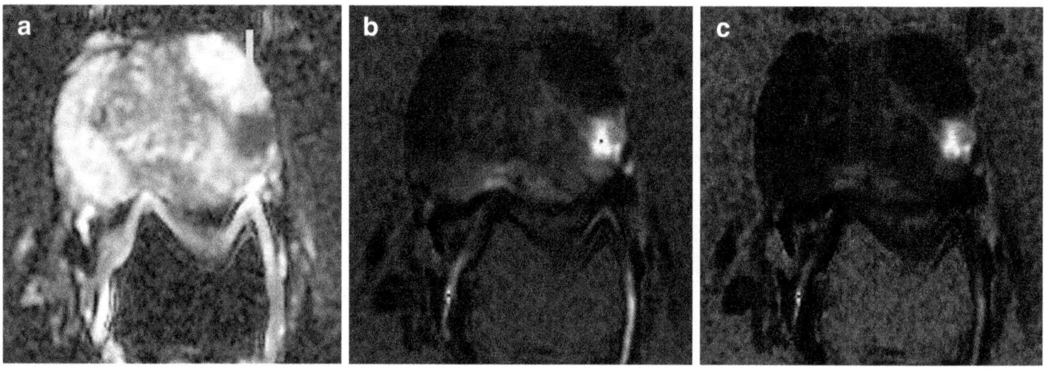

Fig. 5.7 Images from a 75-year-old man with biopsy-proven prostate cancer. (**a**) The area suspicious for cancer (decreased ADC) is shown with the arrow on the ADC map generated using b = 0 and 1000 s/mm². Computed diffusion maps generated from the same diffusion data at (**b**) b = 1500 s/mm² and (**c**) b = 2000 s/mm²

Image Synthesis

There are methods to compute or synthesize high *b*-factor images using only low and intermediate *b*-factor scans through voxel-by-voxel extrapolation of the fitted signal decay curves (Fig. 5.7). Computed DW-MR imaging was introduced by Blackledge to improve tumor detection in oncologic cases [44]. Subsequently, Maas et al. showed that computed DW-MR images calculated from measured images between 0 and 800 s/mm² resulted in higher effective contrast-to-noise ratio than measured DW-MR images and suggested that such imaging may be of clinical aid in the management of prostate cancer [45]. The diagnostic value of computed DW-MRI has been evaluated in several reports including [46, 47]. A comparison of computed DW-MRI and acquired high *b*-value DW-MRI found that computed DW-MR images using IVIM model detected approximately the same number of lesions as acquired high *b*-value DW-MRI [46]. Another report presented a divergent finding that computed DW-MRI improves lesion contrast and conspicuity in PCa [47].

5.3 PI-RADS (Prostate Imaging Reporting and Data System) Recommendations

In 2012, the European Society of Urogenital Radiology published the first version of the Prostate Imaging Reporting and Data System (PI-RADS) [48]. One of the aims was to provide clear and easily understandable guidelines regarding the clinical role of prostate MRI and to design a reporting system. PI-RADS guidelines are excellent steps in the right direction, although details regarding MRI protocol development and implementation are sparse. The Prostate Imaging Reporting and Data System (PI-RADS) Version 2 [49] has recommended following imaging parameters: TE $\leq$ 90 ms; TR $\geq$ 3000 ms; in-plane dimension of $\leq$2.5 mm; slice thickness $\leq$4 mm with no gap; field of view [FOV] = 16–22 cm. The minor revision to PI-RADS (v2.1) was published in 2019 [50]. In this version, it is recommended to use one low *b*-value set at 0–100 s/mm² (preferably 50–100 s/mm²) and one intermediate *b*-value set at 800–1000 s/mm². The maximum *b*-value used to calculate ADC is recommended to be $\leq$1000 s/mm² to avoid diffusion kurtosis effects that have been described at higher *b*-values [51]. Nonetheless, a high *b*-value ($\geq$1400 s/mm²) image set is also mandatory and preferably should be obtained from a separate acquisition or calculated from the low and intermediate *b*-value images. Additional *b*-values between 100 and 1000 may provide more accurate ADC calculations and estimations of calculated high *b*-value images (>1400 s/mm²).

5.4 Conclusions and Future Directions

DW-MRI has an important role in the diagnosis, the assessment of aggressiveness, and the assessment of treatment response of prostate cancer. Improved acquisition strategies will have a major impact in higher image quality and more reliable imaging strategies. Advanced signal analysis models provide an opportunity to more accurately evaluate the disease and provide a more comprehensive assessment of the treatment strategies. Technical development of DW-MRI is an active area of research and promises to provide improved understanding of tissue microstructure and disease status.

References

1. Siegel RL, Miller KD, Jemal A. Cancer statistics, 2019. CA Cancer J Clin. 2019;69(1):7–34.
2. Hricak H, White S, Vigneron D, Kurhanewicz J, Kosco A, Levin D, et al. Carcinoma of the prostate gland: MR imaging with pelvic phased-array coils versus integrated endorectal pelvic phased-array coils. Radiology. 1994;193(3):703–9.
3. Akin O, Sala E, Moskowitz CS, Kuroiwa K, Ishill NM, Pucar D, et al. Transition zone prostate cancers: features, detection, localization, and staging at endorectal MR imaging. Radiology. 2006;239(3):784–92.
4. Hricak H, Choyke PL, Eberhardt SC, Leibel SA, Scardino PT. Imaging prostate cancer: a multidisciplinary perspective. Radiology. 2007;243(1):28–53.
5. Hricak H. Given the improvement in pelvic coils for MR, is an endorectal coil necessary to evaluate prostate carcinoma? AJR Am J Roentgenol. 1995;165(3):733–4.
6. Noworolski SM, Crane JC, Vigneron DB, Kurhanewicz J. A clinical comparison of rigid and inflatable endorectal-coil probes for MRI and 3D MR spectroscopic imaging (MRSI) of the prostate. J Magn Reson Imaging. 2008;27(5):1077–82.
7. Rosen Y, Bloch BN, Lenkinski RE, Greenman RL, Marquis RP, Rofsky NM. 3T MR of the prostate: reducing susceptibility gradients by inflating the endorectal coil with a barium sulfate suspension. Magn Reson Med. 2007;57(5):898–904.
8. Noworolski SM, Reed GD, Kurhanewicz J, Vigneron DB. Post-processing correction of the endorectal coil reception effects in MR spectroscopic imaging of the prostate. J Magn Reson Imaging. 2010;32(3):654–62.
9. Soher BJ, Dale BM, Merkle EM. A review of MR physics: 3T versus 1.5T. Magn Reson Imaging Clin N Am. 2007;15(3):277–90. v
10. Bloch BN, Rofsky NM, Baroni RH, Marquis RP, Pedrosa I, Lenkinski RE. 3 tesla magnetic resonance imaging of the prostate with combined pelvic phased-array and endorectal coils; initial experience(1). Acad Radiol. 2004;11(8):863–7.
11. Sosna J, Pedrosa I, Dewolf WC, Mahallati H, Lenkinski RE, Rofsky NM. MR imaging of the prostate at 3 tesla: comparison of an external phased-array coil to imaging with an endorectal coil at 1.5 tesla. Acad Radiol. 2004;11(8):857–62.
12. Park BK, Kim B, Kim CK, Lee HM, Kwon GY. Comparison of phased-array 3.0-T and endorectal 1.5-T magnetic resonance imaging in the evaluation of local staging accuracy for prostate cancer. J Comput Assist Tomogr. 2007;31(4):534–8.
13. Chang KJ, Kamel IR, Macura KJ, Bluemke DA. 3.0-T MR imaging of the abdomen: comparison with 1.5 T. Radiographics. 2008;28(7):1983–98.
14. Turkbey B, Merino MJ, Gallardo EC, Shah V, Aras O, Bernardo M, et al. Comparison of endorectal coil and nonendorectal coil T2W and diffusion-weighted MRI at 3 tesla for localizing prostate cancer: correlation with whole-mount histopathology. J Magn Reson Imaging. 2014;39(6):1443–8.
15. Starobinets O, Korn N, Iqbal S, Noworolski SM, Zagoria R, Kurhanewicz J, et al. Practical aspects of prostate MRI: hardware and software considerations, protocols, and patient preparation. Abdom Radiol (NY). 2016;41(5):817–30.
16. Saritas EU, Cunningham CH, Lee JH, Han ET, Nishimura DG. DWI of the spinal cord with reduced FOV single-shot EPI. Magn Reson Med. 2008;60(2):468–73.
17. Holdsworth SJ, Skare S, Newbould RD, Guzmann R, Blevins NH, Bammer R. Readout-segmented EPI for rapid high resolution diffusion imaging at 3 T. Eur J Radiol. 2008;65(1):36–46.
18. Porter DA, Heidemann RM. High resolution diffusion-weighted imaging using readout-segmented echo-planar imaging, parallel imaging and a two-dimensional navigator-based reacquisition. Magn Reson Med. 2009;62(2):468–75.
19. Chen NK, Guidon A, Chang HC, Song AW. A robust multi-shot scan strategy for high-resolution diffusion weighted MRI enabled by multiplexed sensitivity-encoding (MUSE). NeuroImage. 2013;72:41–7.
20. Alsop DC. Phase insensitive preparation of single-shot RARE: application to diffusion imaging in humans. Magn Reson Med. 1997;38(4):527–33.
21. Pipe JG. Motion correction with PROPELLER MRI: application to head motion and free-breathing cardiac imaging. Magn Reson Med. 1999;42(5):963–9.
22. Kim DH, Adalsteinsson E, Spielman DM. Simple analytic variable density spiral design. Magn Reson Med. 2003;50(1):214–9.
23. Zhang Y, Holmes J, Rabanillo I, Guidon A, Wells S, Hernando D. Quantitative diffusion MRI using reduced field-of-view and multi-shot acquisition techniques: validation in phantoms and prostate imaging. Magn Reson Imaging. 2018;51:173–81.
24. Chatterjee A, Watson G, Myint E, Sved P, McEntee M, Bourne R. Changes in epithelium, stroma, and lumen space correlate more strongly with Gleason pattern and are stronger predictors of prostate ADC changes than cellularity metrics. Radiology. 2015;277(3):751–62.
25. Le Bihan D, Breton E, Lallemand D, Grenier P, Cabanis E, Laval-Jeantet M. MR imaging of intravoxel incoherent motions: application to diffusion

and perfusion in neurologic disorders. Radiology. 1986;161(2):401–7.
26. Le Bihan D, Turner R, MacFall JR. Effects of intravoxel incoherent motions (IVIM) in steady-state free precession (SSFP) imaging: application to molecular diffusion imaging. Magn Reson Med. 1989;10(3):324–37.
27. King MD, van Bruggen N, Busza AL, Houseman J, Williams SR, Gadian DG. Perfusion and diffusion MR imaging. Magn Reson Med. 1992;24(2):288–301.
28. Le Bihan D, Breton E, Lallemand D, Aubin ML, Vignaud J, Laval-Jeantet M. Separation of diffusion and perfusion in intravoxel incoherent motion MR imaging. Radiology. 1988;168(2):497–505.
29. Riches SF, Hawtin K, Charles-Edwards EM, de Souza NM. Diffusion-weighted imaging of the prostate and rectal wall: comparison of biexponential and monoexponential modelled diffusion and associated perfusion coefficients. NMR Biomed. 2009;22(3):318–25.
30. Kuru TH, Roethke MC, Stieltjes B, Maier-Hein K, Schlemmer HP, Hadaschik BA, et al. Intravoxel incoherent motion (IVIM) diffusion imaging in prostate cancer what does it add? J Comput Assist Tomogr. 2014;38(4):558–64.
31. Mazzoni LN, Lucarini S, Chiti S, Busoni S, Gori C, Menchi I. Diffusion-weighted signal models in healthy and cancerous peripheral prostate tissues: comparison of outcomes obtained at different b-values. J Magn Reson Imaging. 2014;39(3):512–8.
32. Dopfert J, Lemke A, Weidner A, Schad LR. Investigation of prostate cancer using diffusion-weighted intravoxel incoherent motion imaging. Magn Reson Imaging. 2011;29(8):1053–8.
33. Shinmoto H, Tamura C, Soga S, Shiomi E, Yoshihara N, Kaji T, et al. An intravoxel incoherent motion diffusion-weighted imaging study of prostate cancer. AJR Am J Roentgenol. 2012;199(4):W496–500.
34. Pang Y, Turkbey B, Bernardo M, Kruecker J, Kadoury S, Merino MJ, et al. Intravoxel incoherent motion MR imaging for prostate cancer: an evaluation of perfusion fraction and diffusion coefficient derived from different b-value combinations. Magn Reson Med. 2013;69(2):553–62.
35. Mulkern RV, Barnes AS, Haker SJ, Hung YP, Rybicki FJ, Maier SE, et al. Biexponential characterization of prostate tissue water diffusion decay curves over an extended b-factor range. Magn Reson Imaging. 2006;24(5):563–8.
36. Shinmoto H, Oshio K, Tanimoto A, Higuchi N, Okuda S, Kuribayashi S, et al. Biexponential apparent diffusion coefficients in prostate cancer. Magn Reson Imaging. 2009;27(3):355–9.
37. Rosenkrantz AB, Sigmund EE, Johnson G, Babb JS, Mussi TC, Melamed J, et al. Prostate cancer: feasibility and preliminary experience of a diffusional kurtosis model for detection and assessment of aggressiveness of peripheral zone cancer. Radiology. 2012;264(1):126–35.
38. Liu X, Zhou L, Peng W, Wang H, Zhang Y. Comparison of stretched-exponential and monoexponential model diffusion-weighted imaging in prostate cancer and normal tissues. J Magn Reson Imaging. 2015;42(4):1078–85.
39. Tamura C, Shinmoto H, Soga S, Okamura T, Sato H, Okuaki T, et al. Diffusion kurtosis imaging study of prostate cancer: preliminary findings. J Magn Reson Imaging. 2014;40(3):723–9.
40. Jensen JH, Helpern JA, Ramani A, Lu H, Kaczynski K. Diffusional kurtosis imaging: the quantification of non-Gaussian water diffusion by means of magnetic resonance imaging. Magn Reson Med. 2005;53(6):1432–40.
41. Bennett KM, Schmainda KM, Bennett RT, Rowe DB, Lu H, Hyde JS. Characterization of continuously distributed cortical water diffusion rates with a stretched-exponential model. Magn Reson Med. 2003;50(4):727–34.
42. Kim CK, Park BK, Kim B. High-b-value diffusion-weighted imaging at 3 T to detect prostate cancer: comparisons between b values of 1,000 and 2,000 s/mm2. AJR Am J Roentgenol. 2010;194(1):W33–7.
43. Wetter A, Nensa F, Lipponer C, Guberina N, Olbricht T, Schenck M, et al. High and ultra-high b-value diffusion-weighted imaging in prostate cancer: a quantitative analysis. Acta Radiol. 2015;56(8):1009–15.
44. Blackledge MD, Leach MO, Collins DJ, Koh DM. Computed diffusion-weighted MR imaging may improve tumor detection. Radiology. 2011;261(2):573–81.
45. Maas MC, Futterer JJ, Scheenen TW. Quantitative evaluation of computed high B value diffusion-weighted magnetic resonance imaging of the prostate. Investig Radiol. 2013;48(11):779–86.
46. Grant KB, Agarwal HK, Shih JH, Bernardo M, Pang Y, Daar D, et al. Comparison of calculated and acquired high b value diffusion-weighted imaging in prostate cancer. Abdom Imaging. 2015;40(3):578–86.
47. Feuerlein S, Davenport MS, Krishnaraj A, Merkle EM, Gupta RT. Computed high b-value diffusion-weighted imaging improves lesion contrast and conspicuity in prostate cancer. Prostate Cancer Prostatic Dis. 2015;18(2):155–60.
48. Barentsz JO, Richenberg J, Clements R, Choyke P, Verma S, Villeirs G, et al. ESUR prostate MR guidelines 2012. Eur Radiol. 2012;22(4):746–57.
49. Weinreb JC, Barentsz JO, Choyke PL, Cornud F, Haider MA, Macura KJ, et al. PI-RADS prostate imaging reporting and data system: 2015, version 2. Eur Urol. 2016;69(1):16–40.
50. Turkbey B, Rosenkrantz AB, Haider MA, Padhani AR, Villeirs G, Macura KJ, et al. Prostate imaging reporting and data system version 2.1: 2019 update of prostate imaging reporting and data system version 2. Eur Urol. 2019;76(3):340–51.
51. Rosenkrantz AB, Padhani AR, Chenevert TL, Koh DM, De Keyzer F, Taouli B, et al. Body diffusion kurtosis imaging: basic principles, applications, and considerations for clinical practice. J Magn Reson Imaging. 2015;42(5):1190–202.

Dynamic Contrast-Enhanced Imaging

6

Aritrick Chatterjee, Federico Pineda, Gregory S. Karczmar, and Aytekin Oto

6.1 Introduction

Prostate cancer (PCa) is the most common non-cutaneous cancer (174,650 new diagnoses per year) and is among the leading causes of death (31,620 deaths per year) in the United States [1]. Multiparametric MRI (mpMRI) is increasingly being used for diagnosis of PCa. Prostate mpMRI consists of T2-weighted imaging (T2WI), diffusion-weighted imaging (DWI), pre-contrast T1-weighted imaging (T1WI), and dynamic contrast-enhanced (DCE) imaging. MRI has good diagnostic accuracy for PCa, especially a high negative predictive value [2] and good sensitivity and specificity [3]. It can reliably grade the PCa and provide information about location and volume for the selection of optimum therapy and guidance for targeted biopsies.

In PI-RADS v2, DCE-MRI was a required component of mpMRI examinations undertaken for the detection of clinically significant PCa (csPCa), although it had a limited role and was used only to elevate the PI-RADS T2 score of a lesion in the peripheral zone (PZ) from 3 to 4. It did not have any formal role in scoring or assessment category of findings in the TZ. However, experience has shown that, in selected cases, DCE may assist in the detection of csPCa. DCE in practice has been a "safety-net" sequence, especially when either T2WI or DWI is degraded by artifacts or inadequate SNR [4].

6.2 DCE-MRI Imaging Technique and Technical Considerations

Since its earliest days, numerous studies have improved DCE-MRI with new data acquisition methods, use of higher temporal resolution, use of higher-relaxivity contrast agents, and newer methods for quantitative analysis of DCE-MRI data [5–9]. DCE-MRI involves the acquisition of serial T1-weighted images (fast/spoiled gradient echo sequence with fat suppression) of the prostate before and after the bolus injection of a low-molecular-weight chelated gadolinium molecule. Because of its paramagnetic properties, gadolinium contrast agent shortens T1 relaxation time of tissues in which it accumulates. Prostate cancers show early focal signal enhancement and washout due to increased vascularity or angiogenesis [10, 11]. Increased capillary permeability leads to higher uptake of contrast agent that further shortens T1 relaxation time. The combination of

A. Chatterjee · G. S. Karczmar · A. Oto (✉)
University of Chicago, Department of Radiology, Chicago, IL, USA

University of Chicago, Sanford J. Grossman Center of Excellence in Prostate Imaging and Image Guided Therapy, Chicago, IL, USA
e-mail: aritrick@uchicago.edu; gskarczm@uchicago.edu; aoto@radiology.bsd.uchicago.edu

F. Pineda
University of Chicago, Department of Radiology, Chicago, IL, USA
e-mail: fdp@uchicago.edu

T. Tirkes (ed.), *Prostate MRI Essentials*, https://doi.org/10.1007/978-3-030-45935-2_6

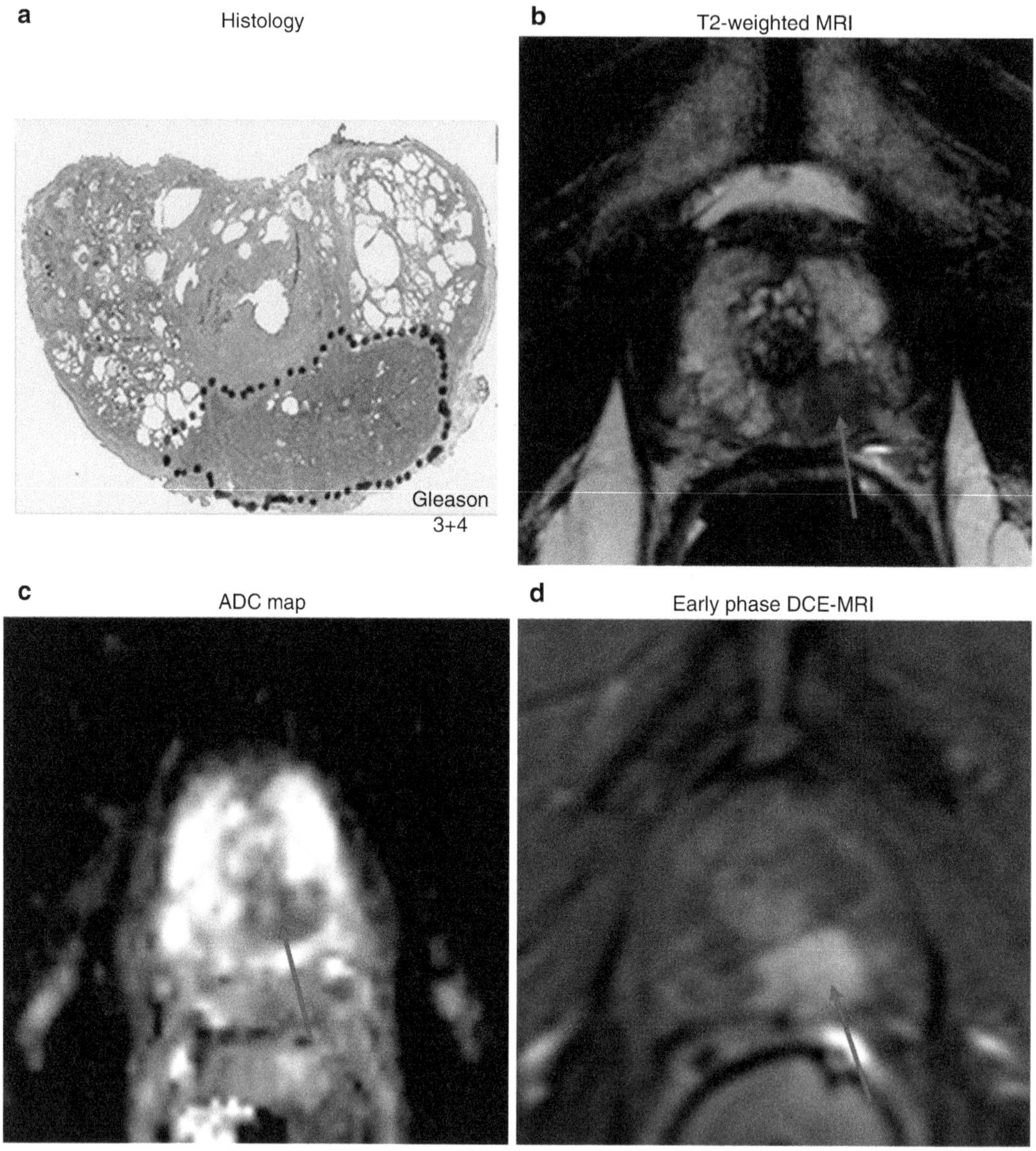

Fig. 6.1 56-year-old patient with Gleason 3 + 4 cancer in the left apex on whole-mount prostatectomy image (**a**). There is a PI-RADS 5 lesion (arrows) which is well-defined, round, and hypointense on T2W (**b**) and ADC map (**c**) and shows early focal enhancement on DCE-MRI (**d**)

high blood flow and high capillary permeability in prostate cancer results in lesions showing up as enhancing foci with respect to surrounding tissues. Representative images from prostate DCE-MRI can be seen in Figs. 6.1 and 6.2.

The standardization is critical for DCE-MRI; therefore PI-RADS v2 guideline published detailed imaging parameters (Table 6.1) [4]. DCE-MRI is performed using either 2D or 3D T1-weighted gradient echo (GRE) sequences. Current MRI scanners allow 3D T1W GRE with excellent image quality which is the widely accepted method. The PI-RADS v2 guidelines recommend a field of view that encompasses the entire prostate gland and seminal vesicles. Images are recommended to be acquired with an in-plane

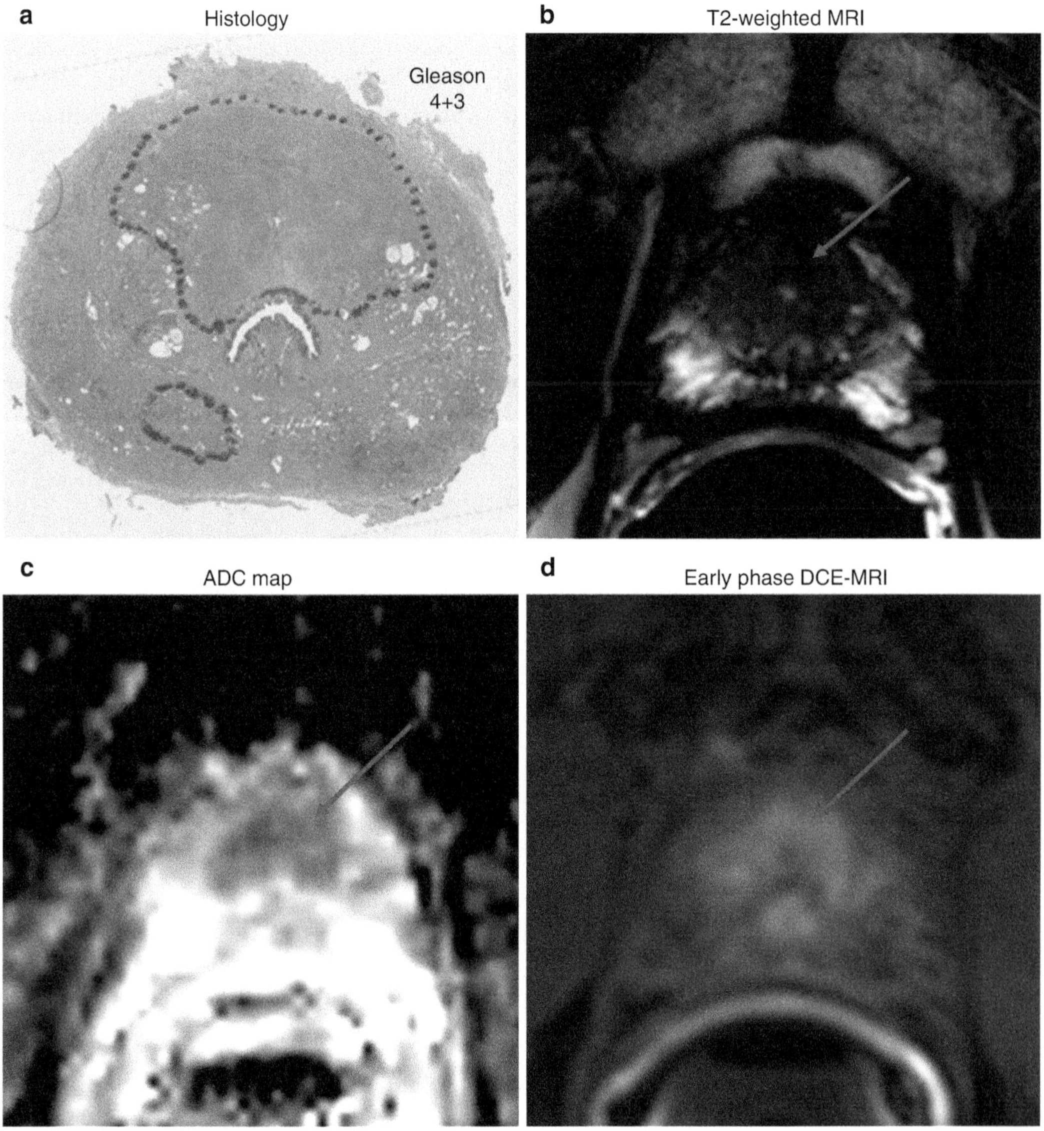

Fig. 6.2 51-year-old patient with Gleason 4 + 3 anterior cancer on prostatectomy (**a**). While the PI-RADS 4 lesion (arrows) is not clearly distant on T2W (**b**), it is hypointense on ADC map (**c**) and is clearly visible as early focally enhancing region on DCE-MRI (**d**)

resolution ≤2 × 2 mm and 3 mm slice thickness without any gaps between slices. The same imaging planes as DWI are recommended to be used for DCE-MRI. The minimum temporal resolution for serial images is ≤15 s per image, with ≤7 s preferred. The recommended dose is 0.1 mmol/kg of gadolinium-based contrast agent with a 2–3 cc/s injection rate. The total time recommended for sampling contrast media uptake and washout is over 2 min, with continuous imaging (without any gaps in acquisition).

Higher MR magnetic field strength (3T) increases signal-to-noise ratio (SNR), spatial resolution, and temporal resolution and reduces acquisition time for DCE-MRI. T1 relaxation times are longer at 3T compared to 1.5T scanners. The relaxivity of low molecular contrast agents is somewhat reduced at 3T relative to

Table 6.1 Recommended DCE-MRI imaging parameters per PI-RADS v2 guidelines

DCE imaging parameters	Recommendations
T1W gradient echo (GRE)	While both 2D and 3D sequences have been described in the literature, 3D T1W GRE is generally available using modern systems and is preferred
TR/TE	<100 ms/<5 ms
Slice thickness	3 mm, no gap. Imaging planes should be the same as those used for DWI and DCE
Field of view (FOV)	Encompass the entire prostate gland and seminal vesicles
In-plane dimension	$\leq 2 \times \leq 2$ mm
Temporal resolution	≤15 s (≤7 preferred)
Gadolinium dose	0.1 mmol/kg
Gadolinium injection rate	2–3 cc/s starting with continuous image data acquisition
Fat suppression	Recommended

1.5T. In addition, tissues that have modest blood flow and capillary permeability have very low signal on T1-weighted images at high field. This leads to excellent contrast between PCa and surrounding tissues due to improved background suppression [12]. Use of higher field strength also allows improved signal-to-noise ratio (SNR) which can be used to improve spatial and temporal resolution. High temporal resolution improves the diagnostic performance of DCE-MRI [9, 13], and therefore PI-RADS v2 recommends temporal resolution to be less than 7 s.

Another consideration is the use of endorectal coils. Endorectal coils significantly improve image quality, particularly in the peripheral zone near the rectal wall, and increase PCa detection rate [14–17]. However, due to additional cost and patients' discomfort, most imaging centers prefer not to use endorectal coils.

T1 relaxivity is the critical property of MRI contrast agents and determines the change in T1 as a function of contrast agent concentration and therefore has effect on image analysis. Gadolinium-based contrast agents with higher T1 relaxivity are optimal for detecting enhancement on T1-weighted images. Some studies have recommended use of macrocyclic agents over linear agents, due to lower likelihood of deposition in the body [18] and relatively fewer adverse reactions [19] compared to linear gadolinium-based contrast agents.

6.3 Prostate DCE-MRI Evaluation

Interpretation of the DCE-MRI per PI-RADS v2.1 guidelines will be discussed in Chap. 7. PI-RADS recommends that DCE-MRI always be interpreted in conjunction with other mpMRI sequences: T2W and DWI/ADC. Any region showing early focal enhancement compared to adjacent benign tissue on DCE-MRI and corresponding to similar suspicious finding on T2-weighted and diffusion-weighted imaging is considered suspicious for cancer. Diffuse enhancement on DCE is usually attributed to inflammation (e.g., prostatitis). Analysis of the DCE-MRI can be done qualitatively, semiquantitatively, or quantitatively.

6.3.1 Qualitative DCE-MRI Analysis

A qualitative visual assessment of DCE-MRI is based on identifying foci that exhibit early and brisk contrast enhancement (Fig. 6.3). Due to the high permeability of tumor-related vessels, contrast media is also expected to wash out faster than normal tissue. The characteristic signal versus time curve for a malignant lesion is early peak in enhancement, followed by a relatively fast decline. In contrast, the signal time curve for normal tissue is expected to have a slower, steady rise followed by a slow decline or no washout at all. PI-RADS v1 defined four types of DCE time curves: type 1 (progressive), type 2 (plateau), type 3 (wash-in and washout), and type 0 (nondiagnostic). Type 3 curve was described as the most suggestive of malignancy.

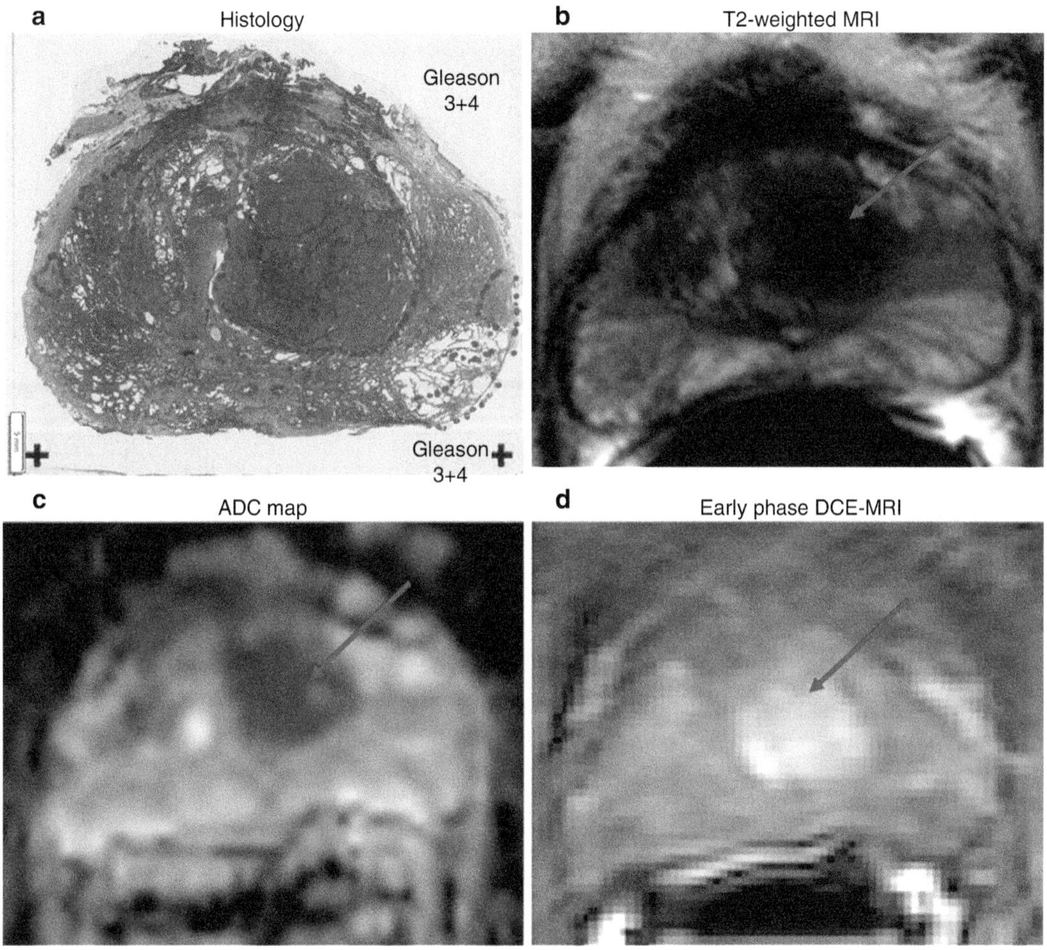

Fig. 6.3 67-year-old patient with transition zone Gleason 3 + 4 cancer on prostatectomy (**a**). While the PI-RADS 5 lesion (arrows) is clearly distant on T2W (**b**), it is hypointense on ADC map (**c**) and is clearly visible as early focally enhancing region on DCE-MRI (**d**). The Gleason 3 + 4 lesion in the left posterolateral peripheral zone was not identified on mpMRI

6.3.2 Semiquantitative DCE-MRI Analysis

An alternative to qualitative kinetic curve type classification is semiquantitative analysis methods that rely on the mathematical description of the signal versus time curve. These pure mathematical models make no assumptions about the underlying physiology of a tumor but simply use functions with limited parameters to characterize the important features of contrast agent uptake and washout curves as a function of time. The mathematical models are used as a tool to smooth the signal enhancement versus time curves, interpolate the data, and produce diagnostically useful kinetic parameters. This approach may be advantageous because normal prostatic tissue and prostate cancers are extremely heterogeneous and the commonly used compartmental models may not be consistent with the true spatiotemporal distribution of contrast agent molecules in the tumor microenvironment [20]. A representative case of semiquantitative DCE-MRI analysis using empirical mathematical model (EMM) parameters is shown on Fig. 6.4.

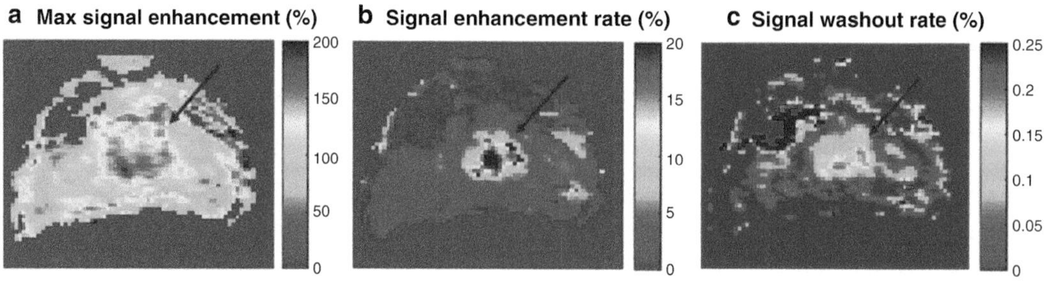

Fig. 6.4 Empirical mathematical model (EMM) parameters for the Gleason 3 + 4 lesion (arrows) for the patient (same MR slice) as shown in Fig. 6.3. Cancer lesions shows increased maximum signal enhancement (**a**), signal enhancement rate (**b**), and signal washout rate (**c**) compared to surrounding benign tissue

6.3.3 Quantitative Analysis of DCE-MRI

Semiquantitative analysis of DCE-MRI removes the subjective aspect of qualitative curve type analysis (eliminating intra-observer variability), but it does not yield parameters directly related to the underlying physiology that drives contrast media uptake and washout. The main advantage of quantitative analysis of DCE-MRI is to provide measures that relate to physiological parameters such as permeability and blood flow. Quantitative analysis relies on models that mathematically describe the distribution of contrast media from the vasculature into tumors and normal tissue. Many of the models used for quantitative analysis were initially developed to describe tracer kinetics in nuclear medicine and adapted for DCE-MRI [21].

A crucial and often challenging step in quantitative analysis of DCE data is accurate measurement of the arterial input function (AIF). The AIF is the contrast media concentration as a function of time in the arterial blood supply following intravenous injection. The local AIF is the concentration in the local arteries feeding a suspicious lesion or specific portion of the body. The gold-standard method of measuring a patient-specific AIF is by serial blood draws following the administration of contrast media. However, this method is too invasive and difficult to implement during every DCE-MRI acquisition. A common approach is to use population AIFs that have been constructed from measurements of the arterial concentration of contrast media in multiple patients and expressed via a convenient functional form. Contrast media AIF can vary significantly for a single subject scanned at different times and between subjects [22–24]. Variations in cardiac output are also a major contributor to the variability in the AIF. Representative cases of signal enhancement curve and Tofts model parameters are shown in Figs. 6.5 and 6.6, respectively.

6.4 Detection of Prostate Cancer Using DCE-MRI

Qualitative analysis of DCE-MRI alone has reported sensitivity and specificity ranges of 46–96 and 74–96%, respectively, for detecting PCa [25–30]. A meta-analysis by Tan et al. [31] consisting of 22 previous studies from 1997 to 2013 based on qualitative assessment by radiologists found that DCE-MRI (AUC = 0.82–0.86) and DWI (AUC = 0.84–0.88) outperformed T2W (AUC = 0.68–0.77). However, Turkbey et al. [30] using a more accurate imaging-pathology correlation (using custom sectioning molds) found that DCE alone (38%) had higher sensitivity than MR spectroscopy (17%) but lower than either DWI (57%) or T2W (65%). On the other hand, DCE had higher positive predictive value (86%) and specificity (97%) than T2W (69%, 90%) and DWI (75%, 93%). Isebaert et al. [32] divided the prostate into 24 sectors and found the sensitivity of DCE-MRI (22.8%) to be much smaller. However, the combination of DCE-MRI to T2W (T2W alone = 25.1 → T2W + DCE = 35.6%) and

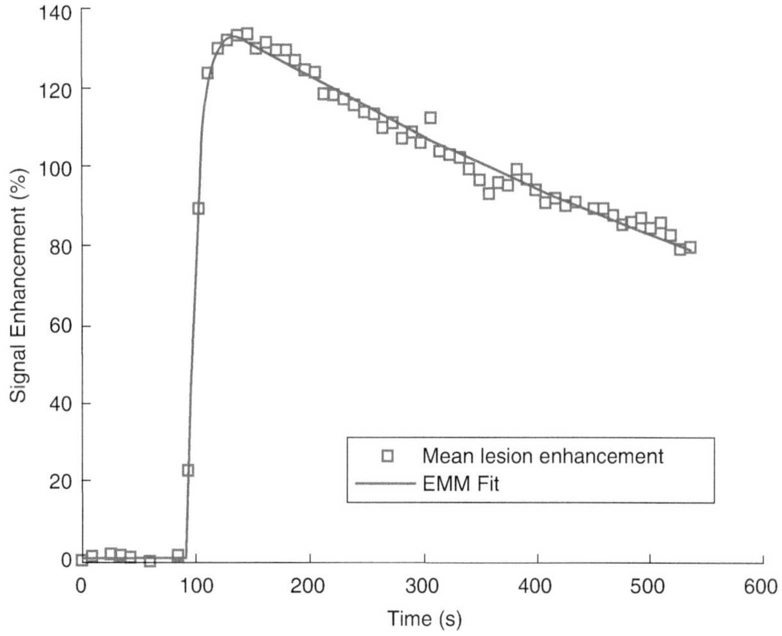

Fig. 6.5 Signal enhancement curve (signal vs time) for the same Gleason 3 + 4 lesion shows a type 3 curve with early focal enhancement and rapid washout

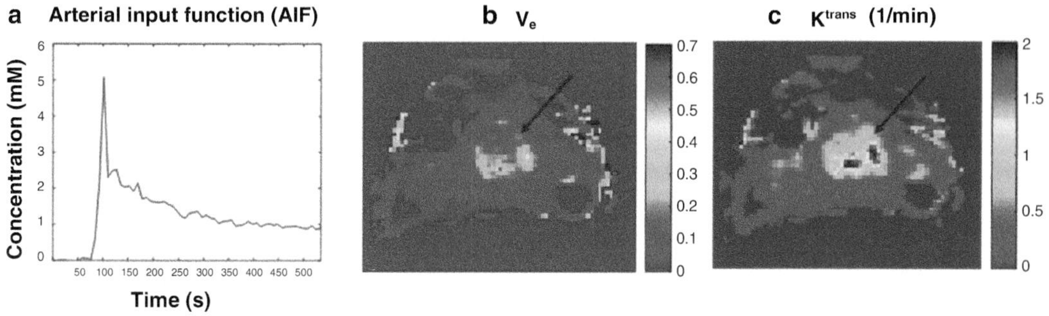

Fig. 6.6 Quantitative analysis using arterial input function (**a**) to derive Tofts model parameter showing cancer (black arrows) as identified as regions with increased v_e (**b**) and K^{trans} (**c**) compared to surrounding benign tissue

DWI (DWI alone = 36.8 → DWI + DCE = 43.7 %) or all three sequences (49.3%) improved PCa detection.

While qualitative analysis is performed and recommended in clinical practice, many studies employ semiquantitative and quantitative DCE-MRI analysis to detect PCa. Rosenkrantz et al. showed that sensitivity for peripheral zone PCa lesions was improved by the use of semiquantitative or quantitative analysis compared with qualitative agreement by radiologists (29). However, they found no difference in performance between semiquantitative and quantitative models. Ocak et al. [25] reported that DCE-MRI can improve specificity and negative predictive value for PCa prostate cancer using qualitative and pharmacokinetic parameters (K^{trans} and k_{ep}) from the two-compartment Tofts model. Also, combination of DCE and T2W improved diagnostic accuracy. Kim et al. showed that contrast uptake (wash-in) rate is useful parameter for prostate cancer detection and localization, with greater sensitivity (96 vs 65%) and specificity (82 vs 60%) than T2W imaging [33]. Similar results were reported by Isebaert et al. [34] where they found that wash-in or contrast media uptake was the best discriminator (AUC = 0.82) between PCa and benign prostatic tissue. Ren et al. found that PCa primarily exhibited curve type 3 (wash-in and washout) [35]. On the other hand, Hansford et al. [36] found that semiquantitative analysis using DCE-MRI signal curve type performed poorly in the differentiation of PCa from benign tissue. Tamada et al. showed that combining DCE-MRI with T2W and DWI improved the detection and management of PCa even in patients with gray zone PSA level (4–10 ng/ml) [37]. The sensitivity and specificity for detecting PCa were 36% and 97% for T2-weighted imaging, 43% and 95% for DCE-MRI, 38% and 96% for DWI, and 53% and 93% for mpMRI. DCE-MRI can play an additional role in PCa management by determining extracapsular extension. Bloch et al. [38] found that DCE-MRI performed better than T2W, while similar performance was found in the detection of seminal vesicle invasion. Overall staging accuracy was higher for DCE (81–84%) compared to T2WI (72%). T2WI (9–19%) tended to underestimate the disease stage more often than DCE (3–9%).

6.4.1 Tumor Aggressiveness

There are concerns regarding the overtreatment of indolent cancer, and therefore determining the aggressiveness of cancer is critical for deciding the optimal treatment option. Numerous studies have used DCE-MRI for determining tumor aggressiveness. An earlier study by Padhani et al. found no correlation between tumor vascular permeability and tumor aggressiveness while showing only weak correlation between tumor stage and permeability [39]. However, more recent studies show DCE-MRI has good diagnostic performance in assessing tumor aggressiveness. Schlemmer et al. found that K^{trans} (exchange rate constant for the pharmacokinetic two-compartment Tofts model) correlates strongly ($r = 0.62$–0.80) with microvessel density (vasculature) and can be used to differentiate low- and high-grade PCa [40]. Franiel et al. showed that high-grade PCa tend to have a higher permeability but lower blood volume and shorter mean transit time than low-grade PCa [41]. Chen et al. used both quantitative and semiquantitative analysis of DCE-MRI data to report that signal washout gradient showed the best correlation ($r = -0.75$) with Gleason score [42]. Vos et al. found that quantitative parameters (K^{trans} and k_{ep} with $\rho = 0.38$–0.43) and semiquantitative parameters (wash-in $\rho = 0.43$ and washout $\rho = -0.39$) correlated with Gleason grade and therefore can be used to assess cancer aggressiveness and distinguish low-grade PCa from intermediate- and high-grade of PCa in the peripheral zone [43]. Hötker et al. studied a larger set of patients ($n = 153$) and found that K^{trans} is higher with higher-grade PCa [44]. Similar results were reported by Low et al. [45], where K^{trans} was found to be higher for higher Gleason grade.

6.5 Challenges and Limitations

The standardization of DCE-MRI is a major challenge and limits establishment of a consensus and reproducibility of this imaging technique. Clinical adoption of DCE-MRI for prostate cancer screening has been limited by the wide range of reported sensitivity and specificity. This variation is due to varying experience of the radiologists, protocols, patient demographics, and diagnostic criteria.

Motion artifacts caused by rectal peristalsis can cause image degradation as DCE images are acquired over a course of 2–10 min. DCE-MRI signal can be increased in conditions such as hyperpermeability secondary to prostatitis in the peripheral zone and hypervascularity secondary to benign prostatic hyperplasia of the transition zone [46, 47]. DCE-MRI has lower spatial resolution compared to conventional T2-weighted images. DCE-MRI by itself has not been shown to be superior to T2W and DWI in detecting prostate cancers. Hence, its role in determination of PI-RADS 2.1 assessment category is secondary to T2W and DWI [4, 48].

Due to recent reports of complications secondary to deposition of gadolinium in the body, use of gadolinium-based contrast agents and DCE-MRI is currently being debated [18, 49]. Recently, He et al. demonstrated that lower doses of gadolinium (15% of standard dose) are effective for diagnosis of PCa, particularly when quantitative analysis is used [50]. This may provide an important alternative to conventional DCE-MRI that greatly reduces risks associated with gadolinium. Another recent study concurred that DCE-MRI with low gadolinium dose contrast agent [50] or a high relaxivity agent can distinguish PCa from benign prostate tissue as effectively as the standard dose [51]. A representative example showing diagnosis of prostate cancer using low quantities (with 15% of standard clinical contrast media dose) of a high relaxivity contrast agent is shown in Fig. 6.7. In addition to using lower doses of gadolinium, newly synthesized contrast agents such as iron [52] and vanadium-based contrast agents [53] are being investigated and may be utilized in the future.

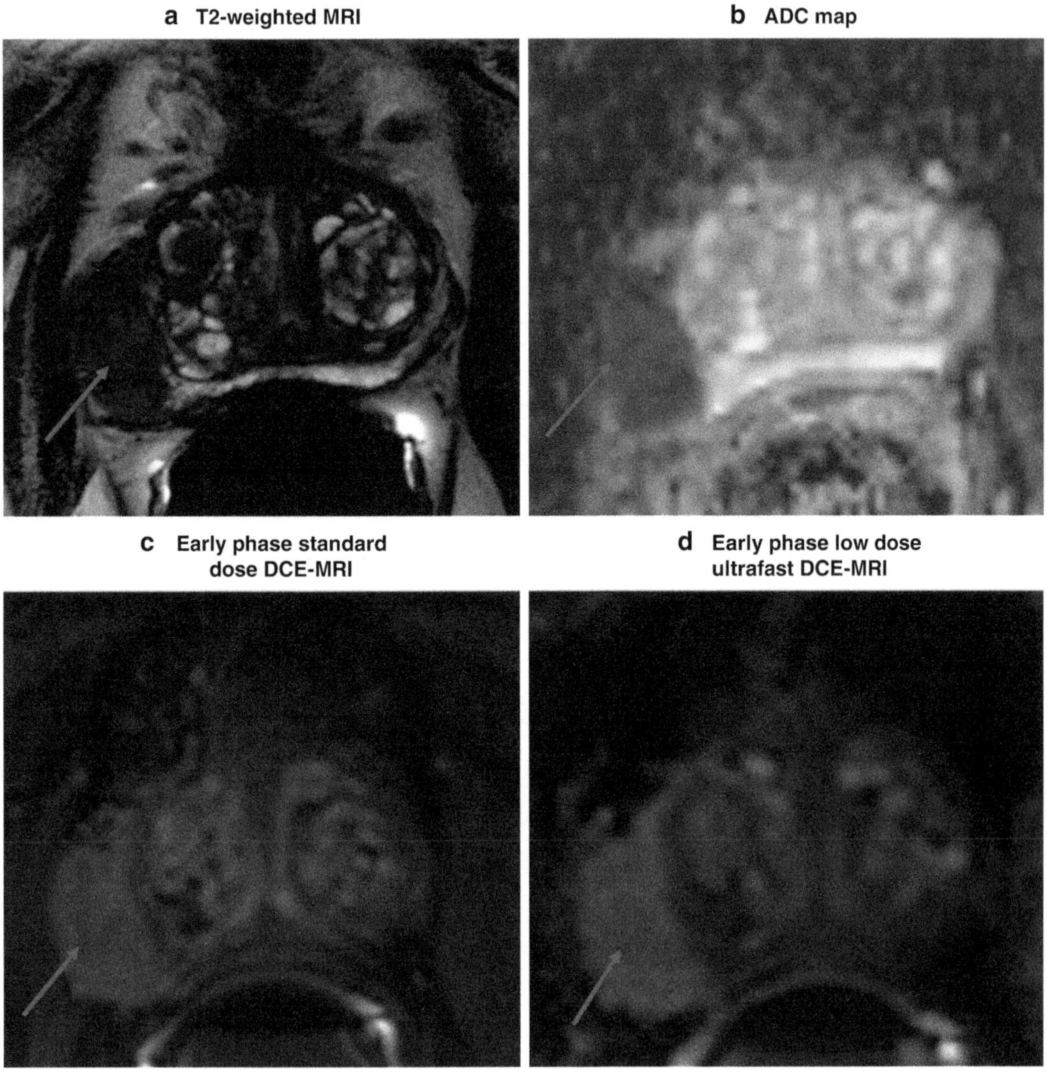

Fig. 6.7 65-year-old patient with Gleason 4 + 5 cancer in the right peripheral zone. This is a PI-RADS 5 lesion with a large hypointense area on T2W (**a**) and ADC map (**b**) with focal enhancement on both early-phase low-dose ultrafast DCE-MRI (**c**) and standard clinical dose DCE-MRI (**d**). The low-dose DCE-MRI used 15% (0.015 mmol/kg) of standard clinical dose (0.1 mmol/kg) and ultrafast sequence with a temporal resolution of 1.5 s. The standard clinical dose DCE-MRI used a temporal resolution of 7.5 s

6.6 PI-RADS v2.1 Update on DCE-MRI

Due to limitations of DCE-MRI discussed above, There is a growing interest in performing prostate MRI without DCE, a procedure termed "biparametric MRI" (bpMRI). A number of recent studies support the utilization of bpMRI for the detection of clinically significant PCa in biopsy-naïve men [54, 55] and those with a prior negative biopsy [56].

The revision 2.1 of PI-RADS committee guidelines was published in 2019 [48] and encouraged continued research about the performance of bpMRI in various clinical scenarios. The committee acknowledges the potential benefits of bpMRI, including (a) elimination of adverse events and gadolinium retention that have been associated with some gadolinium-based contrast agents, (b) shortened examination time, and (c) reduced costs, possibly resulting in increased accessibility and utilization of MRI for biopsy-naïve men with suspected PCa [48].

Recommendations regarding when mpMRI is preferred over bpMRI are:

- Patients with prior negative biopsies and unexplained raised PSA values and those in active surveillance who are being evaluated for fast PSA doubling times or changing clinical/pathologic status
- For men who have previously undergone a bpMRI examination that did not show findings suspicious for clinically significant PCa and those who remain at persistent suspicion of harboring disease
- Prior prostate interventions (TRUS/transrectal resection of the prostate/BPH therapy, radiotherapy, focal therapy, or embolization) and drug/hormonal therapies (testosterone, 5-alpha reductase, etc.) that are known to change prostate morphology
- Biopsy-naïve men with a strong family history, known genetic predispositions, elevated urinary genomic scores, and higher than average risk calculator scores for clinically significant PCa
- Men with a hip implant or other considerations that can be expected to yield degraded DWI

6.7 Summary

DCE-MRI involves the acquisition of serial T1-weighted images of the prostate before and after the bolus injection of a gadolinium-based contrast agent. Prostate cancers show early focal signal enhancement due to increased vascularity or angiogenesis. Increased capillary permeability leads to higher uptake of contrast agent. This shortens the T1 relaxation time, and therefore cancers show up as hyperintense region relative to the surrounding tissue. The recommended image in-plane resolution is $\leq 2 \times 2$ mm with 3 mm slice thickness without any gaps between slices. Image slices from DCE-MRI should match those from diffusion-weighted images. Recommended temporal resolution is <15 s (<7 s is preferred) without any gaps and at least 2 min of acquisition time. In addition to qualitative analysis, semiquantitative (curve type, EMM) and quantitative analysis (Tofts pharmacokinetic model) can be used for PCa diagnosis. Prostate cancers are characterized by increased contrast transfer coefficient (K^{trans}), typically type 3 signal curve type with increased wash-in and washout rate compared to benign tissue. While some concerns and challenges exist with the use of DCE-MRI and gadolinium-based contrast agents, DCE-MRI remains an integral part of the clinical PCa management.

Disclosures Dr Aritrick Chatterjee, Dr Federico Pineda and Dr Gregory Karczmar have no disclosures.

Dr Aytekin Oto has the following disclosures. Research Grant, Koninklijke Philips NV Research Grant, Guerbet SA Research Grant, Profound Medical Inc. Medical Advisory Board, Profound Medical Inc Speaker, Bracco Group.

References

1. Siegel RL, Miller KD, Jemal A. Cancer statistics, 2019. CA Cancer J Clin. 2019;69(1):7–34.
2. Moldovan PC, Van den Broeck T, Sylvester R, Marconi L, Bellmunt J, van den Bergh RCN, et al. What is the negative predictive value of multiparametric magnetic resonance imaging in excluding prostate Cancer at biopsy? A systematic review and meta-analysis from the European Association of Urology prostate Cancer guidelines panel. Eur Urol. 2017;72(2):250–66.

3. Baur AD, Maxeiner A, Franiel T, Kilic E, Huppertz A, Schwenke C, et al. Evaluation of the prostate imaging reporting and data system for the detection of prostate cancer by the results of targeted biopsy of the prostate. Investig Radiol. 2014;49(6):411–20.
4. Weinreb JC, Barentsz JO, Choyke PL, Cornud F, Haider MA, Macura KJ, et al. PI-RADS prostate imaging – reporting and data system: 2015, version 2. Eur Urol. 2016;69(1):16–40.
5. Tofts PS, Brix G, Buckley DL, Evelhoch JL, Henderson E, Knopp MV, et al. Estimating kinetic parameters from dynamic contrast-enhanced t1-weighted MRI of a diffusable tracer: standardized quantities and symbols. J Magn Reson Imaging. 1999;10(3):223–32.
6. Fan X, Medved M, River JN, Zamora M, Corot C, Robert P, et al. New model for analysis of dynamic contrast-enhanced MRI data distinguishes metastatic from nonmetastatic transplanted rodent prostate tumors. Magn Reson Med. 2004;51(3):487–94.
7. Kayhan A, Fan X, Oto A. Dynamic contrast-enhanced magnetic resonance imaging in prostate cancer. Top Magn Reson Imaging. 2009;20(2):105–12.
8. Franiel T, Hamm B, Hricak H. Dynamic contrast-enhanced magnetic resonance imaging and pharmacokinetic models in prostate cancer. Eur Radiol. 2011;21(3):616–26.
9. Othman AE, Falkner F, Weiss J, Kruck S, Grimm R, Martirosian P, et al. Effect of temporal resolution on diagnostic performance of dynamic contrast-enhanced magnetic resonance imaging of the prostate. Investig Radiol. 2016;51(5):290–6.
10. de Rooij M, Hamoen EH, Fütterer JJ, Barentsz JO, Rovers MM. Accuracy of multiparametric MRI for prostate cancer detection: a meta-analysis. Am J Roentgenol. 2014;202(2):343–51.
11. Kozlowski P, Chang SD, Jones EC, Berean KW, Chen H, Goldenberg SL. Combined diffusion-weighted and dynamic contrast-enhanced MRI for prostate cancer diagnosis—correlation with biopsy and histopathology. J Magn Reson Imaging. 2006;24(1):108–13.
12. Hagberg GE, Scheffler K. Effect of r1 and r2 relaxivity of gadolinium-based contrast agents on the T1-weighted MR signal at increasing magnetic field strengths. Contrast Media Mol Imaging. 2013;8(6):456–65.
13. Chatterjee A, He D, Fan X, Wang S, Szasz T, Yousuf A, et al. Performance of ultrafast DCE-MRI for diagnosis of prostate cancer. Acad Radiol. 2018;25(3):349–58.
14. Gawlitza J, Reiss-Zimmermann M, Thörmer G, Schaudinn A, Linder N, Garnov N, et al. Impact of the use of an endorectal coil for 3 T prostate MRI on image quality and cancer detection rate. Sci Rep. 2017;7:40640.
15. Heijmink SWTPJ, Fütterer JJ, Hambrock T, Takahashi S, Scheenen TWJ, Huisman HJ, et al. Prostate cancer: body-array versus endorectal coil MR imaging at 3 T—comparison of image quality, localization, and staging performance. Radiology. 2007;244(1):184–95.
16. Turkbey B, Merino MJ, Gallardo EC, Shah V, Aras O, Bernardo M, et al. Comparison of endorectal coil and nonendorectal coil T2W and diffusion-weighted MRI at 3 Tesla for localizing prostate cancer: correlation with whole-mount histopathology. J Magn Reson Imaging. 2014;39(6):1443–8.
17. Chatterjee A, Devaraj A, Matthew M, Szasz T, Antic T, Karczmar G, et al. Performance of T2 maps in the detection of prostate cancer. Acad Radiol. 2019;26(1):15–21.
18. Kanda T, Ishii K, Kawaguchi H, Kitajima K, Takenaka D. High signal intensity in the dentate nucleus and Globus pallidus on unenhanced T1-weighted MR images: relationship with increasing cumulative dose of a gadolinium-based contrast material. Radiology. 2014;270(3):834–41.
19. McDonald JS, Hunt CH, Kolbe AB, Schmitz JJ, Hartman RP, Maddox DE, et al. Acute adverse events following Gadolinium-based contrast agent administration: a single-center retrospective study of 281 945 injections. Radiology. 2019;292(3):620–7.
20. Port RE, Knopp MV, Hoffmann U, Milker-Zabel S, Brix G. Multicompartment analysis of gadolinium chelate kinetics: blood-tissue exchange in mammary tumors as monitored by dynamic MR imaging. J Magn Reson Imaging. 1999;10(3):233–41.
21. Kety SS. The theory and applications of the exchange of inert gas at the lungs and tissues. Pharmacol Rev. 1951;3(1):1–41.
22. Yang C, Karczmar GS, Medved M, Stadler WM. Multiple reference tissue method for contrast agent arterial input function estimation. Magn Reson Med. 2007;58(6):1266–75.
23. Lavini C, Verhoeff JJC. Reproducibility of the gadolinium concentration measurements and of the fitting parameters of the vascular input function in the superior sagittal sinus in a patient population. Magn Reson Imaging. 2010;28(10):1420–30.
24. Fan X, Haney CR, Mustafi D, Yang C, Zamora M, Markiewicz EJ, et al. Use of a reference tissue and blood vessel to measure the arterial input function in DCEMRI. Magn Reson Med. 2010;64(6):1821–6.
25. Ocak I, Bernardo M, Metzger G, Barrett T, Pinto P, Albert PS, et al. Dynamic contrast-enhanced MRI of prostate cancer at 3 T: a study of pharmacokinetic parameters. Am J Roentgenol. 2007;189(4):W192–201.
26. Tamada T, Sone T, Jo Y, Yamamoto A, Yamashita T, Egashira N, et al. Prostate cancer: relationships between Postbiopsy hemorrhage and tumor detectability at MR diagnosis. Radiology. 2008;248(2):531–9.
27. Villers A, Puech P, Mouton D, Leroy X, Ballereau C, Lemaitre L. Dynamic contrast enhanced, pelvic phased array magnetic resonance imaging of localized prostate cancer for predicting tumor volume: correlation with radical prostatectomy findings. J Urol. 2006;176(6):2432–7.
28. Turkbey B, Pinto PA, Mani H, Bernardo M, Pang Y, McKinney YL, et al. Prostate cancer: value of multiparametric MR imaging at 3 T for detection—histopathologic correlation. Radiology. 2010;255(1):89–99.

29. Rosenkrantz AB, Sabach A, Babb JS, Matza BW, Taneja SS, Deng F-M. Prostate cancer: comparison of dynamic contrast-enhanced MRI techniques for localization of peripheral zone tumor. Am J Roentgenol. 2013;201(3):W471–W8.
30. Turkbey B, McKinney YL, Trivedi H, Chua C, Bratslavsky G, Shih JH, et al. Multiparametric 3T prostate magnetic resonance imaging to detect cancer: histopathological correlation using prostatectomy specimens processed in customized magnetic resonance imaging based molds. J Urol. 2011;186(5):1818–24.
31. Tan CH, Paul Hobbs B, Wei W, Kundra V. Dynamic contrast-enhanced MRI for the detection of prostate cancer: meta-analysis. Am J Roentgenol. 2015;204(4):W439–W48.
32. Isebaert S, Van den Bergh L, Haustermans K, Joniau S, Lerut E, De Wever L, et al. Multiparametric MRI for prostate cancer localization in correlation to whole-mount histopathology. J Magn Reson Imaging. 2013;37(6):1392–401.
33. Kim JK, Hong SS, Choi YJ, Park SH, Ahn H, Kim C-S, et al. Wash-in rate on the basis of dynamic contrast-enhanced MRI: usefulness for prostate cancer detection and localization. J Magn Reson Imaging. 2005;22(5):639–46.
34. Isebaert S, De Keyzer F, Haustermans K, Lerut E, Roskams T, Roebben I, et al. Evaluation of semi-quantitative dynamic contrast-enhanced MRI parameters for prostate cancer in correlation to whole-mount histopathology. Eur J Radiol. 2012;81(3):e217–e22.
35. Ren J, Huan Y, Wang H, Chang YJ, Zhao HT, Ge YL, et al. Dynamic contrast-enhanced MRI of benign prostatic hyperplasia and prostatic carcinoma: correlation with angiogenesis. Clin Radiol. 2008;63(2):153–9.
36. Hansford BG, Peng Y, Jiang Y, Vannier MW, Antic T, Thomas S, et al. Dynamic contrast-enhanced MR imaging curve-type analysis: is it helpful in the differentiation of prostate cancer from healthy peripheral zone? Radiology. 2015;275(2):448–57.
37. Tamada T, Sone T, Higashi H, Jo Y, Yamamoto A, Kanki A, et al. Prostate cancer detection in patients with Total serum prostate-specific antigen levels of 4–10 ng/mL: diagnostic efficacy of diffusion-weighted imaging, dynamic contrast-enhanced MRI, and T2-weighted imaging. Am J Roentgenol. 2011;197(3):664–70.
38. Bloch BN, Furman-Haran E, Helbich TH, Lenkinski RE, Degani H, Kratzik C, et al. Prostate cancer: accurate determination of extracapsular extension with high-spatial-resolution dynamic contrast-enhanced and T2-weighted MR imaging—initial results. Radiology. 2007;245(1):176–85.
39. Padhani AR, Gapinski CJ, Macvicar DA, Parker GJ, Suckling J, Revell PB, et al. Dynamic contrast enhanced MRI of prostate cancer: correlation with morphology and tumour stage, histological grade and PSA. Clin Radiol. 2000;55(2):99–109.
40. Schlemmer H-P, Merkle J, Grobholz R, Jaeger T, Michel MS, Werner A, et al. Can pre-operative contrast-enhanced dynamic MR imaging for prostate cancer predict microvessel density in prostatectomy specimens? Eur Radiol. 2004;14(2):309–17.
41. Franiel T, Lüdemann L, Taupitz M, Rost J, Asbach P, Beyersdorff D. Pharmacokinetic MRI of the prostate: parameters for differentiating low-grade and high-grade prostate cancer. Rofo. 2009;181(6):536–42.
42. Chen Y-J, Chu W-C, Pu Y-S, Chueh S-C, Shun C-T, Tseng W-YI. Washout gradient in dynamic contrast-enhanced MRI is associated with tumor aggressiveness of prostate cancer. J Magn Reson Imaging. 2012;36(4):912–9.
43. Vos EK, Litjens GJS, Kobus T, Hambrock T, Kaa CAH-VD, Barentsz JO, et al. Assessment of prostate cancer aggressiveness using dynamic contrast-enhanced magnetic resonance imaging at 3 T. Eur Urol. 2013;64(3):448–55.
44. Hötker AM, Mazaheri Y, Aras Ö, Zheng J, Moskowitz CS, Gondo T, et al. Assessment of prostate cancer aggressiveness by use of the combination of quantitative DWI and dynamic contrast-enhanced MRI. AJR Am J Roentgenol. 2016;206(4):756–63.
45. Low RN, Fuller DB, Muradyan N. Dynamic gadolinium-enhanced perfusion MRI of prostate cancer: assessment of response to hypofractionated robotic stereotactic body radiation therapy. Am J Roentgenol. 2011;197(4):907–15.
46. Oto A, Yang C, Kayhan A, Tretiakova M, Antic T, Schmid-Tannwald C, et al. Diffusion-weighted and dynamic contrast-enhanced MRI of prostate cancer: correlation of quantitative MR parameters with Gleason score and tumor angiogenesis. Am J Roentgenol. 2011;197(6):1382–90.
47. Chatterjee A, Gallan AJ, He D, Fan X, Mustafi D, Yousuf A, et al. Revisiting quantitative multi-parametric MRI of benign prostatic hyperplasia and its differentiation from transition zone cancer. Abdom Radiol. 2019;44(6):2233–43.
48. Turkbey B, Rosenkrantz AB, Haider MA, Padhani AR, Villeirs G, Macura KJ, et al. Prostate imaging reporting and data system version 2.1: 2019 update of prostate imaging reporting and data system version 2. Eur Urol. 2019;76(3):340–51.
49. Robert P, Frenzel T, Factor C, Jost G, Rasschaert M, Schuetz G, et al. Methodological aspects for preclinical evaluation of gadolinium presence in brain tissue: critical appraisal and suggestions for harmonization—a joint initiative. Investig Radiol. 2018;53(9):499–517.
50. He D, Chatterjee A, Fan X, Wang S, Eggener S, Yousuf A, et al. Feasibility of dynamic contrast-enhanced magnetic resonance imaging using low-dose gadolinium: comparative performance with standard dose in prostate cancer diagnosis. Investig Radiol. 2018;53(10):609–15.
51. Huang B, Liang CH, Liu HJ, Wang GY, Zhang SX. Low-dose contrast-enhanced magnetic resonance imaging of brain metastases at 3.0 T using high-relaxivity contrast agents. Acta Radiol. 2010;51(1):78–84.

52. Boehm-Sturm P, Haeckel A, Hauptmann R, Mueller S, Kuhl CK, Schellenberger EA. Low-molecular-weight Iron chelates may be an alternative to gadolinium-based contrast agents for T1-weighted contrast-enhanced MR imaging. Radiology. 2018;286(2):537–46.
53. Mustafi D, Ward J, Dougherty U, Bissonnette M, Hart J, Vogt S, et al. X-ray fluorescence microscopy demonstrates preferential accumulation of a vanadium-based magnetic resonance imaging contrast agent in murine colonic tumors. Mol Imaging. 2015;14:14.
54. Boesen L, Norgaard N, Logager V, Balslev I, Bisbjerg R, Thestrup KC, et al. Assessment of the diagnostic accuracy of Biparametric magnetic resonance imaging for prostate Cancer in biopsy-naive men: the Biparametric MRI for detection of prostate Cancer (BIDOC) study. JAMA Netw Open. 2018;1(2):e180219.
55. Jambor I, Bostrom PJ, Taimen P, Syvanen K, Kahkonen E, Kallajoki M, et al. Novel biparametric MRI and targeted biopsy improves risk stratification in men with a clinical suspicion of prostate cancer (IMPROD trial). J Magn Reson Imaging. 2017;46(4):1089–95.
56. Krishna S, McInnes M, Lim C, Lim R, Hakim SW, Flood TA, et al. Comparison of prostate imaging reporting and data system versions 1 and 2 for the detection of peripheral zone Gleason score 3 + 4 = 7 cancers. AJR Am J Roentgenol. 2017;209(6):W365–W73.

Interpretation of Multiparametric MRI Using PI-RADS (Prostate Imaging-Reporting and Data System)

7

Bryan R. Foster and Antonio C. Westphalen

7.1 Introduction

Multiparametric prostate magnetic resonance imaging (MRI) has undergone tremendous growth in less than a decade [1]. The impetus for growth is multifactorial but in part reflects great strides made in MRI standardization, image quality, cancer detection, and, importantly, recognition of the value-added outcomes of the exam by urologists. In its infancy prostate MRI consisted of non-standardized sequences, performed mostly in academic, high-volume centers. In time, however, after a significant amount of accumulated international experience, the need for standardization of reporting was recognized, which led to the publication of the first guidelines by the European Society of Urogenital Radiology. This expert-opinion, consensus document was published in 2012 and suggested minimum technical MRI parameters and the first scoring system (Prostate Imaging-Reporting and Data System, PI-RADS v1) for evaluating prostate cancer, modeled on the longstanding and successful breast counterpart, the BI-RADS system [2]. Recognizing the limitations of version 1 [3], specifically the cumbersome nature of the scoring system, the American College of Radiology, European Society of Urogenital Radiology, and the AdMeTech Foundation came together in 2015 to update PI-RADS to version 2 [4]. PI-RADS v2 was an important step forward as it simplified the overall scoring system, eliminated technically challenging spectroscopic imaging, simplified DCE assessment, and recognized that lesions in the peripheral zone and transition zone should be scored differently. More recently, in 2019, because of accumulated data and user experience with PI-RADS v2, a revision was undertaken, again using expert consensus. Because of a more limited scope of the revision it was called PI-RADS v2.1 [5].

PI-RADS has been rapidly adopted, and currently multiparametric MRI is performed in a fairly standardized fashion, not only at major centers but in smaller hospitals and outpatient imaging centers, reaching most of the radiology community. Herein we discuss a practical approach to PI-RADS v2.1, focusing on the important concepts, detailing the scoring system, and providing a framework to interpret multiparametric MRI.

B. R. Foster (✉)
Oregon Health & Science University, Department of Diagnostic Radiology, Portland, OR, USA
e-mail: fosterbr@ohsu.edu

A. C. Westphalen
University of California, San Francisco, Department of Radiology and Biomedical Imaging, and Urology, San Francisco, CA, USA
e-mail: antonio.westphalen@ucsf.edu

T. Tirkes (ed.), *Prostate MRI Essentials*, https://doi.org/10.1007/978-3-030-45935-2_7

7.2 General Concepts of PI-RADS

It is important to understand that PI-RADS v2.1 was designed to detect clinically significant prostate cancers, rather than to detect any and all cancer. There are many published definitions of clinically significant prostate cancer, one which is generally accepted in the clinical and research setting and was adopted by PI-RADS v2.1: Gleason score ≥7, and/or volume ≥0.5 mL, and/or extraprostatic extension [4]. The concept of clinical significance was developed to guide management. Patients with clinically significant cancer typically undergo therapy, such as prostatectomy or radiation therapy, whereas those without clinically significant cancer may be candidates for active surveillance.

PI-RADS recommends scoring up to 4 lesions; however, it is common to identify only 1 or 2 lesions. While prostate cancer is often multifocal, many small and low-grade tumors are often not identified with MRI, and the visible lesion with the highest PI-RADS score is typically the most clinically significant lesion, also characterized as the dominant tumor or index lesion.

The first step in the evaluation of any lesion is to determine from which anatomic portion of the prostate it arises. There are four main anatomic locations with the vast majority of cancers found in the peripheral zone and transition zone (Fig. 7.1).

1. Peripheral zone: gland rich portion lying posteriorly and laterally
2. Transition zone: mixture of glandular and stromal tissue that surrounds the urethra and invariably shows benign prostatic hyperplasia (BPH) in middle age to older men
3. Central zone: a small portion of glandular tissue at the prostate base surrounding the ejaculatory ducts
4. Anterior fibromuscular stroma: T2 dark band of fibrous tissue and muscle along the anterior portion of the gland generally abutting the transition zone

It is critical to accurately identify the anatomic location because lesions in the peripheral zone and transition zone are scored differently. This is known as the dominant sequence concept and was first introduced in PI-RADS v2 after accumulated research experience suggested that diffusion-weighted imaging (DWI) and dynamic contrast-enhanced (DCE) imaging did not add much accuracy to T2-weighted (T2W) imaging for cancer detection in the transition zone [6–9]. BPH nodules may show restricted diffusion and early enhancement patterns typical of prostate cancer. Thus, the evaluation of transition zone lesions is largely dependent on the morphologic assessment on T2W MRI. Conversely, detection of prostate cancer in the peripheral zone is much more accurate with DWI, as most benign peripheral zone lesions do not show marked restricted diffusion. T2W imaging alone in the peripheral zone has poor specificity because many benign lesions such as fibrosis and prostatitis show decreased signal similar to cancer. Therefore, DWI is dominant in the peripheral zone for cancer detection, and this is reflected in the overall PI-RADS assessment.

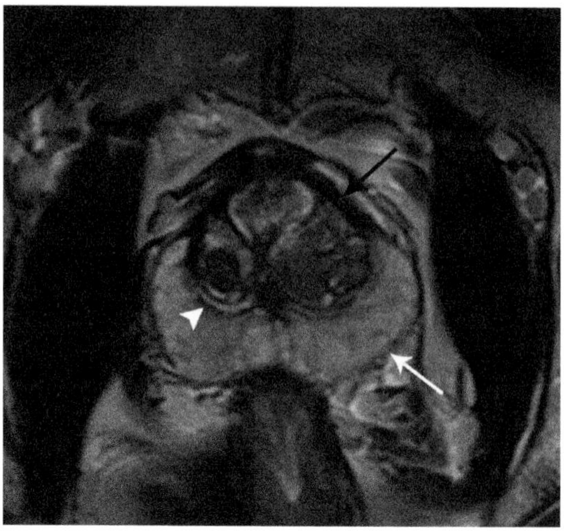

Fig. 7.1 Normal zonal anatomy. Axial T2W image shows the normal high T2 signal intensity of the peripheral zone (white arrow), the heterogenous and nodular transition zone secondary to BPH (arrowhead), and the anterior fibromuscular stroma (black arrow)

The dominant sequence concept implemented in PI-RADS v2 has been evaluated in at least one large study of 654 lesions which found that in the peripheral zone the concept is valid; DWI outperformed T2W imaging in cancer detection.

However in the transition zone, while there was a trend toward T2W MRI outperforming DWI, this was not statistically significant [10]. Subsequent changes made in PI-RADS v2.1 attempt to address these shortcomings, as DWI has a larger role in determining the score of lesions seen in the transition zone [5].

Accurate localization of lesions is important. For example, targeted biopsy is now one of the main indications for MRI, and in many instances the correlation between MRI and transrectal ultrasound (TRUS) findings is done cognitively. At a minimum, lesions should be assigned to 1 or more sextants, by reporting laterality and craniocaudal location (apex, mid or base). However, PI-RADS suggests a more specific mapping of lesions into 38 different sectors which may improve communication with treating physicians prior to biopsy or therapy, improve radiologic-pathologic correlation, and promote research [5]. Notably, it is common that a lesion extends to involve two or more adjacent sectors.

7.3 Overall Assessment

PI-RADS assessment categories are stratified into five likelihoods of malignancy as follows:

7.3.1 PI-RADS v2.1 Assessment Categories

- PI-RADS 1 – Very low (clinically significant cancer is highly unlikely to be present)
- PI-RADS 2 – Low (clinically significant cancer is unlikely to be present)
- PI-RADS 3 – Intermediate (the presence of clinically significant cancer is equivocal)
- PI-RADS 4 – High (clinically significant cancer is likely to be present)
- PI-RADS 5 – Very high (clinically significant cancer is highly likely to be present)

The final PI-RADS category is determined by assessing the T2W imaging, DWI, and DCE imaging scores, starting with the dominant sequence for the zone of the lesion (Table 7.1). A maximum of 2 scores is used to arrive at the final score, though in many cases only one category contributes to the final score. Notably, PI-RADS does not take into account clinical factors or laboratory values, such as prostate-specific antigen (PSA), to assign a score; it is purely an imaging-based scoring system. At this time, unlike BI-RADS, there are no standardized percentages of cancer expected for each category, although many publications have looked at the positivity rate for each category (described below). In the future, with additional research, this may be incorporated into PI-RADS and could be used as a quality control measure, similar to BI-RADS.

Table 7.1 Overall assessment

Peripheral zone			Transition zone	
DWI	DCE	**PI-RADS**	DWI	T2W
1	Any	**1**	Any	1
2	Any	**2**	≤3	2
3	–	**3**	≥4	
			≤4	3
	+	**4**	5	
4	Any		Any	4
5	Any	**5**	Any	5

Note: Table reads from left to middle for peripheral zone and right to middle for transition zone

Adapted from [4, 5, 11]. Reprint of tables from PI-RADS v 2.1. Overall assessment from Section III; https://www.acr.org/-/media/ACR/Files/RADS/Pi-RADS/PIRADS-V2-1.pdf?la=en, with permission from the American College of Radiology [11]

7.4 T2W Assessment

7.4.1 Peripheral Zone

Because of the dominant sequence paradigm, the T2W score in the peripheral zone typically does not determine the overall score unless there is extraprostatic extension (EPE), which is generally best detected on T2W images. As mentioned above, T2W is not the dominant sequence in the peripheral zone because cancers and benign lesions have significant overlap in morphology and signal. However, in general, clinically significant cancers show round or oval morphology

Table 7.2 PI-RADS assessment of T2W [4, 5, 11]

Score	Peripheral zone
1	Uniform hyperintense signal intensity (normal)
2	Linear- or wedge-shaped hypointensity or diffuse mild hypointensity, usually indistinct margin
3	Heterogeneous signal intensity or non-circumscribed, rounded, moderate hypointensity Includes others that do not qualify as 2, 4, or 5
4	Circumscribed, homogenous moderate hypointense focus/mass confined to prostate and <1.5 cm in greatest dimension
5	Same as 4 but ≥1.5 cm in greatest dimension or definite extraprostatic extension/invasive behavior
Score	Transition zone
1	Normal appearing transition zone (rare) or a round, completely encapsulated nodule ("typical nodule")
2	A mostly encapsulated nodule OR a homogeneous circumscribed nodule without encapsulation. ("atypical nodule") OR a homogeneous mildly hypointense area between nodules
3	Heterogeneous signal intensity with obscured margins Includes others that do not qualify as 2, 4, or 5
4	Lenticular or non-circumscribed, homogeneous, moderately hypointense, and <1.5 cm in greatest dimension
5	Same as 4 but ≥1.5 cm in greatest dimension or definite extraprostatic extension/invasive behavior

Reprint of tables from PI-RADS v 2.1 PIRADS assessment for T2W from Section IV, A, #2; https://www.acr.org/-/media/ACR/Files/RADS/Pi-RADS/PIRADS-V2-1.pdf?la=en, with permission from the American College of Radiology [11]

with moderate decreased signal on T2W images and are scored 4 or 5 based on a size cutoff of 1.5 cm (Table 7.2). Benign lesions in the peripheral zone (score 2), on the other hand, generally show vague borders, mild hypointensity, and linear- or wedge-shaped morphology. Another commonly encountered T2W score 2 lesion is diffuse mild hypointensity which is often due to fibrosis or chronic prostatitis, though importantly these lesions show normal DWI or only mild low ADC distinguishing them from a diffuse cancer (Fig. 7.2).

7.4.2 Transition Zone

T2W MRI assessment of the transition zone is perhaps the most challenging part of the PI-RADS scoring due to difficulty in detecting and characterizing malignancy among the inherently heterogeneous and nodular background of BPH. Because of this, multiparametric MRI is less accurate in detecting and characterizing clinically significant prostate cancer in the transition zone compared to the peripheral zone [12]. In the most recent update of PI-RADS to v2.1, the description of the T2W imaging scores in the transition zone has undergone significant reworking and clarification in an attempt to address these difficulties [5].

T2W images remain the dominant sequence for scoring transition zone lesions, and therefore the final PI-RADS score is heavily dependent on the T2W imaging score (Table 7.1). T2W imaging dominates in the transition zone because DWI and DCE features that mimic cancer may be seen in benign BPH nodules. Therefore, T2W imaging morphology of transition zone lesions usually determines the final PI-RADS score. However, this is not to say, that DWI is unimportant in the transition zone as clinically significant cancers often show restricted diffusion similar to cancer in the peripheral zone. Thus, in an attempt to improve accuracy, PI-RADS v2.1 incorporates the DWI score when lesions are assigned a T2W imaging score 2 or 3.

Another important update in PI-RADS v2.1 for the transition zone is guidance on what, if anything, to score in the transition zone, as it is impractical and unnecessary to evaluate and score every nodular area. Only focal lesions in the transition zone that stand out from the background on T2W imaging or DWI need be scored. For instance, on T2W MRI a lesion that is different from the background in shape, low signal, or obscured margins should be scored regardless of DWI appearance. Likewise, a lesion or area that shows features of malignancy (restricted diffusion) on DWI and on the apparent diffusion coefficient (ADC) map should be scored if it stands out from the background appearance of the tran-

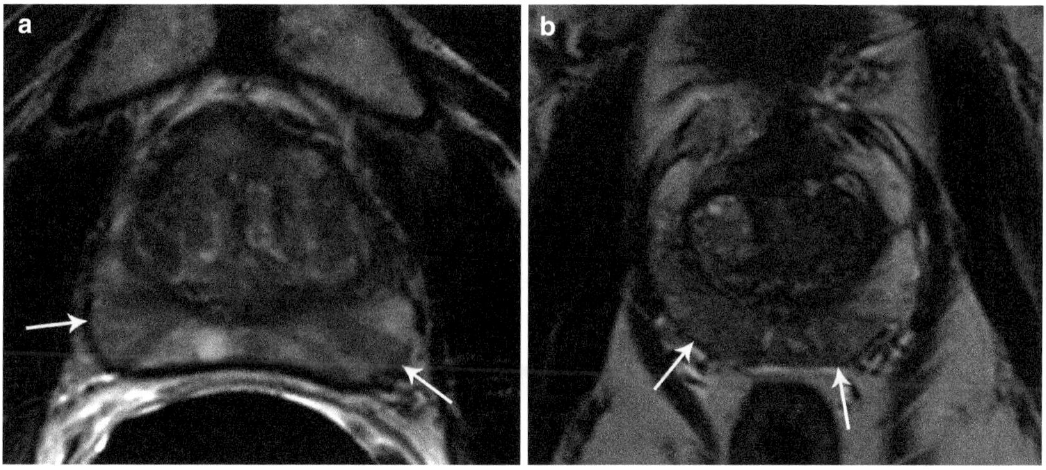

Fig. 7.2 Peripheral zone T2W score 2 lesions. (**a**) Axial T2W image shows linear- and triangular-shaped, streaky areas of low T2 signal intensity (arrows) in the peripheral zone bilaterally in a patient with a history of prostatitis. (**b**) Axial T2W shows diffuse mild low signal throughout the peripheral zone (arrows), in a different patient, without a corresponding abnormality on DWI/ADC (not shown)

sition zone (Fig. 7.3). For instance, a nodule should be scored if it shows moderately high DWI signal and low ADC signal, whereas the background transition zone shows scattered areas of mild high DWI and mild low ADC signal intensities. In contrast, however, if the transition zone shows multiple foci of restricted diffusion, this is considered to be a variant of BPH, and it is not to be scored. As a practicality, one approach for lesion detection at the workstation is to simultaneously assess the DWI and ADC maps along with T2W MRI, looking for areas that stand out and are significantly different from the background BPH.

The T2W MRI assessment for the transition zone is shown in Table 7.2. The following tips and caveats are provided for guidance:

- *Score 1* – Typical BPH nodules appear as round completely encapsulated nodules and often are very heterogeneous with areas of low T2W signal, representing stroma, interspersed with areas of high or very high signal, representing glandular tissue (Fig. 7.3). The capsule should entirely surround the nodule in at least two imaging planes, otherwise it is a score 2. Typical BPH nodules do not need to be assigned a PI-RADS score, though if assigned are considered T2W score 1.
- *Score 2* – Lesions in this category are atypical nodules and are not fully encapsulated or lack a capsule entirely. These lesions may be heterogenous with foci of high T2W signal intensity or may have a homogenously low T2W signal (Fig. 7.4). Importantly, these lesions are distinguished from score 4/5 lesions by circumscribed margins. A homogenous area of low T2W signal intensity between nodules is also considered a T2W score 2.
- *Score 3* – These lesions do not nicely fit into other categories. The term obscured margins is used to describe these lesions which in practicality is similar to non-circumscribed. One distinguishing factor from score 4/5 lesions is that score 3 lesions should be heterogenous, and generally lack a lenticular shape (Fig. 7.5).
- *Score 4/5* – On T2W, score 4 or 5 transition zone lesions are homogenous, have moderately low signal intensity and are lenticular-shaped or non-circumscribed lesions (Fig. 7.6). These lesions are stratified into T2W scores of 4 or 5 depending on a size cut-off of 1.5 cm or the presence of extraprostatic extension (EPE). The "erased charcoal sign" refers to smudging of a charcoal drawing using a finger and is a helpful reminder that the margins of 4/5 lesions are non-circum-

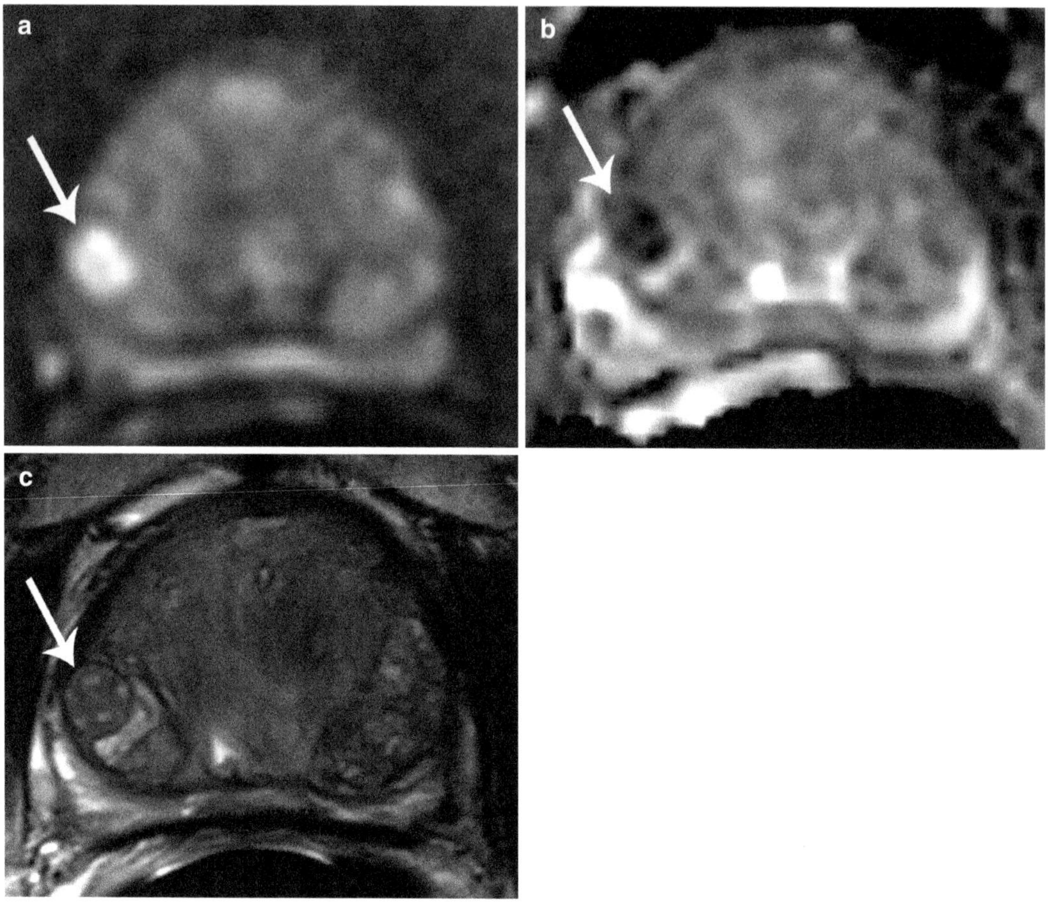

Fig. 7.3 Transition zone T2 score 1 lesion. (**a**) DWI and (**b**) ADC images show a lesion with markedly high and markedly low signal intensity, respectively (arrows). (**c**) The T2W image, though, shows a heterogenous round nodule with a complete capsule (arrow) or a "typical" BPH nodule

scribed or blurred, unlike score 1 and 2 lesions. Though score 4/5 lesions may be found anywhere in the transition zone they are classically found anteriorly abutting the anterior fibromuscular stroma and capsule.

7.5 DWI/ADC Assessment

Most malignancies show restricted diffusion that is thought to be due to increased cell density, disorganized cell arrangement, and/or an abnormal extracellular space [13]. Restricted diffusion is defined as an increase in DWI signal and corresponding decrease in ADC signal on ADC maps, which are generated by software using two or more acquired b-values. In addition to a qualitative assessment, ADC maps allow the user to measure ADC values, which is a measure of diffusion restriction. In fact, ADC values of prostate adenocarcinoma show an inverse correlation with Gleason score. As a rule of thumb, ADC values less than 750–900 $\mu m^2/s$ differentiate malignancy from benign lesions in the peripheral zone. Further, studies suggest ADC values may be used to better characterize lesions assigned a PI-RADS score 4 [14, 15]. Lesions with ADC values at or below the threshold mentioned earlier are as likely as PI-RADS score 5 lesions to represent clinically significant cancer. However, ADC values are not incorporated into PI-RADS scoring as there is significant overlap between individual Gleason scores, benign BPH nodules, as well as lack of a

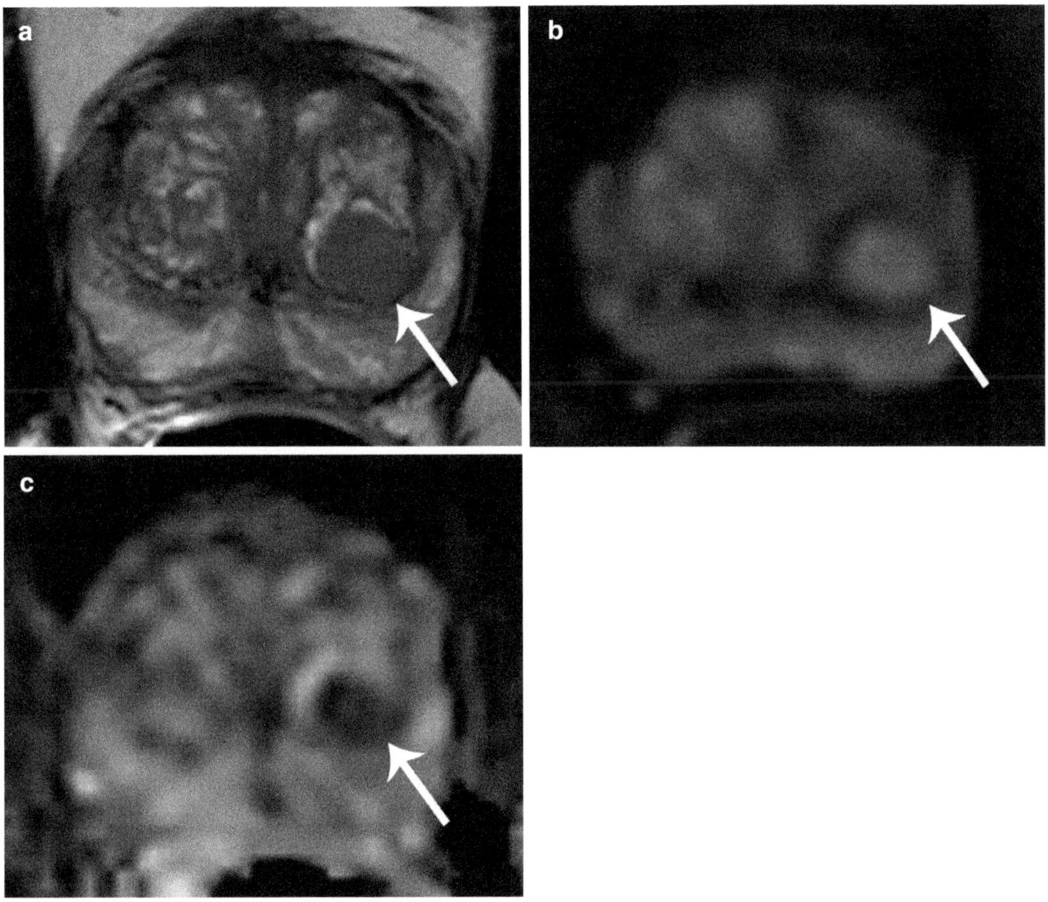

Fig. 7.4 Transition zone T2 score 2 lesion. (**a**) Axial T2W image shows a mostly encapsulated nodule (arrow), while (**b**) DWI shows no increased signal in the nodule (arrow), and (**c**) ADC shows low signal intensity (arrow)

standardized imaging protocol across different MRI scanner models and vendors [4, 16, 17].

Therefore, for PI-RADS DWI scoring, the evaluation remains subjective and based on relative visual intensities. The reference intensity for DWI or ADC is the background prostate gland in the same zone as the lesion [5]. Notably this reference is imperfect as various benign processes can alter the background. Another pitfall in interpretation is failing to adjust the window and level of DWI and ADC images appropriately. The images sent directly from the scanner are not necessarily set at an ideal window and level for interpretation of DWI/ADC (unlike T2W), and, therefore, the radiologist should always optimize the image contrast [18].

The DWI assessment scores are shown in Table 7.3. Importantly, there is no differentiation of scoring by zonal anatomy; the peripheral zone and transition zone are both scored with the same criteria. A DWI score 1 is normal and shows no signal abnormality different than background (Fig. 7.7). PI-RADS v2.1 made minor updates and clarifications to the scoring of DWI 2 and 3 lesions. Score 2 lesions are linear-/wedge-shaped areas of high signal on DWI and/or low signal on ADC. These abnormalities are generally seen in the peripheral zone and represent benign prostatitis or fibrosis. Note, though, that the shape of these lesions is better assessed on T2W images. Score 3 lesions are focal and have low signal on ADC and/or high signal on high b-value

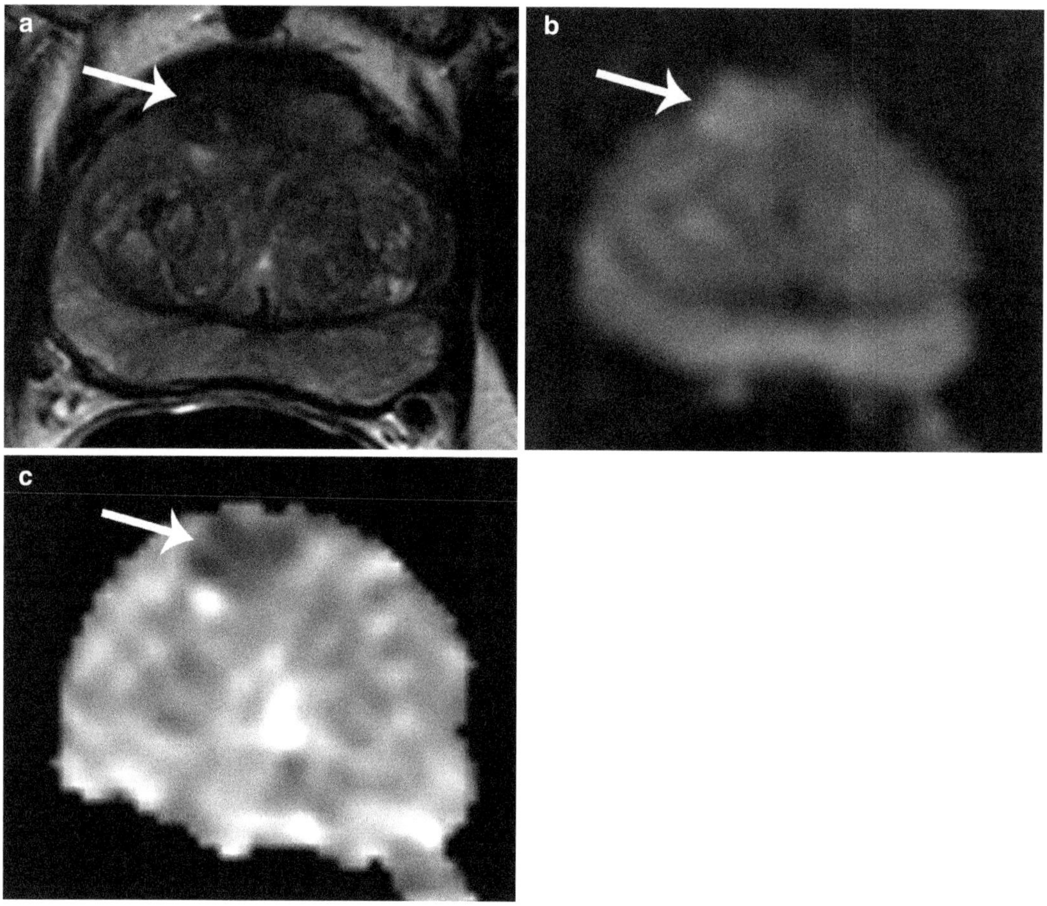

Fig. 7.5 Transition zone T2 score 3 lesion. (**a**) Axial T2W image shows an anterior heterogenous lesion of low signal and obscured margins, consistent with a score 3 (arrow). (**b**) However, DWI and (**c**) ADC show mildly high and (**c**) mildly low signal intensity (arrows). Therefore the overall PI-RADS score is not upgraded and remains 3

DWI. Yet, the lesion should not demonstrate marked abnormality on both sequences; if one sequence shows marked signal abnormality, the other must show mild signal changes. This is in contradistinction to DWI score 4 and 5 lesions which is characterized by both marked high signal intensity on high b-value DWI *and* marked low signal intensity on ADC. The difference between score 4 and 5 lesions is a size cutoff of 1.5 cm or presence of EPE, which is typically assessed on the T2W images.

DWI is the dominant sequence in the peripheral zone, and, therefore, the overall PI-RADS score often equals the DWI score. If the DWI score is 3, then the DCE is used as a tiebreaker. If the lesion is considered to be DCE positive, then the final score is upgraded to an overall score of PI-RADS 4 (Fig. 7.8). On the other hand, DCE negative lesions remain PI-RADS 3 (Table 7.1).

Benign BPH nodules may show restricted diffusion; therefore, DWI has a secondary role in scoring the transition zone. In PI-RADS v2.1, though, this role has increased. A transition zone lesion that is assigned a T2W score 2 is upgraded to an overall PI-RADS 3 lesion if it displays DWI scores of 4 or 5, i.e., if it demonstrates marked restricted diffusion. Similarly, if a T2W score 3 lesion displays DWI score of 5, it is upgraded to an overall PI-RADS 4 (Table 7.1).

7.6 DCE Assessment

Dynamic contrast enhancement is only utilized in the assessment of peripheral zone lesions and is relegated to a secondary role to DWI. It is used as a tiebreaker for DWI score 3 lesions, but it has no role in determining the score of lesions assigned other DWI scores (Table 7.1, Fig. 7.8).

Unlike T2W and DWI scores, the assessment of DCE is not numerical, rather it is classified as "positive" or "negative" (Table 7.4). A classification of "positive" is assigned when there is focal enhancement which is early than or at the same time as adjacent normal prostatic tissues, and, importantly, corresponds to a suspicious finding on T2W MRI and/or DWI (Fig. 7.8). A "negative" status is assigned in the absence of early or simultaneous enhancement. DCE is also considered to be negative when there is diffuse enhancement that does not correspond to a focal lesion on

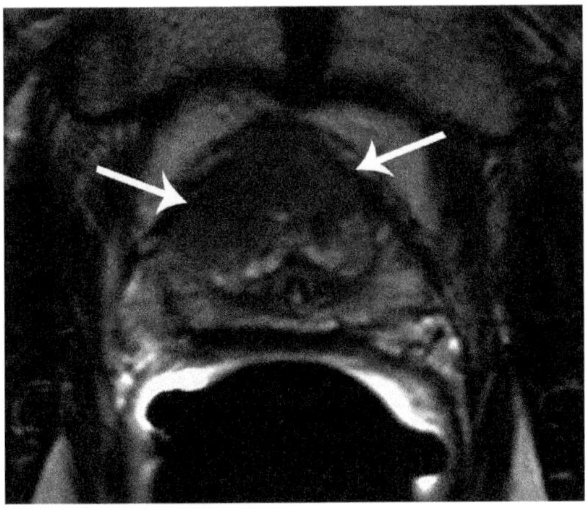

Fig. 7.6 Transition zone T2 score 5 lesion. Axial T2W image shows an anterior lesion that is non-circumscribed, demonstrates homogenous low signal intensity, (arrows) and measures more than 1.5 cm

Table 7.3 PI-RADS assessment of DWI [4, 5, 11]

Score	Peripheral zone or transition zone
1	Normal or no signal abnormality different than background
2	Linear-/wedge-shaped hypointense on ADC and/or linear-/wedge-shaped hyperintense on high b-value DWI
3	Focal (discrete and different from the background) hypointense on ADC and/or focal hyperintense on high b-value DWI. May be markedly hypointense on ADC or markedly hyperintense on high b-value DWI, but not both
4	Focal markedly hypointense on ADC and markedly hyperintense on high b-value DWI; <1.5 cm in greatest dimension
5	Same as 4 but ≥1.5 cm in greatest dimension or definite extraprostatic extension/invasive behavior

Reprint of table from PI-RADS v 2.1 PI-RADS assessment of DWI from Section IV, B, #2; https://www.acr.org/-/media/ACR/Files/RADS/Pi-RADS/PIRADS-V2-1.pdf?la=en, with permission from the American College of Radiology [11]

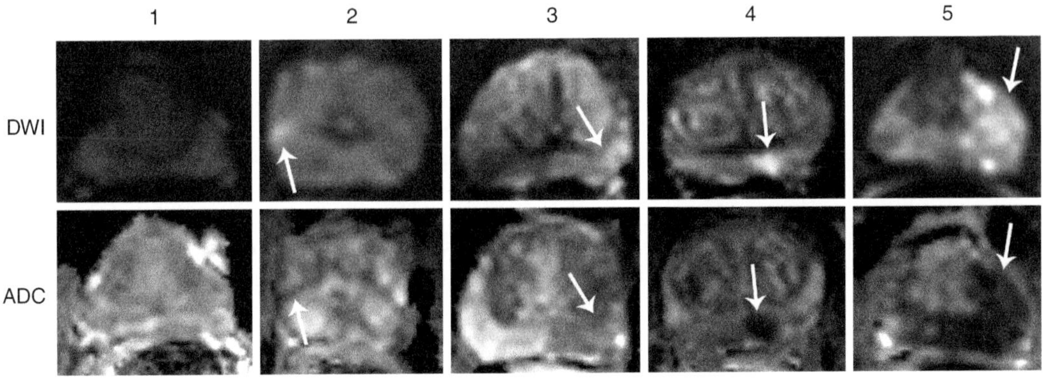

Fig. 7.7 Photomontage of DWI scores in the peripheral zone. DWI score 1 = no abnormalities identified. DWI score 2 = streaky areas of mild signal abnormality (arrow). DWI score 3 = focal mildly high signal intensity on DWI and mildly low signal intensity on ADC (arrow). DWI score 4 = focal markedly high signal intensity on DWI and markedly low signal intensity on ADC with diameter <1.5 cm (arrow). DWI score 5 = same as score 4 but with a diameter ≥1.5 cm

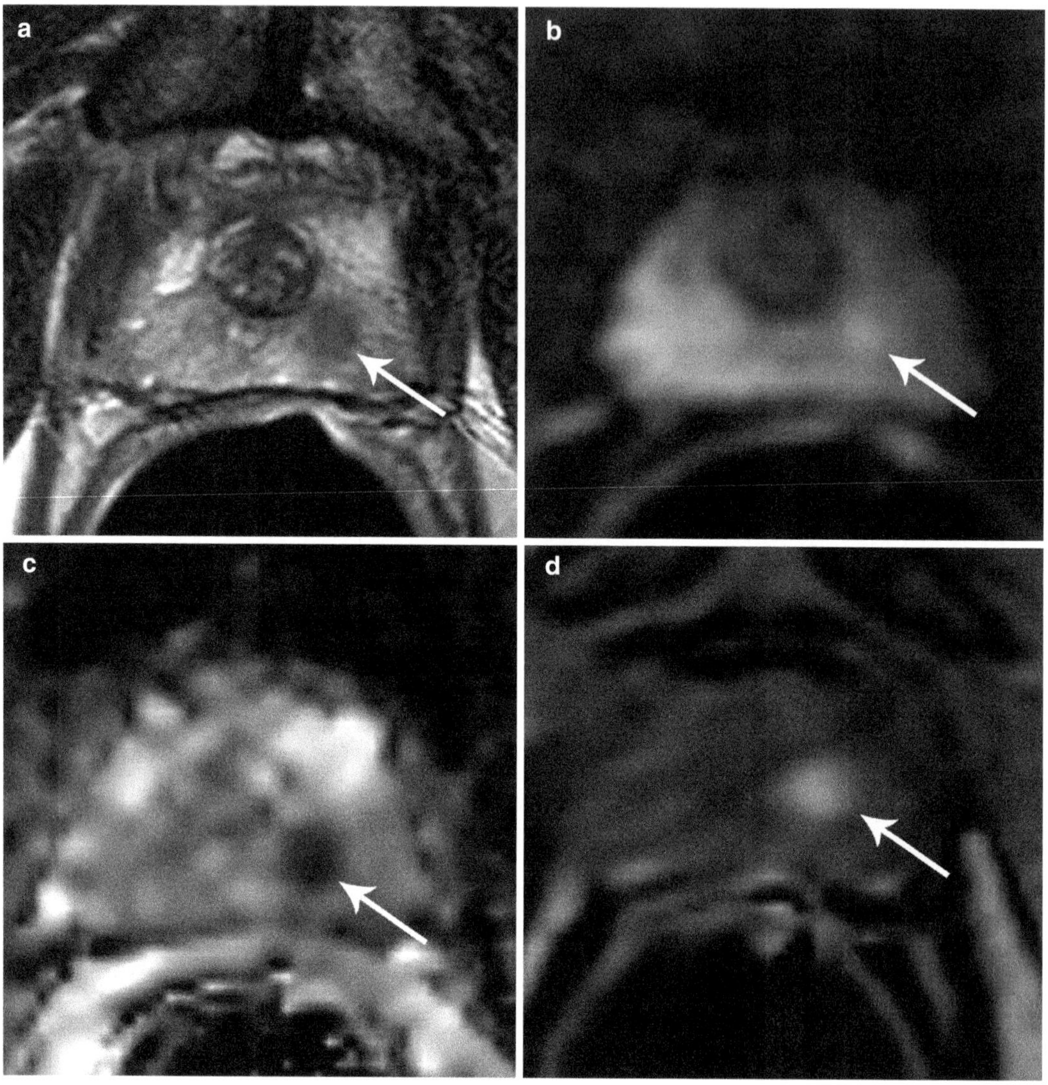

Fig. 7.8 Peripheral zone DWI score 3. (**a**) Axial T2W image shows a round nodule in the left apex peripheral zone (arrow). (**b**) Axial DWI shows focal mildly high signal intensity (arrow) while (**c**) ADC shows markedly low signal intensity (arrow), consistent with a DWI score of 3. (**d**) DCE shows avid focal enhancement earlier than other prostatic tissue (arrow). The overall PI-RADS score is, therefore, upgraded to 4

T2W MRI or DWI. Diffuse enhancement in the peripheral zone is commonly seen and is thought to be due to prostatitis. This should not be mistaken for cancer and generally lacks a correlate on DWI and shows typical linear-, wedge-shaped, or diffuse mild decreased signal without a circumscribed focus of moderate low signal on T2W MRI.

In the transition zone, DCE is not used as part of the overall assessment because BPH nodules can show a similar pattern of early enhancement and washout. Cancers in the transition zone will generally show rapid, strong enhancement and washout, with peak enhancement occurring slightly earlier than BPH nodules. This feature, while not used in the overall assessment, can be helpful to confirm a lesion is malignant.

Although DCE is relegated to a tiebreaker status in the overall assessment for PI-RADS score,

Table 7.4 PI-RADS assessment of DCE [4, 5, 11]

Score	Peripheral zone or transition zone
+	Focal; earlier than or contemporaneously with enhancement of adjacent normal prostatic tissues; and corresponds to suspicious finding on T2W and/or DWI
–	No early or contemporaneous enhancement; or diffuse multifocal enhancement NOT corresponding to a focal finding on T2W and/or DWI; or focal enhancement corresponding to a lesion demonstrating features of BPH on T2WI (including features of extruded BPH in the peripheral zone)

Reprint of tables from PI-RADS v 2.1 PI-RADS assessment for DCE from Section IV, C, #2; https://www.acr.org/-/media/ACR/Files/RADS/Pi-RADS/PIRADS-V2-1.pdf?la=en, with permission from the American College of Radiology [11]

it should be noted that some radiologists find it useful to detect small lesions that are initially missed on evaluation of T2W images and DWI [10, 19]. Careful evaluation and cross-referencing of areas of early, strong enhancement to T2W and DWI images may help the radiologist detect, but not necessarily score, a lesion that was overlooked.

In order to use DCE as a detection tool, the spatial resolution must be reasonably high so that small focal lesions can be seen as discrete areas of enhancement. The trade-off between increasing the spatial resolution is typically a decrease in the temporal resolution. The newest PI-RADS v2.1 guidelines allow for lengthening the temporal resolution to a maximum of 15 s which can allow optimization of the spatial resolution [5].

While there are a variety of ways to view and post-process a DCE dataset, one of the easiest methods of viewing is to scroll through the raw images on PACS. In our experience, cinematically displaying all time points for a given slice location allows for best assessment of the perfusion of the gland and therefore detection of lesions. Various parametric maps and enhancement curves can be generated on independent workstations, and some radiologists prefer to use these methods to detect focal lesions. These tools are not incorporated into PI-RADS, and there are no standardized viewing parameters.

Although not specified in PI-RADS, washout can be a sign of malignancy. Washout is seen as a rapid de-enhancement of a hypervascular focus corresponding to a focal lesion on T2W MRI or DWI. Benign findings can also exhibit washout, such as BPH nodules and prostatitis; however, when seen in conjunction with other PI-RADS score 4 and 5 characteristics, it can lend confidence to the interpreting radiologist. Lastly, initial data on large tumors suggest that men with hypoenhancing tumors may have worse prognosis and develop metastases or die of prostate cancer at an earlier time point than men whose tumors are not hypoenhancing [14].

7.7 Extraprostatic Extension

MRI is reasonably accurate to locally stage prostate cancer. A detailed discussion of prostate cancer staging can be found in Chap. 8 of this book. A cancer confined to the prostate gland is assigned a stage T2 accordingly to the TNM classification. Extraprostatic extension of cancer is classified as stage T3 and generally indicates a worse prognosis compared to organ-confined T2 disease. In fact, in one study, men with obvious extraprostatic extension on MRI had a worse prognosis than D'Amico risk classification matched controls [20]. Extraprostatic extension is defined as tumor invading locally beyond the prostate and may be extracapsular extension of tumor (T3a) or seminal vesicle invasion (T3b). Because an invasive lesion is highly likely to be clinically significant prostate cancer, detection of this feature is scored 5 in both T2W and DWI assessments, irrespective of the lesion size (though these cancers are typically over 1.5 cm).

7.8 Assessment with Inadequate Imaging

PI-RADS v2.1 [5] gives guidance on how to score lesions when image quality is degraded or omitted. This should be rare, as the majority of patients complete the exam with good image quality. Perhaps the most frequently encountered scenario is inadequate DWI imaging due to image distortion from unilateral or bilateral metallic hip prosthesis. In this scenario, the overall score for both the peripheral zone and transition zone is based primarily on the T2W score except for T2W score 3 lesions which are elevated to an overall score of PI-RADS 4 when the DCE score is positive. In a small number of cases, the DCE sequence may be inadequate or unavailable for scoring, because of history of allergy, IV infiltration, or severe image artifact. Yet, concerns about the deposition of gadolinium in various tissues have led to increasing support for abbreviated imaging protocols and, consequently, to a larger number of patients who decline to receive or cannot receive contrast due to poor renal function. In these cases the overall score in the peripheral zone is determined by the DWI score alone. In the transition zone, the scoring approach remains the same as DCE does not play a role in the overall assessment.

7.9 Special Considerations

Several normal anatomic structures and benign lesions may show focal markedly low signal on the ADC map and mimic cancer at first glance. For instance, the anatomic central zone, anterior fibromuscular stroma and gland calcifications generally show low ADC signal because of lack of intrinsic T2 signal. However, on high b-value DWI, the signal intensity of these structures is lower, the same, or only slightly higher than the signal intensity of the gland background. Furthermore, correlation with T2W images will usually show a typical appearance and low signal.

One of the most common pitfalls to the inexperienced reader is the central zone, which is often characterized as a PI-RADS 4 or 5 lesion because of its appearance on the ADC map. The normal central zone is an oval or dumbbell-shaped area that has low T2 signal and surrounds the ejaculatory ducts where they insert at the base of the prostate. As mentioned before, on DWI it generally demonstrates a signal intensity that is equal to or slightly higher than the gland background. On DCE, it lacks early enhancement, presumably because of its high stromal content (Fig. 7.9). Central zone cancers, on the other hand, are rare, show similar features to cancers elsewhere, e.g., marked restricted diffusion, and are more likely to present as locally advanced disease at diagnosis [18, 21].

Another important pitfall is the exophytic BPH nodule, which protrude into the peripheral zone from the transition zone (Fig. 7.10). These nodules abut the prostatic surgical pseudocapsule (the thin T2 dark line between the peripheral zone and transition zone), a feature that can sometimes be used to make the correct diagnosis. Similar to other BPH nodules, exophytic ones may demonstrate markedly low signal on the ADC map and high signal on DWI and at first glance appear to represent a PI-RADS 4 or 5 lesion in the peripheral zone. Evaluation of the T2W images, though, may show that the lesion is encapsulated and heterogeneous, like typical BPH nodules elsewhere, allowing for accurate diagnosis. Accordingly, if a PI-RADS score is deemed necessary, these BPH nodules should be classified as transition zone lesions [18].

Detailed discussion of pitfalls in prostate imaging and interpretation can be found in Chap. 14 of this book.

7.10 Diagnostic Accuracy

PI-RADS v2.1 [5] made minor changes to the scoring schema in 2019. Thus, at the time of this writing there is no published data on the performance of v2.1 compared to v2. However, much work has been done to validate PI-RADS v2 since it was published in 2015. Pooled data from several studies shows good performance with a sensitivity of 89% and a specificity of 73% for clinically significant cancer detection using PI-RADS v2. Head-to-head studies comparing PI-RADS v2 to v1 have also shown a statistically significant improvement in sensitivity [22].

Several studies have been published evaluating the clinically significant cancer detection rate per PI-RADS category using targeted biopsy or

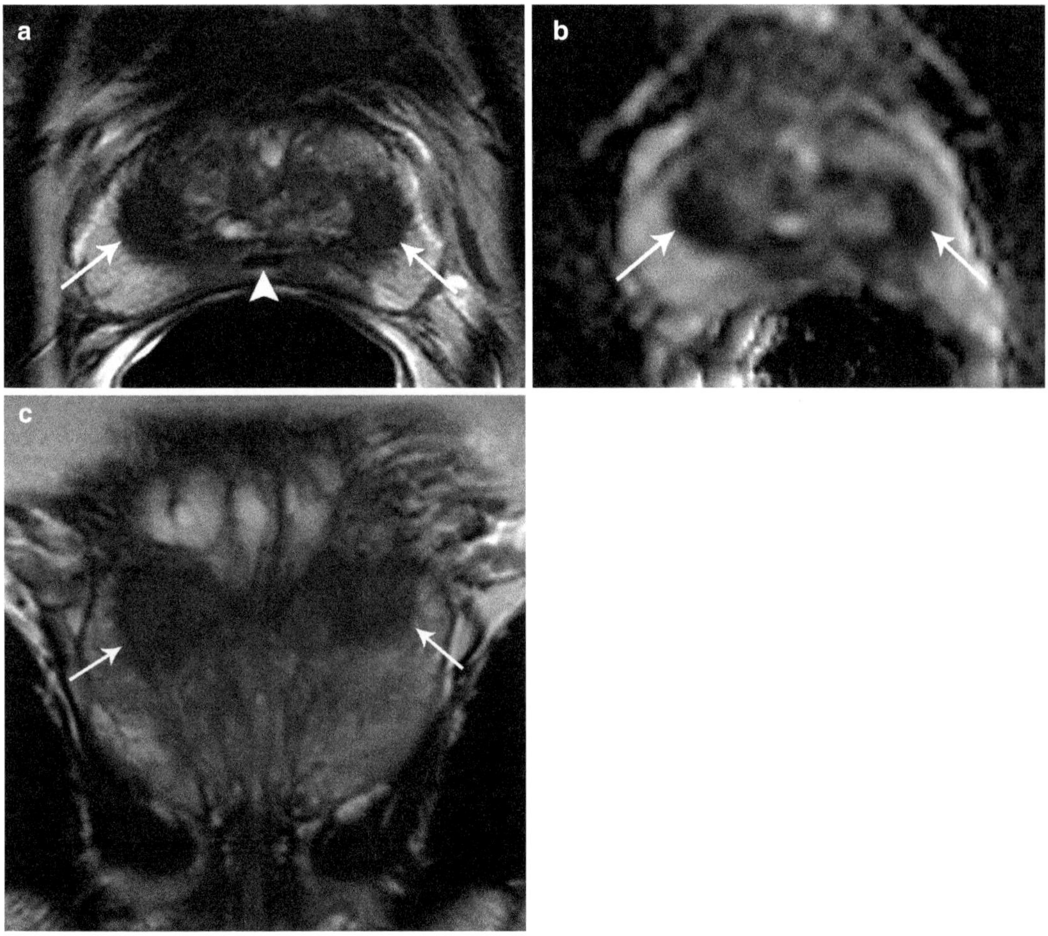

Fig. 7.9 Normal central zone. (**a**) Axial T2W image shows symmetric rounded areas of low signal intensity (arrows) at the base of the prostate on either side of the paired ejaculatory ducts (arrowhead). (**b**) ADC map at the same level shows markedly low signal intensity of the central zone (arrows). DWI images (not shown) showed only slightly increased signal. (**c**) Coronal T2W images show typical dumbbell-shaped appearance of the central zone (arrows)

prostatectomy specimens as the reference standard. The range of cancer detection in these studies was 0–16%, 10–33%, 12–33%, 22–71%, and 67–91% in PI-RADS categories 1, 2, 3, 4, and 5, respectively [10, 23, 24]. The pooled estimates of a recent meta-analysis published by Barkovich et al. found that lesions classified as PI-RADS 1 or 2, 3, 4, and 5 represented high-grade disease in approximately 6%, 12%, 48%, and 72% of patients [25].

Studies evaluating interobserver variability of PI-RADS scoring generally show moderate to substantial agreement for the overall score and scores assigned to lesions seen in the peripheral zone, but only fair agreement when a lesion is located in the transition zone [26–28]. For instance, one study found that the specific transition zone descriptor of a "circumscribed nodule" (T2W MRI score 2) vs. "obscured margins" (T2W MRI score 3) showed a poor Kappa statistic of 0.267 [26]. This reflects the difficult and subjective nature of the scoring in the transition zone.

Missed cancers seem to be common on a per lesion basis when analysis is performed using whole mount histology or combined MRI-guided

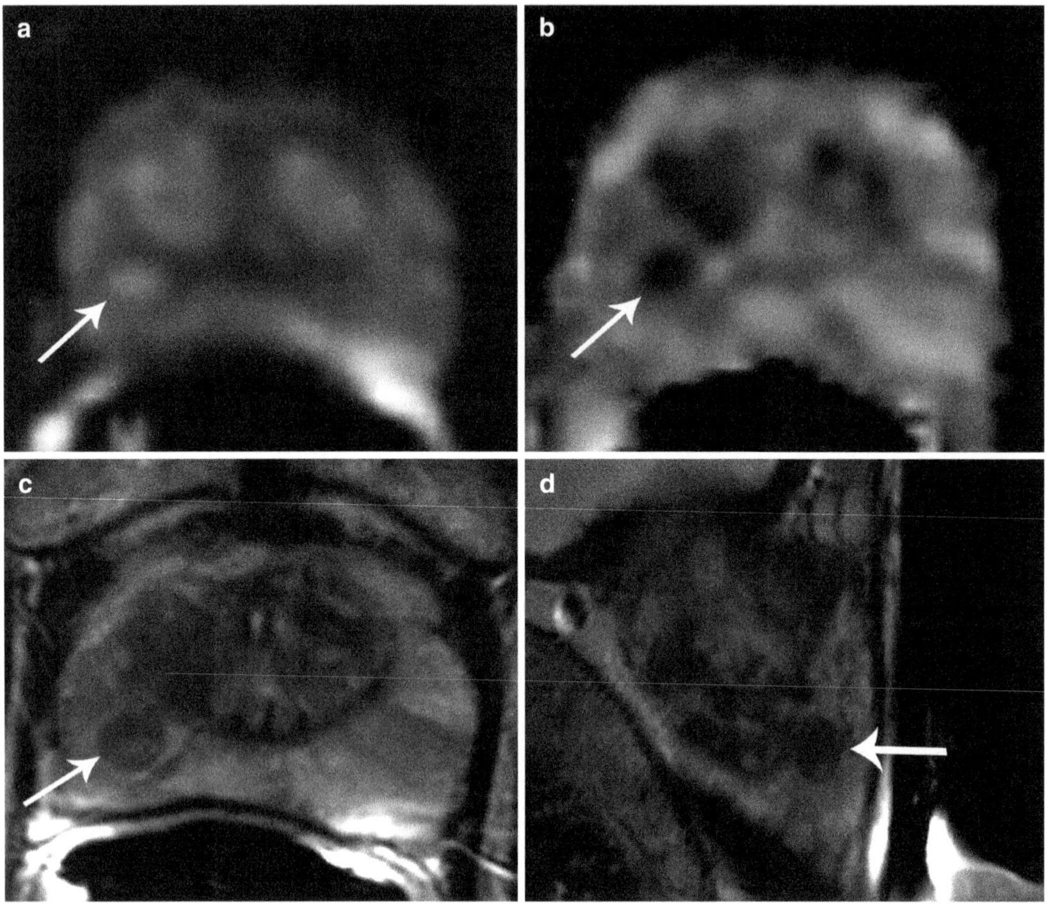

Fig. 7.10 Exophytic BPH nodule. (**a**) Axial DWI and (**b**) ADC map show a focal area in the right peripheral zone with markedly high and low signal intensity, respectively (arrow), which at first appears to represent a PI-RADS 4 lesion. However, on (**c**) axial and (**d**) sagittal T2W images the lesion is round and heterogenous, abuts the surgical capsule, and shows a thin dark capsule (arrows), typical findings of an exophytic BPH nodule

and systematic biopsy [29]. This fact has supported the argument from the urologic community against proposals to restrict the biopsy procedure only to areas in which targets are identified on MRI. However, on a per patient basis, the sensitivity is high and clinically significant cancer is unlikely to be missed [30]. This may be particularly true if targeted biopsies are directed to lesions seen on MRI and/or TRUS. Garcia-Reyes et al. found that only 33 (3.2%) of 1,024 nontargeted systematic cores diagnosed clinically significant prostate cancer. Yet, these 33 tumors represented approximately 1/3 of the total number of clinically significant disease [31]. The use of PSA density may help to identify who are the men with negative MRI who may avoid or need a systematic biopsy [14].

7.11 Management

PI-RADS v2.1 does not provide management recommendations based on PI-RADS score. Specifically, there is no recommendation to perform targeted MRI-guided biopsies on certain categories and to avoid biopsy for others. This is because several clinical factors need to be taken into account prior to biopsy, such as PSA, prior biopsy results, prior therapies, and local practices. However, in general PI-RADS 4 and 5 lesions should be considered for MRI-guided biopsy depending on the clinical scenario [32]. For instance, in men who have undergone prior TRUS biopsy with negative pathology, biopsy should be strongly considered as these lesions often harbor clinically significant cancers [33]. Similarly, men who are on active surveillance for very low-risk or low-risk prostate cancer but are found to have PI-RADS 4 or 5 lesion are also good candidates for MRI-guided biopsy [34]. On the other hand, men who have a known diagnosis of clinically significant prostate cancer and are undergoing MRI for staging purposes prior to therapy generally do not need an additional biopsy.

Because of the fairly low rate of positive biopsies, PI-RADS 3 lesions present a problem in deciding on a biopsy approach. Therefore, local practices, patient preference, and laboratory values such as PSA and PSA density may be taken into account when deciding on a targeted biopsy [14].

7.12 Summary

Multiparametric MRI of the prostate incorporates both anatomical sequences and functional imaging to optimize detection of prostate cancer. PI-RADS was developed to standardize the technical performance and interpretation of multiparametric MRI and has been an important step forward, becoming rapidly adopted as the preferred prostate MRI scoring system. Experience has shown good diagnostic accuracy, and the latest version of PI-RADS attempts to improve on historical lower accuracy in the transition zone. Overall the scoring system is straightforward and is meant to be readily implemented into a busy clinical practice.

References

1. Oberlin DT, Casalino DD, Miller FH, Meeks JJ. Dramatic increase in the utilization of multiparametric magnetic resonance imaging for detection and management of prostate cancer. Abdom Radiol. 2017;42(4):1255–8.
2. Barentsz JO, Richenberg J, Clements R, Choyke P, Verma S, Villeirs G, et al. ESUR prostate MR guidelines 2012. Eur Radiol. 2012;22(4):746–57.
3. Westphalen AC, Rosenkrantz AB. Prostate imaging reporting and data system (PI-RADS): reflections on early experience with a standardized interpretation scheme for multiparametric prostate MRI. AJR Am J Roentgenol. 2014;202(1):121–3.
4. Weinreb JC, Barentsz JO, Choyke PL, Cornud F, Haider MA, Macura KJ, et al. PI-RADS prostate imaging reporting and data system: 2015, version 2. Eur Urol. 2016;69(1):16–40.
5. Turkbey B, Rosenkrantz AB, Haider MA, Padhani AR, Villeirs G, Macura KJ, et al. Prostate imaging reporting and data system version 2.1: 2019 update of prostate imaging reporting and data system version 2. Eur Urol. 2019;76(3):340–51.
6. Vache T, Bratan F, Mege-Lechevallier F, Roche S, Rabilloud M, Rouviere O. Characterization of prostate lesions as benign or malignant at multiparametric MR imaging: comparison of three scoring systems in patients treated with radical prostatectomy. Radiology. 2014;272(2):446–55.
7. Akin O, Sala E, Moskowitz CS, Kuroiwa K, Ishill NM, Pucar D, et al. Transition zone prostate cancers: features, detection, localization, and staging at endorectal MR imaging. Radiology. 2006;239(3):784–92.
8. Hoeks CM, Hambrock T, Yakar D, Hulsbergen-van de Kaa CA, Feuth T, Witjes JA, et al. Transition zone prostate cancer: detection and localization with 3-T multiparametric MR imaging. Radiology. 2013;266(1):207–17.
9. Rosenkrantz AB, Kim S, Lim RP, Hindman N, Deng FM, Babb JS, et al. Prostate cancer localization using multiparametric MR imaging: comparison of prostate imaging reporting and data system (PI-RADS) and Likert scales. Radiology. 2013;269(2):482–92.
10. Greer MD, Shih JH, Lay N, Barrett T, Kayat Bittencourt L, Borofsky S, et al. Validation of the dominant sequence paradigm and role of dynamic contrast-enhanced imaging in PI-RADS version 2. Radiology. 2017;285(3):859–69.
11. ACR® American College of Radiology. PI-RADS® Prostate Imaging-Reporting and Data System. 2019 V 2.1. https://www.acr.org/-/media/ACR/Files/RADS/Pi-RADS/PIRADS-V2-1.pdf?la=en
12. Jordan EJ, Fiske C, Zagoria RJ, Westphalen AC. Evaluating the performance of PI-RADS v2 in the non-academic setting. Abdom Radiol. 2017;42(11):2725–31.
13. Padhani AR, Liu G, Koh DM, Chenevert TL, Thoeny HC, Takahara T, et al. Diffusion-weighted magnetic resonance imaging as a cancer biomarker: consensus and recommendations. Neoplasia. 2009;11(2):102–25.
14. Westphalen AC, Fazel F, Nguyen H, Cabarrus M, Hanley-Knutson K, Shinohara K, et al. Detection of clinically signifi cant prostate cancer with PIRADS v2 scores, PSA density, and ADC values in regions with and without mpMRI visible lesions. Int Braz J Urol. 2019;45:713–23.

15. Jordan EJ, Fiske C, Zagoria R, Westphalen AC. PI-RADS v2 and ADC values: is there room for improvement? Abdom Radiol. 2018;43(11):3109–16.
16. Turkbey B, Shah VP, Pang Y, Bernardo M, Xu S, Kruecker J, et al. Is apparent diffusion coefficient associated with clinical risk scores for prostate cancers that are visible on 3-T MR images? Radiology. 2011;258(2):488–95.
17. Donati OF, Mazaheri Y, Afaq A, Vargas HA, Zheng J, Moskowitz CS, et al. Prostate cancer aggressiveness: assessment with whole-lesion histogram analysis of the apparent diffusion coefficient. Radiology. 2014;271(1):143–52.
18. Rosenkrantz AB, Taneja SS. Radiologist, be aware: ten pitfalls that confound the interpretation of multiparametric prostate MRI. AJR Am J Roentgenol. 2014;202(1):109–20.
19. Rosenkrantz AB, Babb JS, Taneja SS, Ream JM. Proposed adjustments to PI-RADS version 2 decision rules: impact on prostate Cancer detection. Radiology. 2017;283(1):119–29.
20. Muglia VF, Westphalen AC, Wang ZJ, Kurhanewicz J, Carroll PR, Coakley FV. Endorectal MRI of prostate cancer: incremental prognostic importance of gross locally advanced disease. AJR Am J Roentgenol. 2011;197(6):1369–74.
21. Vargas HA, Akin O, Franiel T, Goldman DA, Udo K, Touijer KA, et al. Normal central zone of the prostate and central zone involvement by prostate cancer: clinical and MR imaging implications. Radiology. 2012;262(3):894–902.
22. Woo S, Suh CH, Kim SY, Cho JY, Kim SH. Diagnostic performance of prostate imaging reporting and data system version 2 for detection of prostate Cancer: a systematic review and diagnostic meta-analysis. Eur Urol. 2017;72(2):177–88.
23. Venderink W, van Luijtelaar A, Bomers JG, van der Leest M, Hulsbergen-van de Kaa C, Barentsz JO, et al. Results of targeted biopsy in men with magnetic resonance imaging lesions classified equivocal, likely or highly likely to be clinically significant prostate cancer. Eur Urol. 2017;73:353–60.
24. Mehralivand S, Bednarova S, Shih JH, Mertan FV, Gaur S, Merino MJ, et al. Prospective evaluation of PI-RADS version 2 using the International Society of Urological Pathology Prostate Cancer Grade Group System. J Urol. 2017;198(3):583–90.
25. Barkovich EJ, Shankar PR, Westphalen AC. A systematic review of the existing prostate imaging reporting and data system version 2 (PI-RADSv2) literature and subset meta-analysis of PI-RADSv2 categories stratified by Gleason scores. AJR Am J Roentgenol. 2019;212(4):847–54.
26. Rosenkrantz AB, Ginocchio LA, Cornfeld D, Froemming AT, Gupta RT, Turkbey B, et al. Interobserver reproducibility of the PI-RADS version 2 lexicon: a multicenter study of six experienced prostate radiologists. Radiology. 2016;280(3):793–804.
27. Lin WC, Muglia VF, Silva GE, Chodraui Filho S, Reis RB, Westphalen AC. Multiparametric MRI of the prostate: diagnostic performance and interreader agreement of two scoring systems. Br J Radiol. 2016;89(1062):20151056.
28. Greer MD, Shih JH, Lay N, Barrett T, Bittencourt L, Borofsky S, et al. Interreader variability of prostate imaging reporting and data system version 2 in detecting and assessing prostate Cancer lesions at prostate MRI. AJR Am J Roentgenol. 2019;212:1197–205. 10.2214/AJR.18.20536.
29. Tran GN, Leapman MS, Nguyen HG, Cowan JE, Shinohara K, Westphalen AC, et al. Magnetic resonance imaging-ultrasound fusion biopsy during prostate cancer active surveillance. Eur Urol. 2017;72(2):275–81.
30. Borofsky S, George AK, Gaur S, Bernardo M, Greer MD, Mertan FV, et al. What are we missing? False-negative cancers at multiparametric MR imaging of the prostate. Radiology. 2018;286(1):186–95.
31. Garcia-Reyes K, Nguyen HG, Zagoria RJ, Shinohara K, Carroll PR, Behr SC, et al. Impact of lesion visibility on Transrectal ultrasound on the prediction of clinically significant prostate cancer (Gleason score 3 + 4 or greater) with transrectal ultrasound-magnetic resonance imaging fusion biopsy. J Urol. 2018;199(3):699–705.
32. Meermeier NP, Foster BR, Liu JJ, Amling CL, Coakley FV. Impact of direct MRI-guided biopsy of the prostate on clinical management. AJR Am J Roentgenol. 2019:213(2):371–6.
33. Rosenkrantz AB, Verma S, Choyke P, Eberhardt SC, Eggener SE, Gaitonde K, et al. Prostate magnetic resonance imaging and magnetic resonance imaging targeted biopsy in patients with a prior negative biopsy: a consensus statement by AUA and SAR. J Urol. 2016;196(6):1613–8.
34. Sanda MG, Chen RC, Crispino T, Freedland S, Greene K, Klotz LH, Makarov DV, Nelson JB, Reston J, Rodrigues G, Sandler HM, Taplin ME, Cadeddu JA. Clinically localized prostate cancer: AUA/ASTRO/SUO Guideline 2017. Available from: https://www.auanet.org/guidelines/prostate-cancer-clinically-localized-guideline

Local Staging of Prostate Cancer with MRI

8

Steven C. Eberhardt and Martha F. Terrazas

8.1 Introduction

Prostate cancer is the second most common cancer in men in the United States and the second leading cause of cancer-related deaths among men of all races [1]. Patient prognosis and individual survival are influenced by the cancer histology and the stage of the disease when diagnosed. Accurate local staging of prostate cancer is useful for guiding management choices. MR imaging features of locally advanced prostate cancer or regional lymph node metastases can influence choice of treatment [2]. The presence of extra prostatic extension has been shown to confer greater risk of a positive surgical margin, decreased survival, and increased need for additional treatment [3]. Seminal vesicle invasion is also a marker for poor prognosis, and patients will be at higher risk for biochemical recurrence [3]. The detection of lymph node metastases has prognostic significance and can be an early indicator of systemic disease and overall worse prognosis [4].

Multiparametric magnetic resonance imaging (mpMRI) of the prostate with T2-weighted imaging always in conjunction with diffusion-weighted MRI, and sometimes also with dynamic contrast-enhanced imaging and/or MRI spectroscopy, has become commonplace over the last decade for detection of prostate cancer and prostate cancer surveillance. MRI for local staging is primarily accomplished using the high-resolution small field of view T2-weighted images and has been an indication for MRI of prostate cancer for even longer [5]. In addition to MRI staging, allowing for risk stratification to help patients and treating physicians weigh the risks and benefits of therapeutic options, when surgical management is pursued MRI staging information can facilitate surgical margin planning prior to radical prostatectomy [6, 7].

S. C. Eberhardt (✉) · M. F. Terrazas
University of New Mexico Hospital, Department of Radiology, Albuquerque, NM, USA

University of New Mexico, Albuquerque, NM, USA
e-mail: seberhardt@salud.unm.edu; MFTerrazas@salud.unm.edu

8.2 Technical Aspects Impacting MRI Staging

8.2.1 Protocols for mpMRI

The American College of Radiology Prostate Imaging Reporting & Data System (PI-RADS) Steering Committee published PI-RADS version 2.1 in 2019. The document includes best practice technical specifications for mpMRI [8]. Confident detection of significant prostate cancer requires high-quality diffusion-weighted imaging which allows strong reader confidence about presence of significant cancer. Local staging is achieved with simultaneous review of fast T2-weighted images, also according to specifications, with small field of view (around 15 cm) and thin slices (3 mm), in 3D or multiplanar acquisitions (Fig. 8.1).

T. Tirkes (ed.), *Prostate MRI Essentials*, https://doi.org/10.1007/978-3-030-45935-2_8

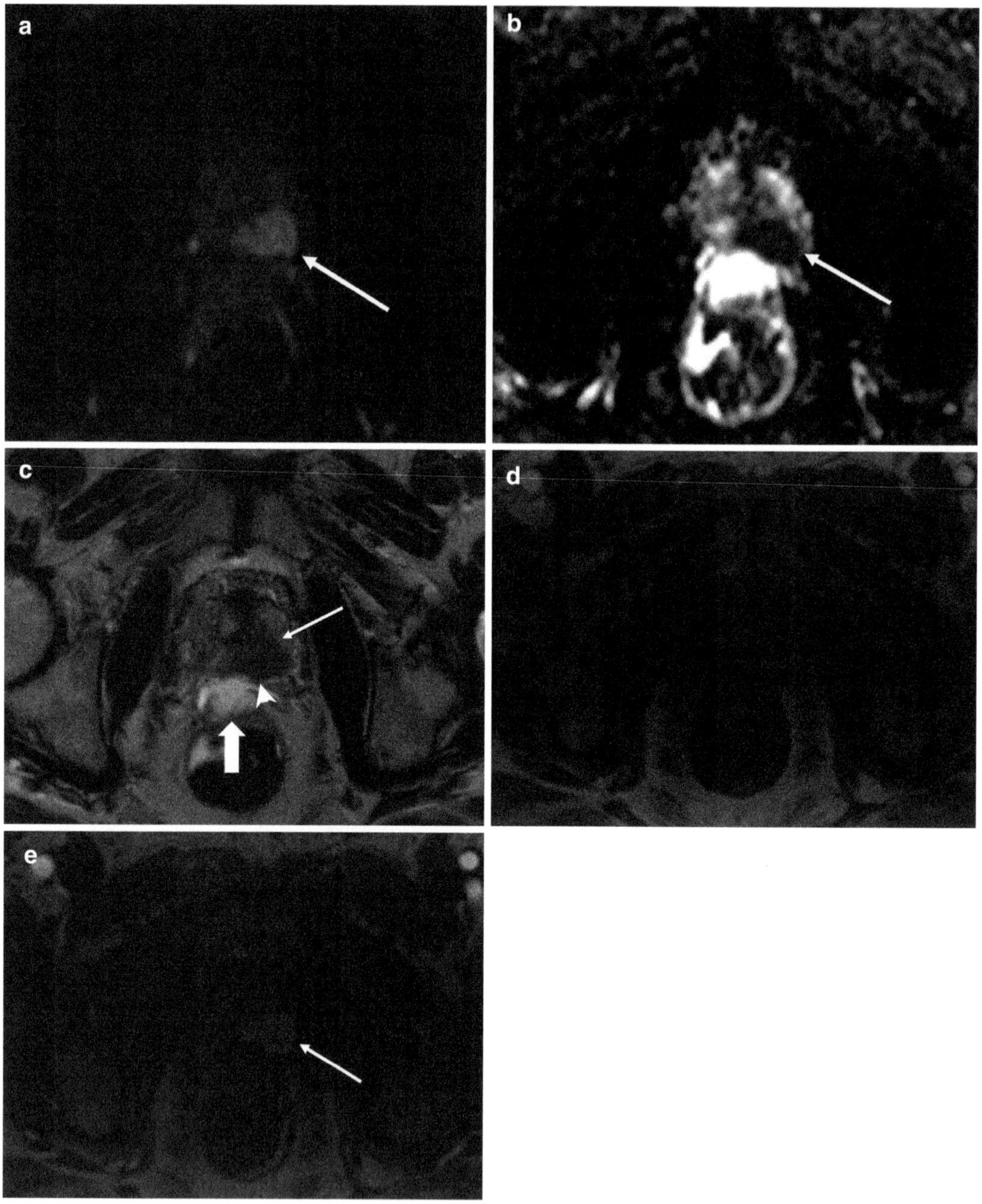

Fig. 8.1 (**a**) Axial DWI MR (b = 1400 s/mm^2). A 2.0 cm hyperintense lesion centered in the left mid gland peripheral zone posterolaterally (arrow), corresponding to biopsy-proven prostate adenocarcinoma, Gleason pattern 4. (**b**) Axial ADC map – corresponding 2.0 cm hypointense lesion centered in the left mid gland peripheral zone demonstrates low-signal intensity, indicative of restricted diffusion, highly suspicious for clinically significant prostate cancer. (**c**) Axial high-resolution T2W image through the prostate gland. A 2.0 cm T2 hypointense homogenous signal lesion (thin arrow) in the posterolateral left mid gland peripheral zone corresponds to the site of restricted diffusion. Incidental note is made of hydrogel spacer between the posterior prostate and anterior rectum (block arrow). Prostate tumor shows broad extension along glandular margin and focal irregular bulging posteriorly (arrowhead), features suspect for early, small volume, and extra glandular spread. (**d**) T1-wieghted dynamic sequence prior to contrast shows homogeneous low-signal character prostate. (**e**) Later time period than (**d**) shows arterial phase of enhancement. Prostate cancer (arrow) shows marked early contrast enhancement compared to surrounding normal gland

8.2.2 Magnetic Field Strength

Although 3.0 T and 1.5 T whole-body MRI systems can provide diagnostic exams when optimized, most members of the PI-RADS Steering Committee prefer and recommend 3.0 T for prostate MRI, if available [8].

8.2.3 Endorectal Coils

Endorectal coils (ERCs) increase the signal to noise ratio (SNR) in the prostate, regardless of the magnetic field strength. In larger patients where SNR is decreased, ERCs can help increase the quality of the MRI [9]. However, ERCs increase exam time and cost, and although they increase SNR, they can introduce artifacts and distort the gland. Additionally, ERCs may be uncomfortable and cause patient anxiety or aversion to imaging. It is important to note that some older 1.5 T MRI systems require the use of an ERC to achieve SNR optimal for prostate cancer staging. 3.0 T MRI exams without an ERC are considered comparable to 1.5 T with an ERC in terms of image quality [8].

8.2.4 Post-biopsy Hemorrhage

Hemorrhage is identified as T1W hyperintense signal and is most commonly seen in the peripheral zone and seminal vesicles when MRI follows transrectal ultrasound-guided systematic (TRUS) biopsy [10, 11]. Post-biopsy hemorrhage and inflammation can confound mpMRI interpretation and may persist for many months. The usual recommendation is to wait 6 weeks or more between biopsy and MRI [11]. However, this issue is controversial, since when MRI is performed after a TRUS biopsy, the likelihood of clinically significant prostate cancer becoming undetectable due to hemorrhage is low. Also, if high-signal hemorrhage remains to be present, a clinically significant cancer may be outlined by the T1-hyperintense hemorrhage, making the lesion more conspicuous. Thus, delaying MRI may not be necessary to adequately characterize clinically significant cancer [8].

8.2.5 Patient Preparation

The use of antispasmodic agents (such as glucagon or sublingual hyoscyamine sulfate) to reduce bowel motion peristalsis artifact may be useful in some patients. However, since preparation is costly and risk of potential drug reactions, antispasmodic agents are not routinely recommended. The patient should be instructed to evacuate the rectum prior to the MRI exam. Air and stool within the rectum may result in artifact and significantly degrade DWI quality. A simple over the counter cleansing enema administered by the patient hours before the MRI exam may be beneficial without the use of antispasmodic agents (especially if patient was called back secondary to bowel gas artifact) [8, 12]. Lastly, it has been recommended that patients refrain from ejaculation for 3 days prior to the MRI exam to ensure distention of the seminal vesicles. However, this recommendation has not been firmly established as a benefit for accurate staging [8].

8.3 Patient Information to Assist Staging

The most recent serum prostate-specific antigen (PSA) level and the PSA history inform the interpreting radiologist on the patient risk of locally advanced cancer. Results from prostate biopsies and biopsy dates, including number of cores, locations, Gleason scores of positive biopsies, and other relevant clinical history such as a digital rectal exam, should be provided to or sought by the radiologist [8]. Though there are not many well-performed studies to support it, most radiologists interpreting MRI of prostate believe this information can aid confidence and accuracy in detection and staging assessments, as is true for other diagnostic imaging tests [13, 14].

8.4 Histology

The traditional histologic diagnosis of prostate cancer from biopsy samples is the Gleason score (or sum). The aggressiveness and dedifferentiation increase from low cancer grade (or histologic pattern) 3 to highest grade, 5. The pathologist assigns a Gleason grade to the tissue, including the dominant pattern in the biopsy sample added to the lesser component. The score may be formed by the same number if the tissue sample is all of one type (i.e., 3 + 3). Thus, Gleason sums assigned prostate cancer range from 6 to 10 (with 6 being the lowest-grade cancer and 10 the highest). Additionally, the individual numbers and order are important in predicting prognosis [15]. For example, a patient with a Gleason score of 3 + 4 = 7 has a better prognosis as a patient with 4 + 3 = 7. Pathology guidelines are in transition from this system to an alternative grading system, called Grade Group, where Group 1 is equivalent to Gleason 3 + 3 = 6, Group 2 is Gleason 3 + 4, Group 3 is Gleason 4 + 3, Group 4 is Gleason 4 + 4, and Group 5 for any pattern 5 (Gleason sum 9 or 10) [16]. More detailed information on this topic can be found in Chap. 1 of this book.

8.5 Anatomy Relevant to Staging

8.5.1 Prostate Capsule

Although the prostate does not have a true capsule histologically, the prostate is partially surrounded by a T2W-hypointense margin which has been referred to as the prostate capsule and which should be scrutinized during assessment for extra prostatic or "extracapsular" extension of cancer (ECE) [7, 17] (Fig. 8.2).

8.5.2 Prostate Zones

The peripheral zone (PZ) is along the posterior and lateral aspects of the prostate gland and at the

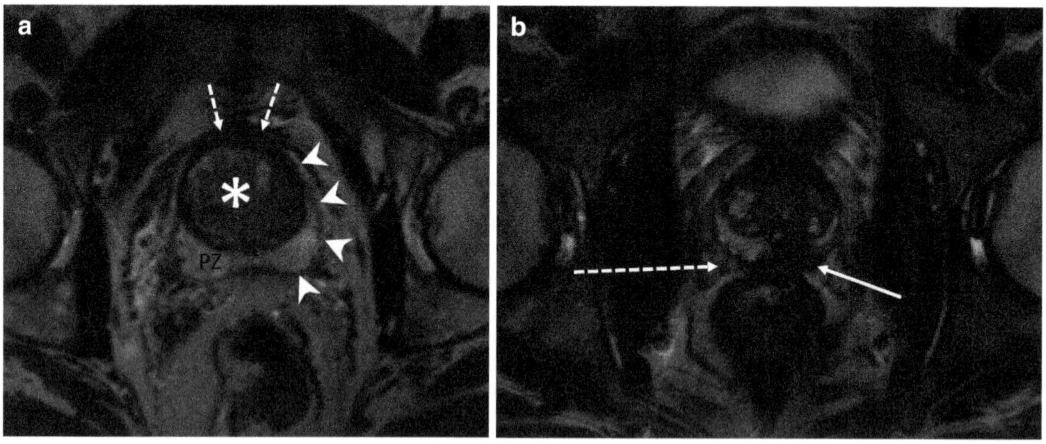

Fig. 8.2 Anatomy relevant to staging. (**a**) Trans axial high-resolution T2-weighted image of the mid prostate, non-cancerous gland with BPH in the TZ (asterisk). Zonal anatomy is well depicted, with the peripheral zone (PZ) high in signal intensity. The gland margin shows a smooth T1-dark border (arrowheads) with adipose tissue and veins outside of this. This border, commonly referred to as a "capsule" despite no true capsule present histologically, defines the prostate glandular surface. Anterior fibromuscular stroma runs along the anterior aspect (dashed arrows). (**b**) Trans axial T2-weighted image in a different patient with biopsy-proven cancer. Lesion centered in left posterior PZ (consistent with significant prostate cancer on DWI, not shown). Right recto-prostatic angle (location of neurovascular bundle) preserved (dashed arrow). Left posterior side shows tumor bulge at margin abutting recto-prostatic angle (arrow). Pathology from prostatectomy showed perineural invasion beyond gland margin, but otherwise not extra glandular disease

apex. Posteriorly, this portion of the gland closely abuts the rectal wall. Most prostate cancers originate in the PZ (approximately 70–80%). On mpMRI, lesions in the peripheral zone should be measured on ADC [8]. Prostate cancers arising in the peripheral zone are generally more aggressive and with worse prognosis (for similar size) than those arising in the transition zone [18].

The transition zone (TZ) surrounds the urethra and is the site of almost all benign prostatic hyperplasia (BPH). Approximately 20% of prostate cancers occur in the TZ. On mpMRI, prostate lesions should be assessed primarily and measured on T2W sequence. TZ cancers are generally more challenging to identify secondary to heterogeneous signal intensity including low T2 signal nodules from BPH [8]. Prostate cancers arising in the transition zone are generally less aggressive and with better prognosis (for similar size) than those arising in the transition zone [18].

The central zone (CZ) is the prostate tissue which surrounds the ejaculatory ducts. A small percentage of prostate cancers arise in the CZ (less than 5%). Frequently the central zone is involved by tumors also involving and indistinguishable from adjacent peripheral zone cancers [19]. Due to anatomic location, cancers involving or originating in the CZ are more likely to have aggressive features and invade the seminal vesicles [7, 19]. More information on prostate zonal anatomy can be found in Chap. 3 of this book.

8.5.3 Neurovascular Bundles and Recto-prostatic Angle (Fig. 8.2)

The posterolateral aspect of the prostate gland has important anatomic features which are relevant to staging. Paired neurovascular bundles (NVBs) reside along the posterolateral margin of the gland, arising from S2–S4 nerve roots and the pelvic plexus of sympathetic and parasympathetic fibers along the lateral aspects of the rectum [20]. The inferior division of the pelvic plexus forms the NVB and innervates the prostate, as individual nerve fibers extend from this tract along with vessels into the posterolateral gland. In addition, NVB fibers extending more caudally include cavernosal nerves involved in erectile function. When prostate cancer develops, there is a tendency of the cancer to invade the perineural sheath within the prostate and to exit the prostate along nerves and vessels at the NVB [21]. Loss of erectile function is a known complication of radical prostatectomy, and surgical techniques have developed to preserve or spare the NVB [22]. Information from MRI staging can aid this decision, and radiologists interpreting MRI should pay attention to and report cancer proximity to the posterolateral gland margin and extension beyond the gland margin (ECE) at the NVB [7]. The NVB resides within an anatomical triangle on trans axial cross-sectional images, surrounded by thin fascial investments, bound anteromedially by the prostate, posterolaterally by the rectum, and laterally by the pelvic floor musculature including levator ani. The medial corner of this interface had been called the recto-prostatic angle, and obliteration of this space by bulging or invading tumor is a described sign of extra prostatic disease [23].

8.5.4 Additional Gland Margins

In addition to the posterior and lateral "capsule" margins at the edges of the peripheral zone, the anterior, apical, and basal gland margins have anatomical features pertinent to staging. Anteriorly the margin of the gland is bordered by anterior fibromuscular stroma (FMS) which contains no glandular tissue and is contiguous with the bladder neck at the prostate base. On T2W images, FMS appears as a dark band of tissue usually 2–3 mm thick, darker, and thicker than the PZ "capsule" laterally and posteriorly, and in older men, the FMS margin largely abuts BPH in the TZ [24]. Cancer in the TZ may be more resistant to extra prostatic spread due to this, and tumor extension into the FMS does not constitute extra prostatic disease, but extension through the FMS is extra prostatic extension [25]. Lentiform- or semilunar-shaped anterior cancers along or within the anterior FMS in some studies have been subclassified as a separate tumor type [26, 27].

The apex of the gland constitutes peripheral zone tissue histologically and is a surgical margin for prostatectomy. It has the least well-defined margin, better depicted in coronal than trans axial images due to the conical shape of the prostate apex, and oblique angles relative to trans axial plane. Cancer in this region can spread beyond the prostate, along periurethral tissues, leading to positive surgical margins at prostatectomy [28], so analysis and description of tumors in this region on MRI reporting can have implications for surgical technique and treatment selection.

The base of the prostate is complex and contains portions of peripheral, transition, and central zones along the prostatic margin. Medially and posteriorly, central and peripheral zones are contiguous with the ejaculatory ducts leading to the vas deferens and seminal vesicles. Periurethral transition zone tissue is contiguous with the bladder neck, and more laterally peripheral zone tissue lies adjacent a thin periprostatic space separating the gland from the lateral parts of the seminal vesicles. As a result, the direct spread of cancer from the base of the prostate includes cases with seminal vesicle invasion and bladder muscle involvement [26].

8.6 Multi-parametic Imaging, Contributions to Staging

8.6.1 Diffusion-Weighted Imaging

Over the last decade, the addition of DWI used in conjunction with apparent diffusion coefficient (ADC) mapping to T2WI has become central to accurately staging prostate cancer. DWI is the most important method for the *detection* of tumor, overall assessment of tumor *aggressiveness*, and may aid in correct interpretation of extra prostatic extension [29]. DWI reflects random motion of water molecules (Brownian movement) within and between extracellular to intracellular spaces and changes with increased cellular membrane permeability and cellular density, features that are commonly different in malignancies [29, 30]. Clinically significant prostate cancers show relative restricted diffusion compared to normal tissues and appear hypointense on ADC maps and hyperintense on high b-value images. The effect of restricted diffusion in prostate cancer is more useful in the peripheral zone of the prostate and is the dominant sequence for interpretation of significant cancer in that part of the prostate. In the transition zone and central zone, the normal and hypertrophic tissues can show some degree of diffusion restriction making the detection of significant cancers more challenging, but the diffusion-weighted images and ADC maps remain useful.

DWI must include an ADC map and high b-value images. Two or more b-values are needed to calculate ADC values. Since ADC calculations can vary across different vendors, qualitative visual assessment is recommended to assess if a lesion demonstrates low ADC values (rather than standardized quantitative measurements). Although there is currently no accepted optimal high b-value, it is required to utilize a b-value of at least 1400 sec/mm^2. It is also important to note that SNR decreases as the b-value increases [8, 11]. More detailed discussion on DWI can be found in Chap. 5 of this issue (see Figs. 8.1, 8.3, 8.4, 8.5, and 8.6).

8.6.2 T2-Weighted Imaging

Clinically significant prostate cancers in the PZ are usually focal, round, elliptical, or poorly marginated hypointense lesions on T2W imaging. Other abnormalities of the PZ can also have this appearance, including prostatitis, hemorrhage, and BPH. Clinically significant cancers in the TZ are usually non-circumscribed, homogenous, and moderately hypointense on T2W imaging with loss of usual nodular architecture of BPH within and at the margins (typically described as "erased charcoal" or "smudgy fingerprint") [8]. When

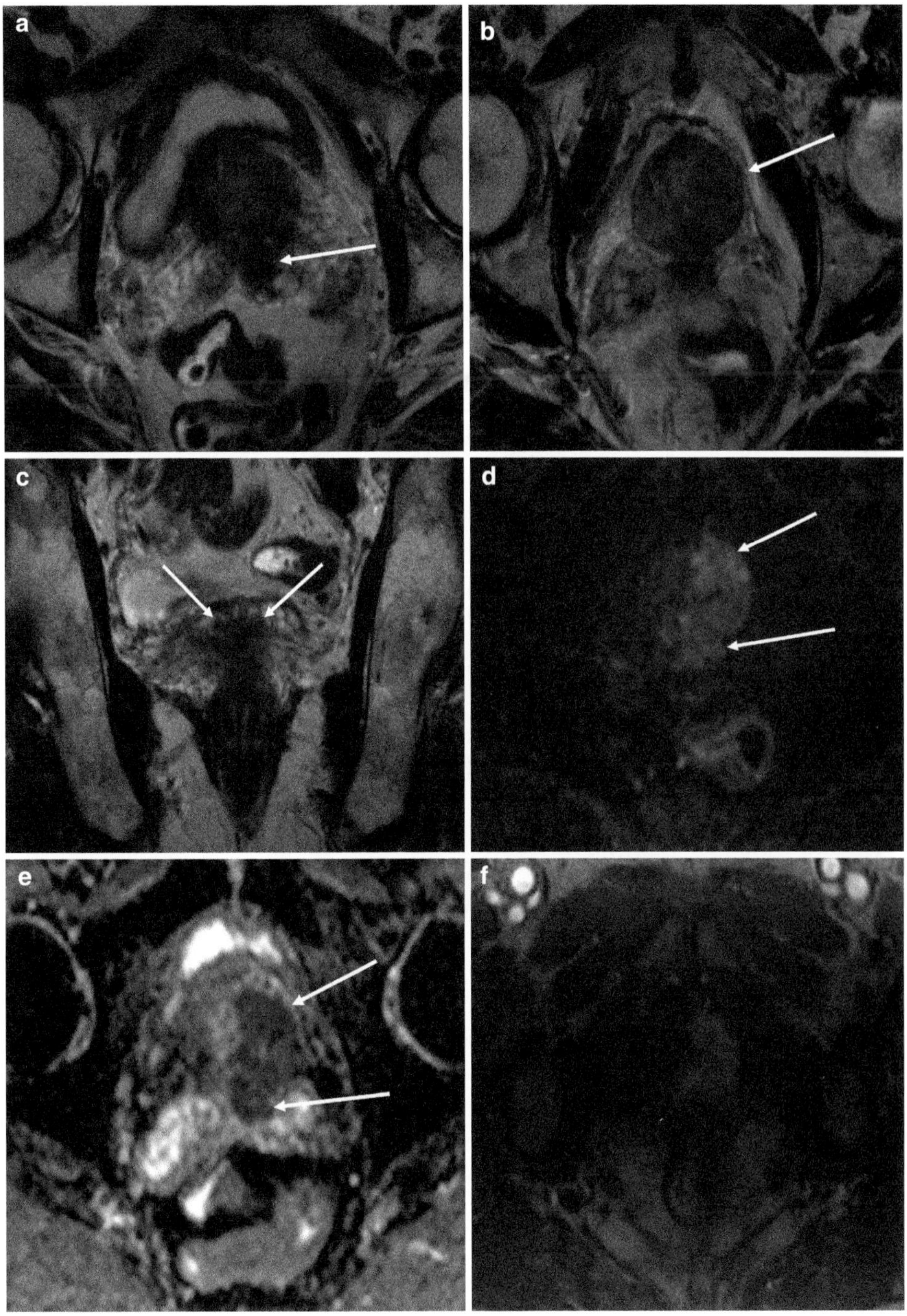

Fig. 8.3 (**a**) Axial high-resolution T2W sequence. A 3.5 cm T2W-hypointense mass in the posterior prostate base shows extension into the medial aspect of the left seminal vesicle (white arrow). (**b**) Caudal to 3A, there is bulging and irregularity of the capsule at the left anterolateral prostate base and tumor abutment along gland margin greater than 1.0 cm, features suspect for extra glandular extension (white arrow). (**c**) Coronal T2W sequence – also depicts direct extension of T2W-hypointense tumor into the seminal vesicles (arrows). (**d**) Axial DWI MR (b = 1400 s/mm^2) and ADC map – tumor with restricted diffusion (high-signal character, arrow) extending into the seminal vesicles has corresponding restricted diffusion (low ADC signal, arrow). (**e**) Axial DWI MR (b = 1400 s/mm^2) and ADC map – tumor with restricted diffusion (high-signal character, arrow) extending into the seminal vesicles has corresponding restricted diffusion (low ADC signal, arrow). (**f**) Axial DCE. Positive early contrast enhancement directly corresponds to the 2.5 cm T2W-hypointense mass with restricted diffusion

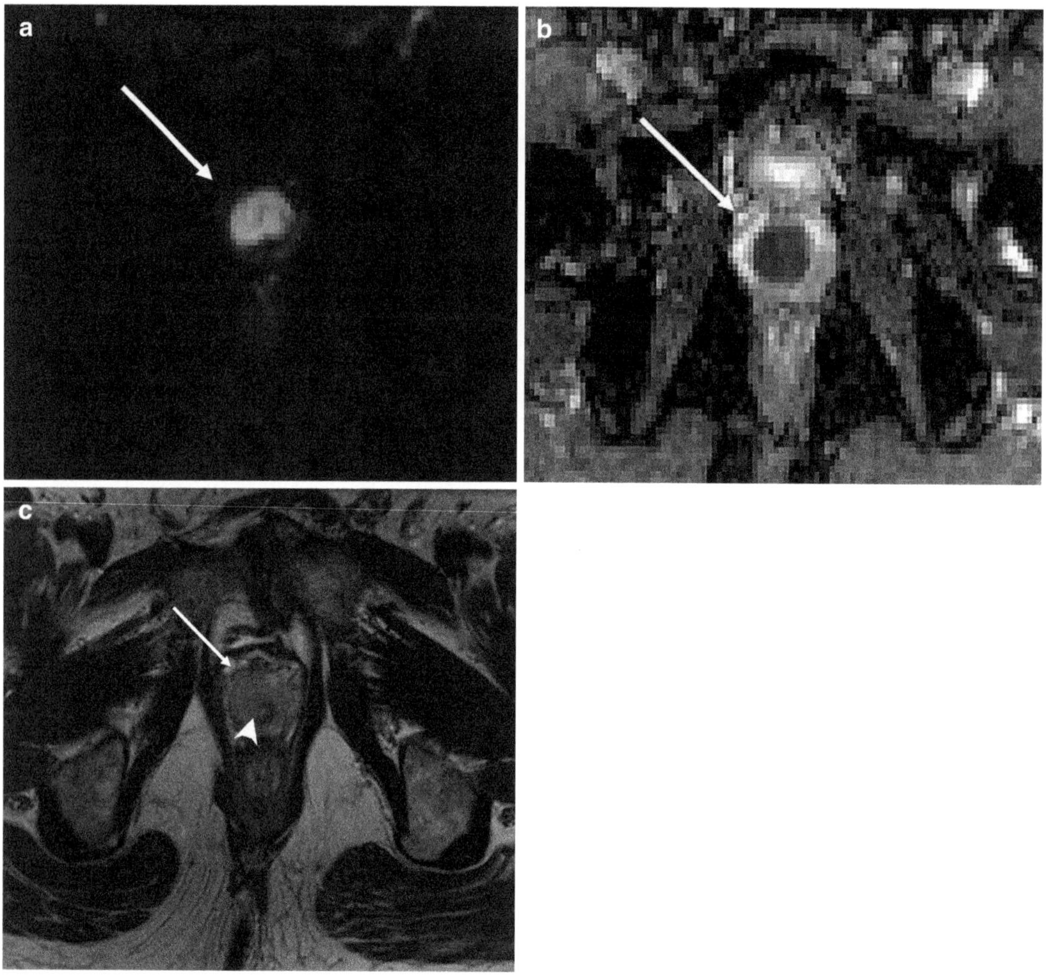

Fig. 8.4 (**a**) Axial DWI MR (b = 1600 s/mm^2) show hyperintense high b-value image tumor in prostate (arrow). (**b**) ADC map through prostate apex, 2.5 cm with restricted diffusion (arrow), consistent with clinically significant cancer. (**c**) Axial high-resolution T2W sequence. Focal T2W homogenous relatively hypointense mass in the apex involving both the PZ and TZ. There is tumor extension into the T2W relatively even more hypointense urethra on the right side, suspicious for invasion of the urethral sphincter (arrowhead). Bulging and irregularity of contour anteriorly on the right also are suspected extra glandular spread

significant cancers advance locally, features of extra prostatic growth of tumor are best depicted anatomically on the high-resolution T2-weighted images (Fig. 8.7).

8.6.3 Dynamic Contrast Enhancement (DCE) mpMRI

DCE is characterized by the acquisition of rapid T1W imaging during and after the administration of intravenous contrast. DCE is considered positive when there is focal early enhancement that corresponds to a suspicious lesion with abnormal T2W and DWI [31]. More detailed discussion on DCE can be found in Chap. 6 of this book. In general, prostate cancers usually demonstrate early enhancement compared to normal adjacent prostatic tissue. The kinetics of prostate cancer can be variable with some clinically significant cancers demonstrating typical early washout, while other tumors retain contrast [8]. Importantly, enhancement is not definitive for clinically significant cancer in the absence

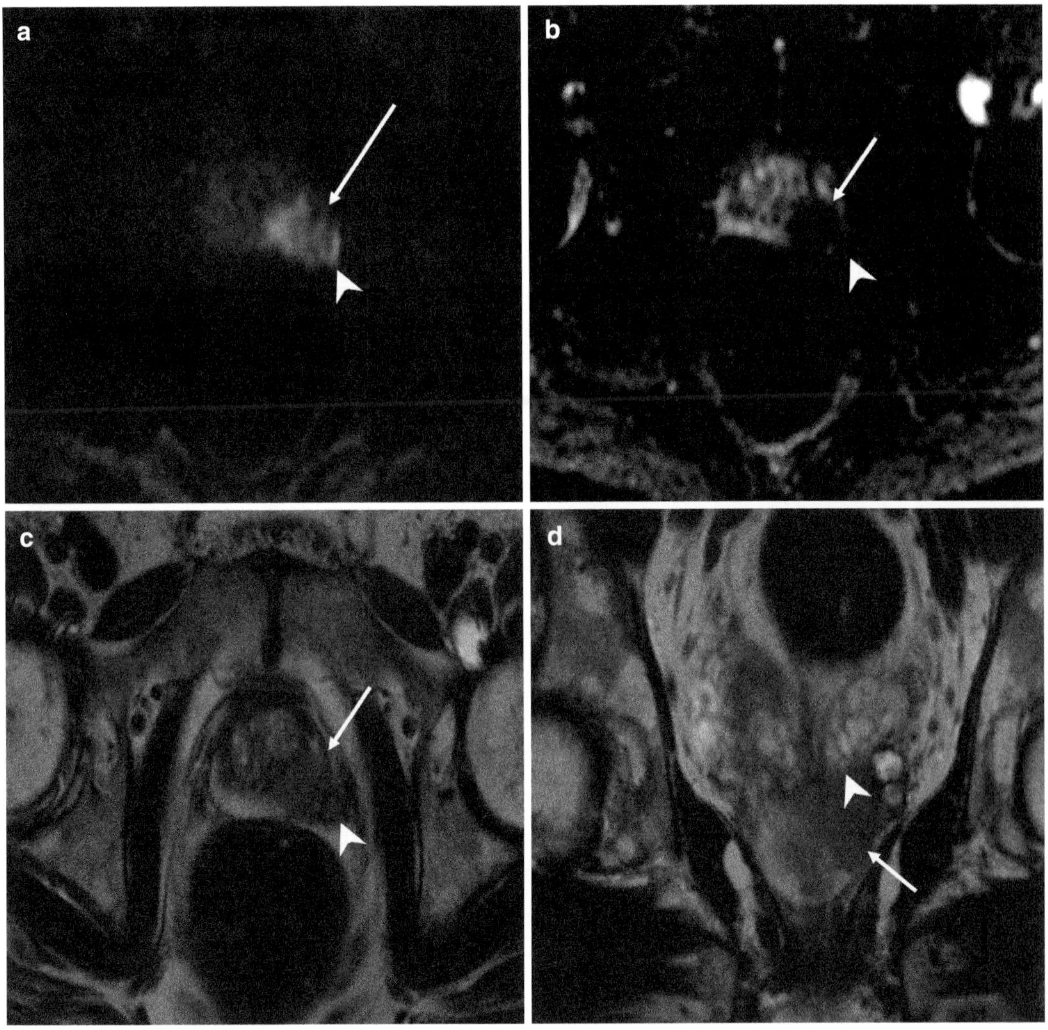

Fig. 8.5 (**a**) Axial DWI MR (b = 1400 s/mm^2) and (**b**) ADC map. Images show features of restricted diffusion consistent with significant cancer 3.0 cm in size in the left base PZ (arrows). The posterolateral aspect is irregular (arrowheads) and also demonstrates restricted diffusion. (**c**) Axial T2W image shows a 3.0 cm homogenously hypointense mass in the left base of the PZ (arrows). Evidence of gross extra glandular extension with focal 7 to 8 mm extension at the left posterolateral aspect of the base into the region of the left neurovascular bundle (arrowhead). (**d**) Coronal T2W-hypointense tumor (arrow) extends across base of prostate into the adjacent inferior aspect of the left seminal vesicle (SVI, arrowhead)

of other features, such as restricted diffusion or corresponding T2W abnormality. The absence of early enhancement does not exclude clinically significant prostate cancer. The presence of early enhancement in the absence of a corresponding T2W hypointense or DWI signal abnormality can be seen in the setting of prostatitis [8]. Therefore, compared to T2W and DWI, DCE plays a minor role when assigning a PI-RADS score.

8.7 Staging of Prostate Cancer

The most widely used staging system for prostate cancer is the American Joint Committee on Cancer TNM system, which was last (eighth edition) published in 2016 and effective in 2018 [32]. The system is based on five components including anatomic (TNM) and clinical data, extent of the primary tumor (T category), lymph

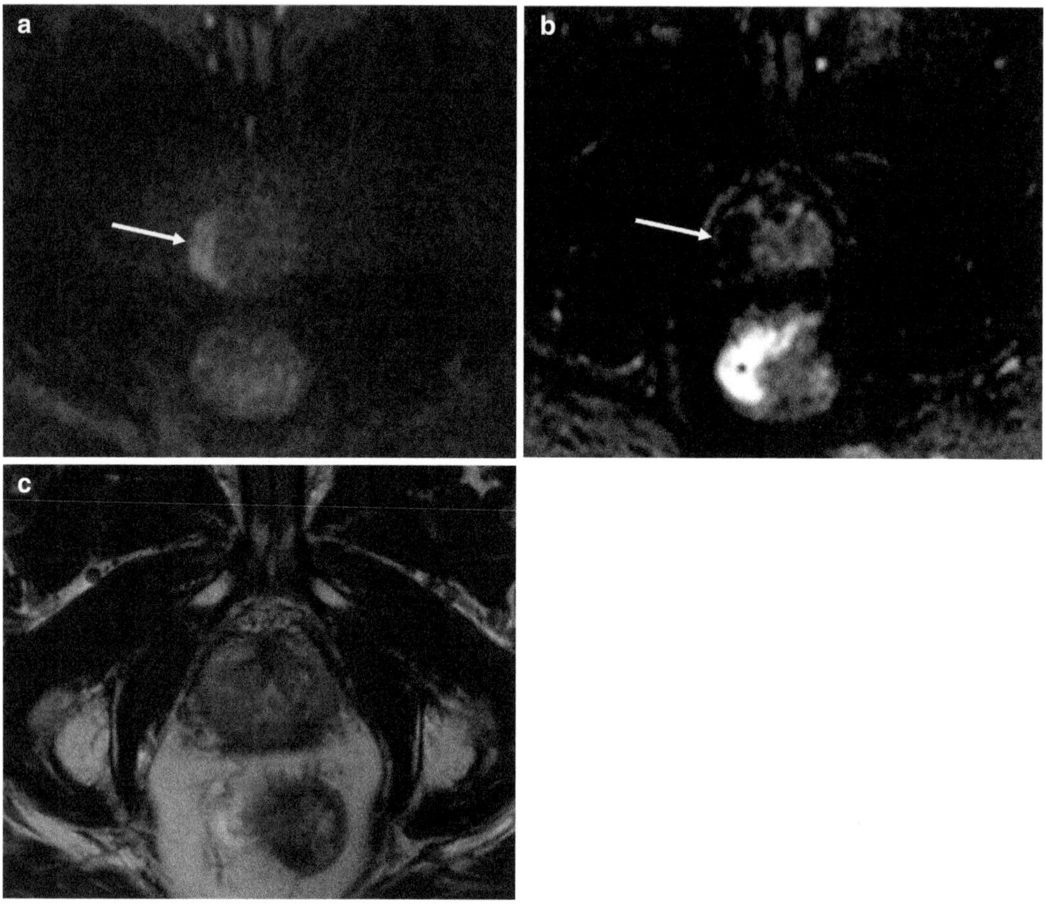

Fig. 8.6 (**a**) Axial DWI MR (b = 1400 s/mm^2) and (**b**) ADC map. Right mid gland lesion (arrows) has features of restricted diffusion indicative of clinically significant prostate cancer, 2.3 cm maximal dimension compatible with a PI-RADS 5. (**c**) Axial high-resolution T2W sequence shows T2-hypointense lesion in the right lateral mid gland. The lesion abuts the gland margin, but smoothly marginated, without features of gross extracapsular extension. Long interface with glandular margin (> 1.5 cm) in a cancer with significant restricted diffusion confers increased risk for extra glandular T3 tumor

node metastasis (N category), distant metastasis (M category), and PSA level at the time of diagnosis, Grade Group (based on Gleason score) that is determined by prostate biopsy [8, 32, 33]. MRI can provide pretreatment details on anatomic staging that help inform decision-making and is particularly useful in patients at higher risk for locally advanced disease based upon clinical factors.

8.8 Extra Prostatic Spread of Prostate Cancer

Prostate mpMRI is the most useful imaging method available to determine the T stage: prostate cancer confined to the gland (T2 disease) or extending outside the gland (T3 disease and greater). The high-spatial resolution T2-weighted acquisition images allow evaluation for features

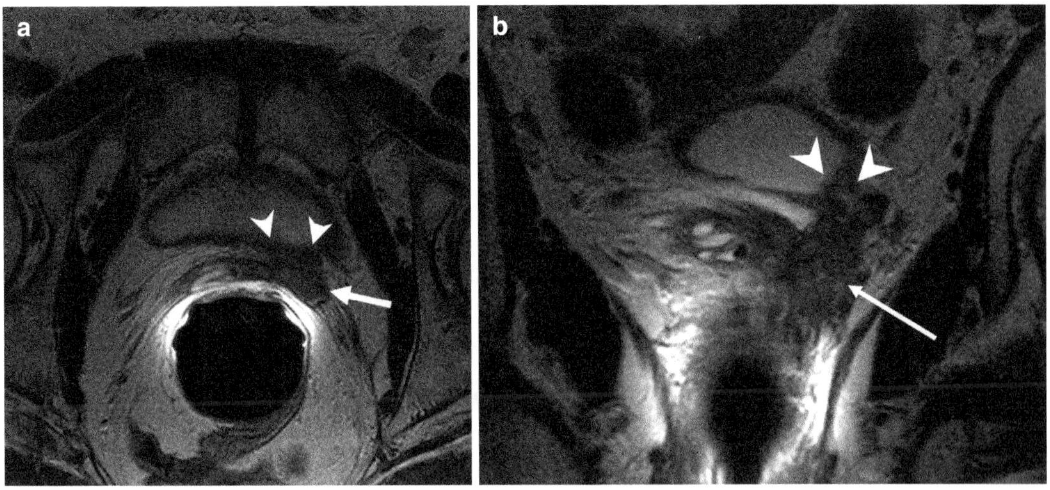

Fig. 8.7 Locally advanced cancer. Large clinically significant prostate cancer based on DWI (not shown) also shows T2-weighted imaging features of T3–T4 disease. (**a**) Trans axial image (performed with ERC) at level of seminal vesicles shows tumor infiltration of left seminal vesicle lumen (arrow) with extension anteriorly to involve urinary bladder wall (arrowheads). (**b**) Coronal T2W image same exam showing involvement of left seminal vesicle (arrow) and urinary bladder (arrow heads)

of extra prostatic extension, including evaluation of the neurovascular bundle, seminal vesicles, bladder neck, and apex.

The accuracy of local staging to determine organ confined versus extra prostatic disease has been widely studied. Contemporary meta-analysis of staging shows that MRI has a high specificity (around 90%) and low sensitivity (around 60%) for extra prostatic spread of cancer, when the standard of reference is histology from prostatectomy, with benefit from endorectal coil use for seminal vesical invasion determination [34]. The low sensitivity is due to the inability of MRI to show microscopic extra prostatic spread demonstrated on histology. Sensitivity appears improved by use of higher field strength and functional techniques to compliment T2-weighted imaging [34].

Table 8.1 Local staging features of extra prostatic disease on MRI

Features associated with extra prostatic extension
Asymmetry (or enlargement) of tumor-associated neurovascular bundle
Bulging of the tumor-associated prostate contour, including into recto-prostatic angle
Irregular/speculated tumor-associated external margin
Tumor interface along gland margin greater than 1.0 cm (or length of contact stratified risk)
Features of direct tumor extension to periprostatic tissues or structures
1. Bladder wall invasion
2. Rectal wall invasion
3. Apical periurethral invasion
Features associated with seminal vesicle invasion
Focal or diffuse T2W hypointense thickening of vesicle walls
Low T2W filling of vesicle lumen(s)
Contrast enhancement of above findings on T1WI, greater than unaffected parts
Positive DWI (low ADC signal and high b-value hyperintensity)
Direct gross tumor extension across the base or up the ducts and through central zone

8.8.1 MRI Features of Extra Prostatic Extension of Disease

Various features present on MRI prostate images have been described as signs of extra prostatic extension and seminal vesicle invasion (Table 8.1), and these signs have been variously assessed for utility, showing sporadic but generally effective results [5, 8, 17, 23, 35–37]. Combined signs are more powerful predictors of extra prostatic spread, so an EPE risk model using several features such as significant cancer (by MRI features) contact length along gland margin, focal bulging, and gross spread (by various associated observations) may ultimately result in a well-tested and widely adopted system of risk-based staging, especially when combined with clinical data from biopsy and PSA [36, 37]. The figures provided give examples of the features which should be reported as either direct evidence or risk-associated findings of local stage.

8.9 Adenopathy and Metastases

High-risk patients (>5% chance of for lymph node metastases) will generally undergo nodal staging. The most reliable staging method is lymph node dissection. However, it is invasive and positive lymph nodes can be found outside the routine and extended lymph node dissection templates [38]. The route of lymphatic spread of prostate cancer should be evaluated at imaging: common femoral, obturator, pararectal, presacral, external iliac, common iliac, paracaval, and para-aortic [8, 39]. At least one sequence for MRI should provide a field of view up to the level of aortic bifurcation. The evaluation and detection of metastatic involved lymph nodes on mpMRI is dependent on size, shape, and MRI features including heterogeneity, diffusion restriction, and enhancement pattern [39]. Size threshold for lymph nodes suspect for cancer involvement varies, with short axis used generally and greater sensitivities for lower thresholds of size and more specificity for greater threshold. A size threshold of 1.5 cm short axis for pelvic and retroperitoneal nodes is almost universally specific for metastatic involvement [38]. A traditional threshold for calling nodes suspect at MRI is 1.0 cm short axis for oval nodes, and 0.8 mm diameter for round nodes [40], while PI-RADS 2.1 uses 0.8 cm short axis as recommended threshold [8]. Lymph nodes of the inguinal region and bilateral common iliac chains are metastatic disease, while internal/external iliac, obturator, and perirectal nodes are regional.

Bone metastases appear as T1-weighted hypointense lesions replacing marrow or T2- heterogeneous versus T2 hyperintense (when fast saturation used) lesions. Bone metastases generally show restricted diffusion and are hyperintense on high b-value diffusion-weighted images [41] (Figs. 8.8 and 8.9).

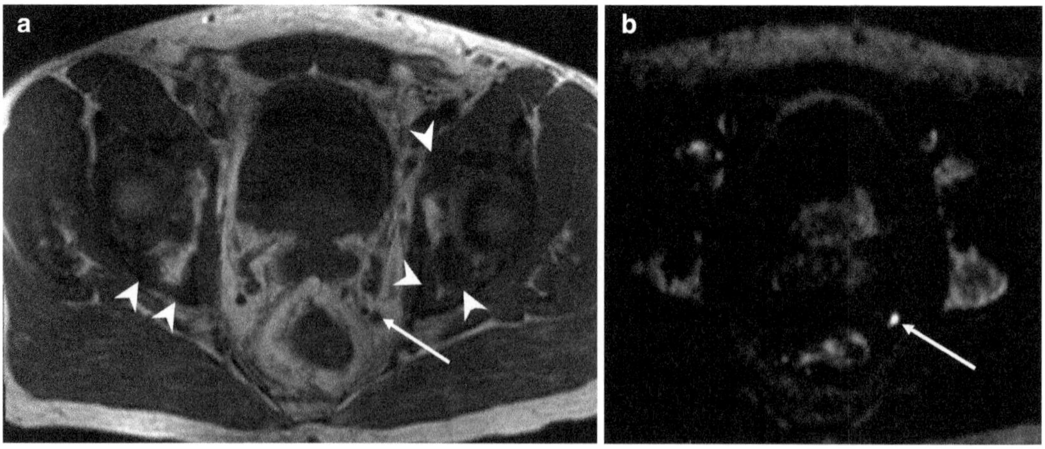

Fig. 8.8 Metastatic disease. (**a**) T1-weighted imaging of the pelvis shows multiple metastatic lesions to bone (arrowheads), appearing as T1-hypointense lesions replacing usually T1 hyperintense predominantly fatty marrow. (**b**) High b-value (b = 1400) diffusion-weighted axial image shows restricted diffusion at sites of osseous metastases. In addition, small left internal iliac node (arrows on Fig. 8.8a, b) shows restricted diffusion in excess of normal inguinal nodes, consistent with metastatic involvement

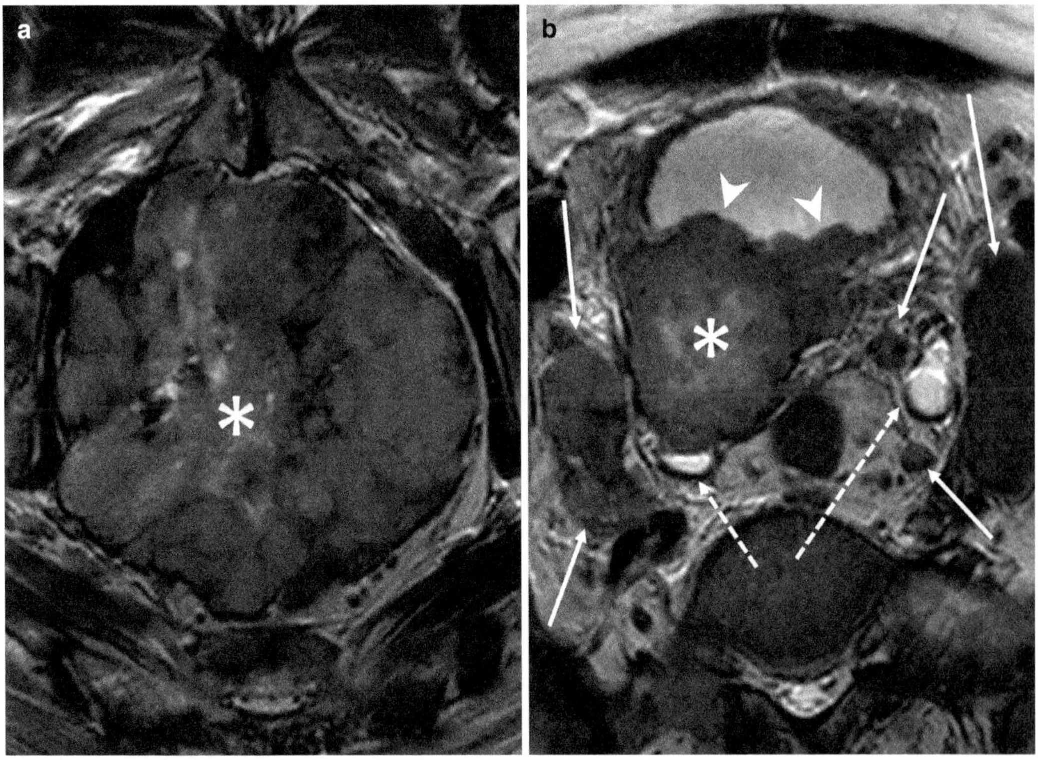

Fig. 8.9 Late-stage metastatic prostate cancer. (**a**) Trans axial T2-weighted image with large mass (asterisk) centered on the prostate with complete loss of internal zonal architecture, effacing surrounding structures. (**b**) Superior to Fig. 8.9a shows tumor involving bladder wall extensively (arrowheads), bilateral enlarged irregular and heterogeneous nodes (arrows), and bilateral obstructed ureters (dashed arrows). Low-signal heterogeneity of bone marrow also due to metastases

8.10 Summary

Multi-parametric prostate MRI is the best imaging method to determine the T stage of prostate cancer and differentiate between cancer confined to gland ($\leq$ T2 disease) and disease that extends beyond the gland ($\geq$T3). High-spatial resolution T2W imaging can demonstrate features of extra prostatic extension, including bulging of the prostate capsule, irregularity or speculated prostate margin, seminal vesicle invasion, or extension to surrounding structures, including involvement of neurovascular bundle. Pelvic and retroperitoneal lymph nodes can be evaluated for metastasis based on size, morphology, and MRI character. In the same setting, larger field of view images allow evaluation for metastases to nodes or bone.

Acknowledgment We are grateful for the assistance of Ms. Ruth Anne A. Bump, University of New Mexico, Department of Radiology, for her assistance with the creation of this chapter.

References

1. Cancer Facts & Figures. Atlanta: American Cancer Society; 2016. cited 2019 21 July 2019.
2. Soylu FN, Eggener S, Oto S. Local staging of prostate cancer with MRI. Diagn Interv Radiol. 2017;8:265–373.
3. Epstein JI, Partin AW, Potter SR, Walsh PC. Seminal vesicle invasion by prostate Cancer: prognostic significance and therapeutic implications. Urology. 2000;56(2):283–8.
4. Datta K, Muders M, Zhang H, Tindall DJ. Mechanism of lymph node metastasis in prostate cancer. Turkish J Urol. 2010;6(5):823–36.

5. Hricak H, Choyke PL, Eberhardt SC, Leibel SA, Scardino PT. Imaging prostate cancer: a multidisciplinary perspective. Radiology. 2007;243(1):28–53.
6. Kozikowski M, Malewski W, Michalak W, Dobruch J. Clinical utility of MRI in the decision-making process before radical prostatectomy: systematic review and meta-analysis. PLoS One. 2019;14(1):e0210194. https://doi.org/10.1371/journal.pone.0210194.
7. Hricak H, Wang L, Wei DC, Coakley FV, Akin O, Reuter VE, et al. The role of preoperative endorectal magnetic resonance imaging in the decision regarding whether to preserve or resect neurovascular bundles during radical retropubic prostatectomy. Cancer. 2004;100(12):2655–63.
8. Turkbey B, Rosenkrantz AB, Haider MA, Padhani AR, Villeirs G, Macura KJ, et al. Prostate Imaging Reporting and Data System Version 2.1: 2019 Update of Prostate Imaging Reporting and Data System Version 2. Eur Urol. 2019. pii: S0302-2838(19)30180–0.
9. Turkbey B, Merinio MJ, Gallardo EC, Shah V, Aras O, et al. Comparison of endorectal and non-endorectal coil T2W and diffusion-weighted MRI at 3 T for localizing prostate cancer: comparison with whole-mount histopathology. J Magn Reson Imaging. 2014;39(6):1443–8. https://doi.org/10.1002/jmri.24317.
10. Rosenkrantz AB, Kopec M, Kong X, Melamed J, Dakwar G, Babb JS, et al. Prostate cancer vs. post-biopsy hemorrhage: diagnosis with T2- and diffusion-weighted imaging. J Magn Reson Imaging. 2010;31(6):1387–94.
11. Park KK, Lee SH, LIm BJ, Kim JH, Chung BH. The effects of the period between biopsy and diffusion-weighted magnetic resonance imaging on cancer staging in localized prostate cancer. BJU Int. 2010;106:1148–51.
12. Wagner M, Rief M, Busch J, Scheuring C, Taupitz M, et al. Effect of butylscopolamine on image quality in MRI of the prostate. Clin Radiol. 2012;65:460–5.
13. Loy CT, Irwig L. Accuracy of diagnostic tests read with and without clinical information: a systematic review. JAMA. 2004;292(13):1602–9.
14. Dhingsa R, Qayyum A, Coakley FV, Lu Y, Jones KD, Swanson MG, et al. Prostate cancer localization with endorectal MR imaging and MR spectroscopic imaging: effect of clinical data on reader accuracy. Radiology. 2004;230(1):215–20.
15. Chen N, Zhou Q. The evolving Gleason grading system. Chin J Cancer Res. 2016;28(1):58–64. https://doi.org/10.3978/j.issn.1000-9604.2016.02.04.
16. Epstein JI, Zelefsky MJ, Sjoberg DD, Nelson JB, Egevad L, Magi-Galluzzi C, et al. A contemporary prostate cancer grading system: a validated alternative to the Gleason score. Eur Urol. 2016;69(3):428–35.
17. Baco E, Rud E, Vlatkovic L, Svindland A, Eggesbø HB, Hung AJ, et al. Predictive value of magnetic resonance imaging determined tumor contact length for extra-capsular extension of prostate cancer. J Urol. 2015;193:466–72.
18. Noguchi M, Stamey TA, NEAL JE, Yemoto CE. An analysis of 148 consecutive transition zone cancers: clinical and histological characteristics. J Urol. 2000;163(6):1751–5.
19. Vargas HA, Akin O, Franiel T, Goldman DA, Udo K, Touijer KA, et al. Normal central zone of the prostate and central zone involvement by prostate cancer: clinical and MR imaging implications. Radiology. 2012;262:894–902.
20. Costello AJ, Brooks M, Cole OJ. Anatomical studies of the neurovascular bundle and cavernosal nerves. BJU Int. 2004;94(7):1071–6.
21. Villers A, McNeal JE, Redwine EA, Freiha FS, Stamey TA. The role of perineural space invasion in the local spread of prostatic adenocarcinoma. J Urol. 1989;142(3):763–8.
22. Geary ES, Dendinger TE, Freiha FS, Stamey TA. Nerve sparing radical prostatectomy: a different view. J Urol. 1995;154(1):145–9.
23. Yu KK, Hricak H, Alagappan R, Chernoff DM, Bacchetti P, Zaloudek CJ. Detection of extracapsular extension of prostate carcinoma with endorectal and phased-array coil MR imaging: multivariate feature analysis. Radiology. 1997;202(3):697–702.
24. Akin O, Sala E, Moskowitz CS, Kuroiwa K, Ishill NM, Pucar D, et al. Transition zone prostate cancers: features, detection, localization, and staging at endorectal MR imaging. Radiology. 2006;239(3):784–92.
25. McNeal JE. Cancer volume and site of origin of adenocarcinoma in the prostate: relationship to local and distant spread. Hum Pathol. 1992;23(3):258–66.
26. Radtke JP, Boxler S, Kuru TH, Wolf MB, Alt CD, Popeneciu IV, et al. Improved detection of anterior fibromuscular stroma and transition zone prostate cancer using biparametric and multiparametric MRI with MRI-targeted biopsy and MRI-US fusion guidance. Prostate Cancer Prostatic Dis. 2015;18(3):288.
27. Bouyé S, Potiron E, Puech P, Leroy X, Lemaitre L, Villers A. Transition zone and anterior stromal prostate cancers: zone of origin and intraprostatic patterns of spread at histopathology. Prostate. 2009;69(1):105–13.
28. Shah O, Melamed J, Lepor H. Analysis of apical soft tissue margins during radical retropubic prostatectomy. J Urol. 2001;165(6 Part 1):1943–9.
29. Tamada T, Prabhu V, Li J, Babb JS, Taneja SS, Rosenkrantz AB. Prostate cancer: diffusion-weighted MR imaging for detection and assessment of aggressive – comparison between conventional and kurtosis models. Genitourinary Imaging. 2017;284(1):100–8.
30. Malayeri AA, El Khouli RH, Zaheer A, Jacobs MA, Corona-Villalobos PC, Kamel IR, Macura KJ. Principles and applications of diffusion-weighted imaging in cancer detection, staging, and treatment follow-up. Radiographics. 2011;31(6):1773–91. https://doi.org/10.1148/rg.316115515.
31. Ream JM, Doshi AM, Dunst D, Parikh N, Kong MX, Babb JS, et al. Dynamic contrast-enhanced MRI of the prostate: an intraindividual assessment of the effect of temporal resolution on qualitative detection and quan-

titative analysis of histopathologically proven prostate cancer. J Magn Reson Imaging. 2017;45:1464–75.
32. Buyyounouski MK, Choyke PL, McKenney JK, Sartor O, Sandler HM, Amin MB, Kattan MW, Lin DW. Prostate cancer–major changes in the American joint committee on Cancer eighth edition cancer staging manual. CA Cancer J Clin. 2017;67(3):245–53.
33. Xiao WJ, Zhu Y, Dai B, Ye DW. Evaluation of clinical staging of the American joint committee on cancers (eighth edition) for prostate cancer. World J Urol. 2018;36(5):769–74.
34. de Rooij M, Hamoen EH, Witjes JA, Barentsz JO, Rovers MM. Accuracy of magnetic resonance imaging for local staging of prostate cancer: a diagnostic meta-analysis. Eur Urol. 2016;70(2):233–45.
35. Grivas N, Hinnen K, de Jong J, Heemsbergen W, Moonen L, Witteveen T, et al. Seminal vesicle invasion on multi-parametric magnetic resonance imaging: correlation with histopathology. Eur J Radiol. 2018;98:107–12.
36. Boesen L, Chabanova E, Løgager V, Balslev I, Mikines K, Thomsen HS. Prostate cancer staging with extracapsular extension risk scoring using multiparametric MRI: a correlation with histopathology. Eur Radiol. 2015;25(6):1776–85.
37. Mehralivand S, Shih JH, Harmon S, Smith C, Bloom J, Czarniecki M, et al. A grading system for the assessment of risk of extraprostatic extension of prostate cancer at multiparametric MRI. Radiology. 2019;290(3):709–19.
38. Hövels AM, Heesakkers RA, Adang EM, Jager GJ, Strum S, Hoogeveen YL, et al. The diagnostic accuracy of CT and MRI in the staging of pelvic lymph nodes in patients with prostate cancer: a meta-analysis. Clin Radiol. 2008;63(4):387–95. https://doi.org/10.1016/j.crad.2007.05.022.
39. Thoeny HC, Froeliich JM, Triantafyllou M, Huesler J, Bains LJ, et al. Metastases in normal-sized pelvic lymph nodes: detection with diffusion-weighted MR imaging. Radiology. 2014;273:125–35.
40. Jager GJ, Barentsz JO, Oosterhof GO, Witjes JA, Ruijs SJ. Pelvic adenopathy in prostatic and urinary bladder carcinoma: MR imaging with a three-dimensional TI-weighted magnetization-prepared-rapid gradient-echo sequence. AJR Am J Roentgenol. 1996;167(6):1503–7.
41. Messiou C, Collins DJ, Giles S, De Bono JS, Bianchini D, de Souza NM. Assessing response in bone metastases in prostate cancer with diffusion weighted MRI. Eur Radiol. 2011;21(10):2169–77.

9 Post-processing of Prostate MRI

Mehmet Coskun and Baris Turkbey

9.1 Introduction

Multiparametric prostate magnetic resonance imaging (mpMRI) is based on three basic pulse sequences: three-plane T2-weighted imaging (T2WI), diffusion-weighted imaging (DWI), and dynamic contrast imaging (DCE). The minimum technical parameters of these three sequences are detailed in the prostate imaging reporting and data system (PI-RADS) versions 2 (v2) and 2.1 (v2.1) [1, 2]. In PI-RADS scoring, all three sequences should be evaluated together. All three sequences need to be obtained in the same geometric plane and with the same cross-section thickness [3]. Such an approach will allow synchronous assessment of T2WI, DWI, and DCE. Synchronized evaluation is critical for accurate localization of the lesion. Accurate description of the lesion location is also necessary for the success of the intervention such as biopsy or focal therapy. In this chapter, we will describe how to do post-processing of prostate MRI and basic reporting requirements for accurate prostate biopsy guidance.

9.2 Minimum Requirement of the Prostate MRI Report

The PI-RADS document described the assessment and reporting of mpMRI in detail [2]. Especially for the standardization of reporting in the active surveillance patients, the panel of Prostate Cancer Radiological Estimation of Change in Sequential Evaluation (PRECISE) presented a series of recommendations in the assessment of mpMRI [4]. According to these two important documents, the prostate MRI report should include prostate-specific antigen (PSA) information and prostate volume. It is useful to specify the PSA density (PSAd) using the formula of PSA/prostate volume. Describing the localization of the lesions is very critical. It is recommended to report maximum number of four lesions. Index lesion, which is highest likelihood of clinically significant cancer (CSC), should be specified as the first lesion [2].

The report should include magnet strength, coil usage, date of scan, and report. PI-RADS scores and maximum diameter of the lesions should be given. In likelihood of CSC and extraprostatic extension, TNM stage can be reported. Reporting the index lesion size using absolute values at

M. Coskun
Health Science University Dr. Behçet Uz Child Disease and Surgery Training and Research Hospital, Department of Radiology, Izmir, Turkey

B. Turkbey (✉)
National Cancer Institute (NIH), Center of Cancer Research, Molecular Imaging Program, Bethesda, MD, USA
e-mail: turkbeyi@mail.nih.gov

T. Tirkes (ed.), *Prostate MRI Essentials*, https://doi.org/10.1007/978-3-030-45935-2_9

baseline and at each subsequent MRI was recommended. The radiologists should assess the likelihood of true change over time (i.e., change in size or change in lesion characteristics on one or more sequences) on a 1–5 scale. There was an agreement and consensus on the use of the Gleason score in active surveillance when reporting of the lesion sampled before. Increase in size, becoming visible on DWI (significant progression), appearance of extracapsular extension, seminal vesicle involvement, or bone metastasis (definite progression) were the criteria which could state radiologic progression [4]. All these criteria and suggestions should be considered in assessment and reporting of the mpMRI.

9.2.1 Lesion Localization and Measurement

Prostate cancer is usually multifocal. The aim of prostate MRI is to detect CSC. Although there is no clear consensus on identification of CSC, Gleason ≥3 + 4, volume ≥ 0.5 cc, and extraprostatic extension tumors were defined as CSC in the PI-RADS document [2].

The prostate MRI tends to underestimate tumor volume. PZ lesions' diameter should be measured on apparent diffusion coefficient (ADC) maps, while TZ lesions' dimension should be measured on T2WI. The PI-RADS v2 proposed that if lesion measurement is difficult or compromised on ADC (for PZ) or T2W (for TZ), measurement should be made on the sequence that shows the lesion best. Lesion size should be measured on axial slices. It can also be evaluated on coronal or sagittal plane if it has larger dimension on coronal or sagittal plane [2].

The size can be measured using volume (by manual planimetry or calculated from three diameters), by biaxial measurement of maximum diameters on an axial slice, or by a single measurement of maximum diameter [2]. The authors of PRECISE panel underlined that there is no definite consensus about measurement of lesion's diameter or volume, but a single diameter may be more reproducible than a volume [4]. The PI-RADS was recommended that the minimum requirement is to report the largest dimension, but alternatively volume may be automatically calculated using a software or manually calculated using ellipse formula [2]. Free-handed volume of interest (VOI) can be used in volume determination. The lesion can be marked with region of interest (ROI) on each slice; 3D volume rendering and volume measurement can be made on workstation (Fig. 9.1).

The sequence and slice number of the lesion with maximum diameter should be indicated in the report. According to PRECISE, a single-axis measurement of a lesion on a functional sequence (e.g., high b-value images) is more reproducible than volume [4]. The PI-RADS proposed that PZ lesions should be measured from ADC, while TZ lesions should be measured from T2WI [2]. Axial T2WI sequence has the highest resolution in mpMRI, and anatomic details are evaluated in T2WI such as neurovas-

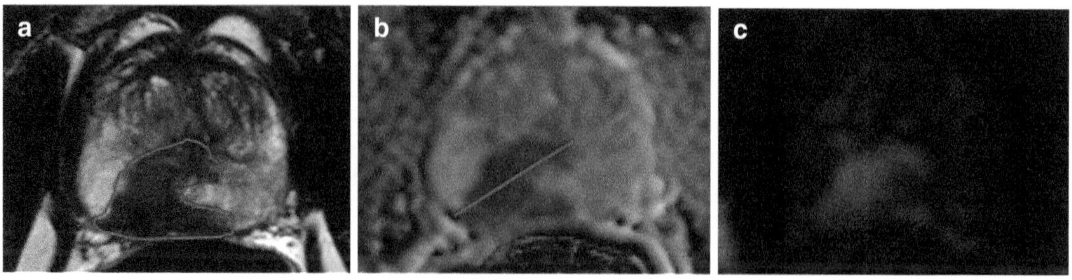

Fig. 9.1 Volume calculation vs single measurement of Gleason 4 + 4 lesion. (**a**) Volume determination with VOI on T2WI (4 ml), (**b**) single maximum diameter on ADC (2 cm), the lesion is also visible on b = 2000s/mm^2 DW MRI (**c**).

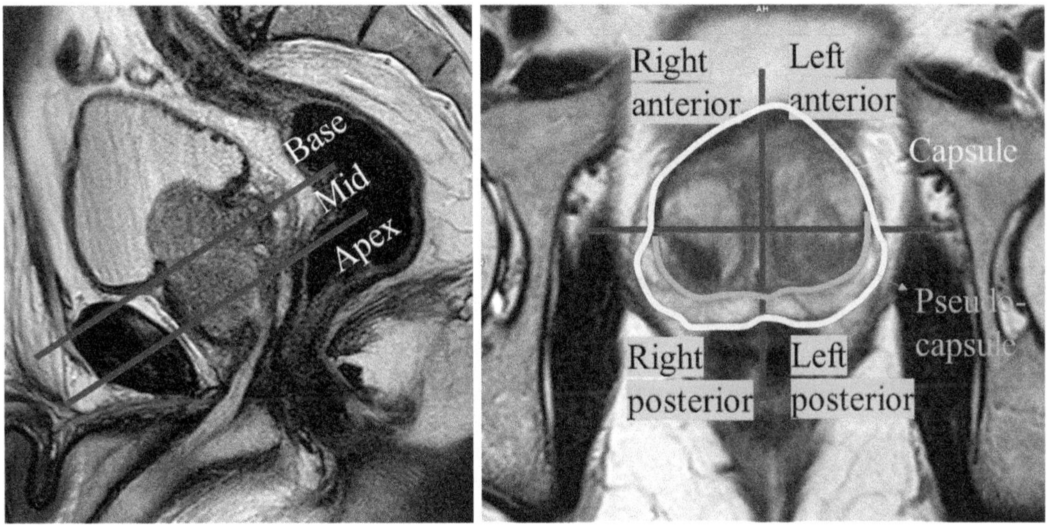

Fig. 9.2 Radiological anatomy of the prostate

cular bundle thickening. Also, extraprostatic extension and differentiation of benign prostate nodules (BPH) and cancer nodules should be assessed on T2WI. Nevertheless, it is somewhat confusing that the measurement was suggested on functional sequences in which spatial resolution is inferior than T2WI. In a study, it is emphasized that the addition of DWI MRI significantly improves the accuracy of prostate tumor volume measurements when compared with T2-weighted MRI alone [5]. It may be more appropriate that the measurement can be done on axial T2WI and providing the largest single dimension since it has highest spatial resolution. However, if DWI provides extra information, both T2WI and DWI can be evaluated together.

Accurate reporting of the lesion's location is critically important. A detailed description of zonal localization was described in the PI-RADS document in Appendix 2 with a title of sector map [2]. In PI-RADS v2.1, the revised sector map contains two additional sectors in the base PZ: right and left posterior PZ medial. With this revision, there are now 38 prostate sectors, plus 2 sectors for the seminal vesicles and 1 for the membranous urethra, amounting to a total 41 sectors [1]. Practically, the prostate is divided into right/left on axial images by the center (prostatic urethra) and into anterior/posterior by a horizontal line through the middle of the gland. The gland also subdivided the TZ and the PZ by pseudocapsule (sometimes referred to as the "surgical capsule). In sagittal plane, it is subdivided into three sections: base, mid, and apex (Fig. 9.2) [2]. So, three-plane evaluation should be the basic principle in proper localization of the lesions.

The central zone is a bandlike tissue around ejaculatory ductus at the base. It exhibits decreased T2 and ADC signal, and it can show diffusion restriction and mimic a tumor in some cases. Coronal T2WI should be used in the evaluation of the central zone [1, 2, 6]. Normal central zone is seen as symmetric triangular-shaped appearance on coronal T2WI (Fig. 9.3). In the presence of asymmetry, the probability of tumor increases. The central zone's symmetry on either side of the midline and classic location surrounding the ejaculatory ducts are helpful features in its proper identification [6]. Less than 5% of prostate cancers arise within central zone [7].

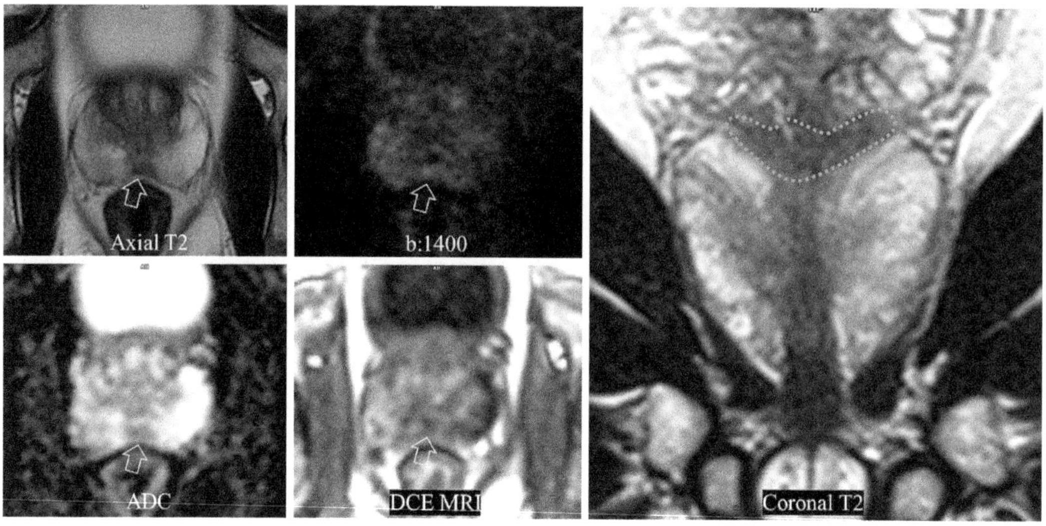

Fig. 9.3 Normal central gland is mimicking a tumor on axial slices. It is triangular symmetric central gland typically located around ejaculatory ducts (blue dash)

9.3 Post-processing of MRI for Targeted Biopsy

MRI data can be utilized in many ways for guiding prostate biopsies. Currently defined techniques include cognitive, in-bore, and TRUS/MRI fusion-guided techniques [8]. Among those, the TRUS/MRI fusion-guided technique requires many steps with MRI data post-processing. These steps can sometimes be tedious and require a consistent and careful approach for a successful MRI-guided biopsy result. The basic steps for post-processing are volumetric segmentation of the prostate gland from the entire imaging field of view, target lesion delineation within the prostate gland, and proper labelling/communication of these detected and delineated target lesions. It should be noted that almost all of the platforms utilize axial T2W images for biopsy guidance since they offer the highest spatial resolution with intraprostatic anatomic details. Therefore, the post-processing for biopsy guidance should be conducted on axial T2W images.

9.3.1 Volume Assessment and Segmentation

Prostate volume should be calculated and reported in all patients. Volume is used to calculate PSAd which can be used as a marker of aggressive cancers. The volume is directly related to the severity of BPH, and change in prostate volume is a more objective measure of BPH treatment [9].

There are some different options to assess volume of the prostate. The basic one is digital rectal examination and is often inaccurate; therefore measurements from US and MRI would be very helpful information. In transabdominal/transrectal US or MRI, triplanar measurements are used to calculate the prostate volume using the ellipsoid formula [9, 10]:

$$\text{Volume} = [\text{maximum AP diameter}] \times [\text{maximum transverse diameter}] \times [\text{maximum longitudinal diameter}] \times 0.52.$$

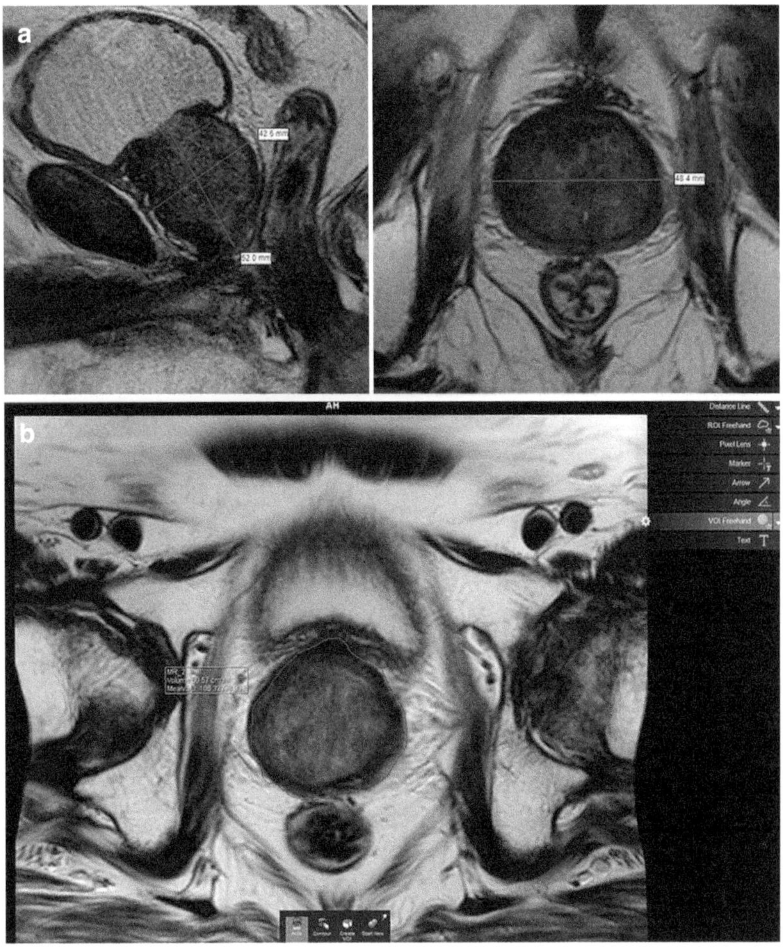

Fig. 9.4 Volume measurement (**a**) using ellipse formula (48 × 43 × 52 mm × 0.52 = 56 ml) on sagittal and axial T2W MRI and (**b**) VOI manually (61 ml) on axial T2W MRI. Radical prostatectomy specimen including seminal vesicles was 67 g

This formula assumes that the object has a regular ovoid shape. In fact, prostate is a cone-shaped rather than ellipsoid, and it has usually eccentrically enlarged median lobe which is not accounted by the ellipsoid formula [10]. The ellipsoid formula method is simple, rapid, and cost-effective, but it may cause inaccurate results as mentioned above. Besides, at least two planes of T2WI were required for this measurement [2].

The other option in the assessment of the prostate volume is segmentation method. It can be done manually, semi-, or full automatically. In manual segmentation, prostate capsule is manually traced in each or desired plane (mostly axial plane) on T2WI [9, 10]. On the workstation, region of interest is selected (ROI), or volume of interest (VOI) is selected, and the capsule is contoured on each slice manually. The computer integrates the slices and calculates the prostate volume, and 3D images are generated. This is an effective but time-consuming and may take up to 10–15 min per patient. This method is also referred to as manual planimetry (Fig. 9.4).

To overcome the inefficiency and subjectivity of planimetry, semiautomated and fully automated segmentation softwares have been developed [9, 10]. Automated segmentation algorithms overcome the limitations imposed by the complexity of shapes and images through the use of shape and appearance models that serve to automatically detect the margin of the prostate [11]. Automated procedures relieve radiologists from time-consuming manual segmentation while maintaining high levels of accuracy and reproducibility, equal to or even greater than those of the manual method [12]. Semiautomated programs still require some manual user input especially at the interface of the prostate with the rectum, which is difficult for most algorithms. In fully automated segmentation, different models used to draw prostate contour with the help of intensity difference, appearance, shape, and topology information of the individual prostate subregion [9, 10]. It does not need any manual input and seems to be more objective.

In a study comparing the ellipsoid formula, manual and fully automated segmentation methods, Pearson correlation coefficients were found to be 0.86–0.90, 0.89–0.91, and 0.88–0.91, respectively. All three methods had a comparable accuracy for estimating the radical prostatectomy volumes [10]. Segmentation methods had some advantages over ellipsoid formula since their end product can be used in fusing the MRI to other modalities such as ultrasound for biopsy or PET for diagnosis. Such segmentations can also be used in focal ablation therapies [9, 10].

9.3.2 Target Lesion Segmentation

A detailed definition of the localization of the intraprostatic lesions is extremely important. Five regions including apical, apical-mid, mid, mid-base, and base can be more accurately defined using the midsagittal plane. The anterior half can be described as anterior gland, and the rest is simply posterior gland. It should be specified as right vs left with reference to the midline. It should also be reported whether the lesion is localized in the TZ, PZ, or both. There is no need to add "posterior" if it is localized in the PZ [2]. However, definition of "anterior" is usually needed for the lesion located in the TZ. Biopsy can be performed more effectively by accurate and consistent specification of the lesion location and its relation to specific landmarks of the prostate such as capsule, urethra, etc.

9.4 Conclusion

Proper post-processing of the prostate MRI is penultimate step in which a diagnostic radiologist directs an MRI-guided fusion biopsy. Segmentation of the prostate and contouring of the target lesion are critical for accurate biopsy guidance. The contour should be drawn on axial T2WI using the free-handed ROI drawing tool. This will appear as target to the physician who will perform the biopsy. Axial T2WI has the highest spatial resolution and is more accurate for localization of the lesion; nevertheless utilization of multi-plane images will increase our accuracy. We should also be aware of partial volume effects which can be detected using three-plane assessment. Finally, trying to add as much information from DWI and DCE will increase accuracy.

References

1. Turkbey B, Rosenkrantz A, Haider M, Padhani A, Villeirs G, Macura K, et al. Prostate imaging reporting and data system version 2.1: 2019 update of prostate imaging reporting and data system version 2. Eur Urol. 2019;76(3):340–51. https://doi.org/10.1016/j.eururo.2019.02.033.
2. Weinreb J, Barentsz J, Choyke P, Cornud F, Haider M, Macura K, et al. PI-RADS prostate imaging – reporting and data system: 2015, version 2. Eur Urol. 2016;69(1):16–40. https://doi.org/10.1016/j.eururo.2015.08.052.
3. Turkbey B, Brown A, Sankineni S, Wood B, Pinto P, Choyke P. Multiparametric prostate magnetic resonance imaging in the evaluation of prostate cancer. CA Cancer J Clin. 2015;66(4):326–36. https://doi.org/10.3322/caac.21333.
4. Moore C, Giganti F, Albertsen P, Allen C, Bangma C, Briganti A, et al. Reporting magnetic resonance imaging in men on active surveillance for prostate Cancer: the PRECISE recommendations—a report of a European School of Oncology task force. Eur Urol. 2017;71(4):648–55. https://doi.org/10.1016/j.eururo.2016.06.011.
5. Mazaheri Y, Hricak H, Fine S, Akin O, Shukla-Dave A, Ishill N, et al. Prostate tumor volume measurement with combined T2-weighted imaging and diffusion-weighted MR: correlation with pathologic tumor volume. Radiology. 2009;252(2):449–57. https://doi.org/10.1148/radiol.2523081423.
6. Rosenkrantz A, Taneja S. Radiologist, be aware: ten pitfalls that confound the interpretation of multiparametric prostate MRI. Am J Roentgenol. 2014;202(1):109–20. https://doi.org/10.2214/AJR.13.10699.
7. Vargas H, Akin O, Franiel T, Goldman D, Udo K, Touijer K, et al. Normal central zone of the prostate and central zone involvement by prostate Cancer: clinical and MR imaging implications. Radiology. 2012;262(3):894–902. https://doi.org/10.1148/radiol.11110663.

8. Mertan F, Berman R, Szajek K, Pinto P, Choyke P, Turkbey B. Evaluating the role of mpMRI in prostate Cancer assessment. Expert Rev Med Devices. 2016;13(2):129–41. https://doi.org/10.1586/17434440.2016.1134311.
9. Garvey B, Türkbey B, Truong H, Bernardo M, Periaswamy S, Choyke PL. Clinical value of prostate segmentation and volume determination on MRI in benign prostatic hyperplasia. Diagn Interv Radiol. 2014;20(3):229–33. https://doi.org/10.5152/dir.2014.13322.
10. Turkbey B, Fotin S, Huang R, Yin Y, Daar D, Aras O, et al. Fully automated prostate segmentation on MRI: comparison with manual segmentation methods and specimen volumes. Am J Roentgenol. 2013;201(5):W720–9. https://doi.org/10.2214/AJR.12.9712.
11. Martin S, Troccaz J, Daanenc V. Automated segmentation of the prostate in 3D MR images using a probabilistic atlas and a spatially constrained deformable model. Med Phys. 2010;37(4):1579–90. https://doi.org/10.1118/1.3315367.
12. Pasquier D, Lacornerie T, Vermandel M, Rousseau J, Lartigau E, Betrouni N. Automatic segmentation of pelvic structures from magnetic resonance images for prostate cancer radiotherapy. Int J Radiat Oncol Biol Phys. 2007;68(2):592–600. https://doi.org/10.1016/j.ijrobp.2007.02.005.

MRI-Guided In-Bore and MRI-Targeted US (Fusion) Biopsy

10

Melina Hosseiny and Steven S. Raman

10.1 Introduction

Systematic transrectal ultrasound-guided biopsy (TRUS bx) of prostate has been regarded as the standard of care for sampling prostate in men with clinical suspicion of prostate cancer (PCa), mainly based on the increased prostate-specific antigen (PSA) or abnormal digital rectal exam (DRE).

While the traditional goal of TRUS bx was cancer detection, the contemporary goal of targeted prostate biopsy is to maximize the detection rate of clinically significant prostate cancer (csPCa) (Gleason score (GS) $\geq$ 7 or Gleason group (GG) $\geq$ 2) and minimize the detection of clinically insignificant cancer (low-volume cancer with Gleason group 1). Long-term cohort studies have shown that patients with low-grade, clinically insignificant prostate cancers do not benefit from invasive therapy, because cancer-related mortality in this subgroup of patients was similar to patients on active surveillance, while they show higher rates of morbidity [1, 2]. Traditional TRUS bx, adopted widely since 1986, has several drawbacks. First, it is a random sampling of the peripheral, posterior half of the prostate gland and may miss clinically significant foci of PCa located outside the biopsy zones. Transition zone and anterior region lesions are often missed on systematic TRUS bx. Out of 121 anterior PCa lesion in the study of Volkin et al., 48.7% would have been missed by TRUS bx alone [3]. Second, it is associated with an unfavorably high detection of low-grade PCa. Third, TRUS bx underestimates PCa grade and leads to error rates in up to 49% in patients on active surveillance [4]. Fourth, the risk of bleeding and infection/sepsis is up to 5% in men undergoing TRUS bx. Other strategies such as transperineal-ultrasound biopsy (TPUS bx) also have these limitations. Overall, despite the simplicity and widespread availability of TRUS bx, the nontargeted nature of the technique undersamples csPCa and oversamples clinically insignificant PCa.

The accuracy of prostate imaging for detection of PCa has significantly increased with the advances in multiparametric MRI (mpMRI) hardware, imaging sequences, and postprocessing software [5]. A standardized method has been developed to increase inter-reader reliability for interpretation of prostate mpMRI. Based in part on prior published single-center scoring systems (e.g., UCLA score, NIH score), the Prostate Imaging-Reporting and Data System (PIRADS) was introduced in 2012 with ongoing updates (PIRADS v2 and v2.1) [6, 7]. The PRECISION trial, a multicenter, randomized trial of 500 men, suggested

M. Hosseiny · S. S. Raman (✉)
Ronald Reagan UCLA Medical Center, Department of Radiology: Abdominal Imaging and Cross Sectional IR, Los Angeles, CA, USA
e-mail: mhosseiny@ucla.edu; sraman@mednet.ucla.edu

T. Tirkes (ed.), *Prostate MRI Essentials*, https://doi.org/10.1007/978-3-030-45935-2_10

that initial assessment with mpMRI and MR-US fusion biopsy (MRUS-Fbx) of MR-positive lesions resulted in 12% increase in detection of csPCa and 13% decrease in detection of clinically insignificant cancers, compared to systematic TRUS bx alone. A retrospective review of 4259 individuals [8] who underwent mpMRI between January 2012 and December 2017 showed that biopsy was precluded in 53% of individuals at risk by using PIRADS assessment scoring. csPCa diagnosis-free survival was 99.6% after 3 years in this group of individuals. The PROMIS study, which was a paired-cohort confirmatory study [9], showed that mpMRI has higher sensitivity and negative predictive value for the detection of clinically significant PCa, compared to TRUS bx. A high negative predictive value is important because a negative mpMRI result would assure that csPCa would be highly unlikely, potentially precluding biopsy in many individuals at risk. The PROMIS study indicated that targeted biopsy in individuals with suspicious mpMRI could potentially avoid biopsy in up to 25% of men at risk. The study reported that targeted biopsy can improve the detection of clinically significant PCa with significant reduction in the number of diagnosed clinically insignificant cancer.

Various strategies for performing MR-targeted biopsy of prostate have been proposed without an absolute consensus on the preferred method. Overall, MR-targeted biopsy might be performed via three approaches including MRUS-Fbx, cognitive guidance (MRUS-Cbx), and direct in-bore MR-guided biopsy (IBMR-Bx). MRUS-Fbx strategy fuses previously acquired MRI data with the real-time TRUS or TPUS images on the day of biopsy. In the MRUS-Cbx, the operator mentally maps the previously acquired MR target on the real-time TRUS or TPUS biopsy images, thus "cognitively fusing" and approximating the MRI target on the real-time US image and guiding the needle to this location. Finally, the IBMR-Bx can be performed using transrectal (TR), transperineal (TP), or transgluteal (TG) approaches with a direct in-bore approach while patient is lying in the MR gantry.

Both MRUS-Fbx and MRUS-Cbx use pre-acquired MRI-based suspicious targets (PIRADS 3–5), while IBMR-Bx uses these pre-acquired targets supplemented by real-time anatomic (T2-weighted) and functional (diffusion-weighted) MR images during biopsy of suspicious targets. A number of studies have shown the significantly higher detection of clinically significant disease with lower required biopsy cores in MR-targeted methods compared to TRUS bx. A systematic review of 43 studies on MR-targeted biopsy of prostate found that omitting TRUS bx would result in missing 10% of csPCa and 50% of clinically insignificant cancers [10].

10.2 MRI-Ultrasound Fusion Biopsy

10.2.1 Biopsy Technique

Prior to a TRUS-bx procedure, the patient is instructed to eat a low-residue diet and undergo a bowel preparation on the day prior to biopsy to ensure no fecal matter remains in the rectum. Transperineal approach doesn't require bowel preparation. MRUS-Fbx using either the TRUS or TPUS route essentially converts a systematic partial organ sampling procedure into a targeted biopsy of suspicious MRI foci with or without systematic TRUS bx. After obtaining either 3-Tesla or 1.5-Tesla mpMRI of the prostate, the outline of the prostate gland and the suspicious targets is contoured on T2-weighted images using one of several automated, semiautomated, or manual software programs (e.g., DynaCAD (InVivo Inc., Gainesville Fl), Profuse ((Artemis Inc., Grass Valley, Ca), SyngoVIA (Siemens Healthineers), Osirix (Osirix)) that enables contouring of the whole gland and individual suspicious lesions. The data is then transferred to one of several MRUS-Fbx platforms (UroNav, Artemis, Koelis, etc.). To perform the TRUS bx, the patient is placed in lateral decubitus position on the operating table. An anesthetic gel (e.g., lidocaine) is administered into the rectum to reduce pain during TRUS probe manipulation. A 2D TRUS probe is then inserted into the rectum to perform an ultrasound sweep, which captures small slices of the prostate. These slices are sent to the fusion platform to generate a 3D segmented model of the prostate. For TPUS biopsy, the patient lies supine with anesthetic gel injected bilaterally to anesthetize the pudendal nerves [11]. The perineum is imaged with a needle guide attached to the probe, and the images are sent to the fusion platform. The vendor-specific software then co-registers ultrasound images on the previously acquired segmented MR images by fusing the contours of the prostate [12, 13]. The platform will create a live "tracking" guidance for prostate biopsy. The platforms for software-assisted MR-ultrasound fusion prostate biopsy mainly differ by the type of image registration, the needle tracking method, and the biopsy approach (TP vs. TR) (Fig. 10.1).

10.2.1.1 Image Registration

Image registration can be either rigid or nonrigid (elastic). In rigid image registration, mpMRI images are superimposed on TRUS or TPUS images without considering the possible prostate deformation by position difference between mpMRI and ultrasound (e.g., supine position for mpMRI and TPUS biopsy vs. left lateral decubitus position for TRUS), ultrasound probe pressure, or possible patient movement. In the elastic image registration, the deformation of prostate by biopsy probe adjusted, and therefore elastic registration supposed to be a more accurate method with the elimination of the residual cognitive fusion for targeting the lesion. Several FDA-approved devices such as Artemis (Eigen, Grass Valley, CA) and UroNav (Philips-InVivo, Gainesville, FL) use a combined elastic and rigid registration. A systematic review by Venderink et al. [15] pooled the results of studies, which compared the performance of MRUS-Fbx to systematic TRUS bx, including 11 studies with elastic and 10 studies with rigid image registration techniques. Venderink et al. reported OR of 1.45 (95% CI: 1.21–1.73, $p < 0.0001$) and 1.40 (95% CI: 1.13–1.75; $p = 0.002$) for elastic and rigid registration subgroups, respectively. They did not find any superiority for either image registration method to detect PCa (P: 0.19) and csPCa (P: 0.83).

10.2.1.2 Transrectal vs. Transperineal Approach

MR-ultrasound fusion-targeted biopsy may be used via the TR or TP approaches. As stated, the incidence of infection, rectal bleeding, and septic shock is reportedly much lower using a TP approach [16] as compared to the dominant TR approach (up to 5% compared to near 0%) [17]. Reasons include tracking of inadequately treated fecal bacteria into the bloodstream or bacterial resistance to ciprofloxacin during biopsy [17]. A comparison between TRUS and TPUS biopsy

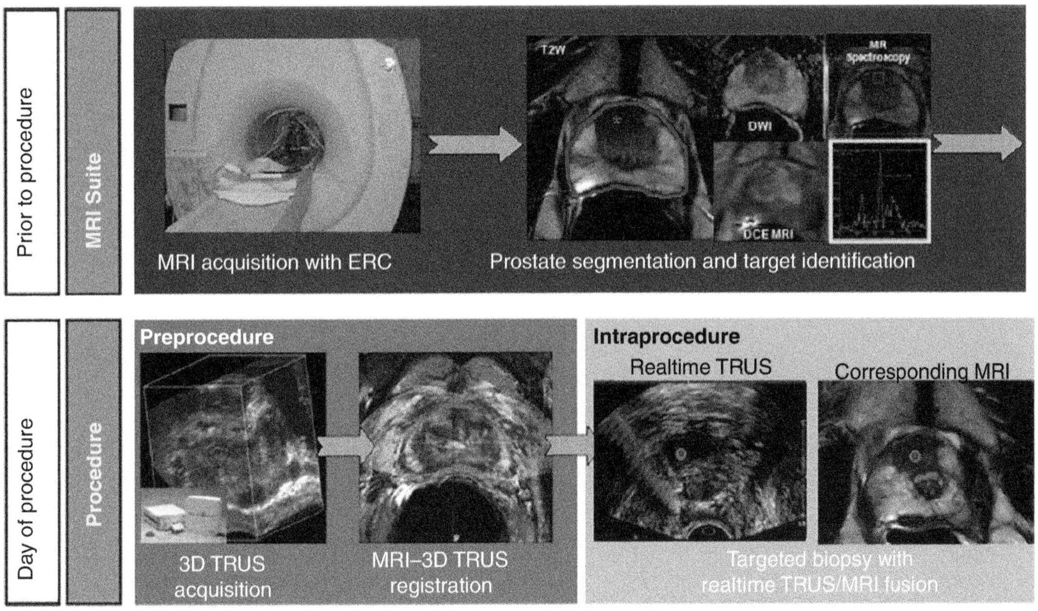

Fig. 10.1 Steps required to obtain an MR-ultrasound fusion-guided biopsy. *ERC* endorectal coil, *T2W* T2 weighted, *DWI* diffusion-weighted imaging, *DCE* dynamic contrast enhanced, *TRUS* transrectal ultrasound, *3D* three dimensional. (Reprinted from Siddiqui et al. [14], with permission from Elsevier)

showed similar minor complication rates for hematuria, lower urinary tract symptoms, and dysuria, while TRUS was associated with significantly higher rate of infection and rectal bleeding [18]. A drawback of TPUS guidance is that it is significantly more painful than TRUS guidance, and, therefore, it requires a pudendal block or spinal anesthesia but can also easily performed under local anesthesia in an outpatient setting [11]. Moreover, TRUS approach is more likely to miss the anterior prostate lesions [19].

10.2.1.3 Fusion Platforms

A number of commercially available platforms have been developed for performing MRUS-Fbx of prostate. These platforms differ based on the needle tracking system (e.g., electromagnetic tracking, position-encoded joints tracking, and image-based software tracking), type of ultrasound probe, the biopsy route, and image registration method [20]. Several examples of common commercially available systems are outlined below.

1. *UroNav (Philips/InVivo, Gainesville, Fl)*: The first and currently the most common MRUS-Fbx platforms for prostate sampling, UroNav uses a passive electromagnetic field generator, similar to global positioning system (GPS), to track the motion of TRUS probe on previously acquired axial MR imaging (Fig. 10.2). This platform allows elastic and rigid image registration and enables freehand ultrasound for prostate biopsy [21]. Another feature of the platform is its documentation of the biopsy location for future reference, to enable repeat biopsy from previous positive targets. The tracking error of this platform is approximately 2–3 mm on average but can be much larger due to many factors. Siddiqui et al. detected 30% more csPCa detection by UroNav device compared to systematic TRUS bx [22].
2. *Artemis (Eigen)*: One of the first commercially available MRUS-Fbx platforms, Artemis uses a fixed mechanical arm to TRUS probe with embedded angle-sensing encoders, which track the position of the probe and needle. This system immobilizes the probe from target acquisition to firing the probe. Similar to UroNav, Artemis utilizes both rigid and nonrigid image registration and has also the advantage of recording the biopsy site for potential future sampling (Fig. 10.3). Studies with this device have shown that PCa detection was three times more likely with Artemis MRUS fusion platform compared to systematic TRUS bx, with 38% of csPCA which were detected only on MRUS-FBx and not on TRUS bx [23].
3. *Urostation (Koelis)*: Widely used in Europe and the United States, this MRUS-Fbx platform uses a TRUS-TRUS registration tracking in which fusion of 3D ultrasound images with previously acquired MRI is performed and then biopsy is taken. Immediately after biopsy, an additional 3D TRUS is obtained to retrospectively determine the accuracy of biopsy needle position (Fig. 10.4). Unlike other fusion biopsy devices, this platform does not provide real-time prospective targeting but enables an automatic TRUS probe rotation and elastic image registration [24]. Mozer et al. showed significantly higher csPCa detection rate (43% vs. 37%), higher csPCa core positivity rate (31% vs. 7.5%), and higher positive cores length (8 mm vs. 4 mm) using Urostation MRUS-Fbx, compared to systematic TRUS bx [25].
4. *HI-RVS/Real-time Virtual Sonography (Hitachi) and Virtual Navigator (Esaote)*: Similar to UroNav, these platforms use a freehand TRUS probe with electromagnetic tracking sensors, enable only rigid image registration. Target delineation can only be performed after MR images are transferred into fusion platform. HI-RVS platform has the advantage of utilizing both TR and TP approaches [20].
5. *BioJet (GeoScan Medical)*: This system is also based on a position-encoded mechanical arm. This platform uses rigid registration and allows for both transrectal and transperineal biopsies. Using this MRUS-Fbx platform, Shoji et al. identified 79% of csPCa using a whole-mount histopathology (WMHP) as reference standard [26].
6. *BiopSee (PiMedical/ MedCom)*: This is a fusion platform for performing TP fusion

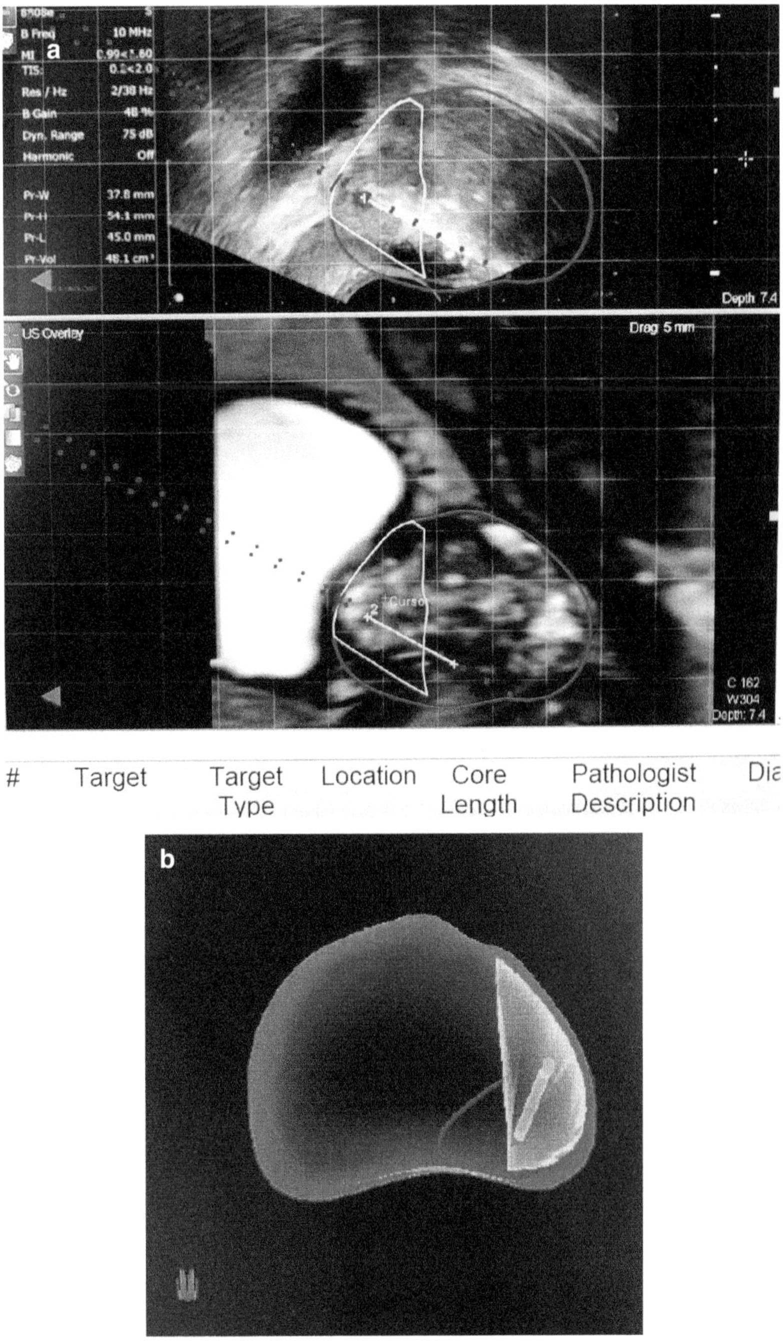

Fig. 10.2 Transrectal MRUS fusion biopsy using UroNav platform. (**a**) The snapshot shows the operator view while performing the procedure with overlay of ultrasound image (upper) and previously acquired MRI (lower). (**b**) This platform allows elastic image registration and freehand manipulation of ultrasound probe. The yellow line shows the position of the biopsy needle. (Image courtesy of Allan J. Pantuck, MD, UCLA Institute of Urologic Oncology, Department of Urology, UCLA)

biopsy. TRUS probe is mounted on a stepper that is fixed to the operating table. A grid mounted on the mechanical stepper is used to place the biopsy needles. In a study of 120 patients who underwent MRUS-Fbx using BiopSee, 79% of csPCa was detected with WMHP correlation [27].

10.2.2 Current Opinions on MRUS Fusion Biopsy

Several studies have found that MRUS-Fbx increases the detection rate of csPCa and decreases the detection of clinically insignificant PCa, compared to systematic TRUS bx. The ability of this

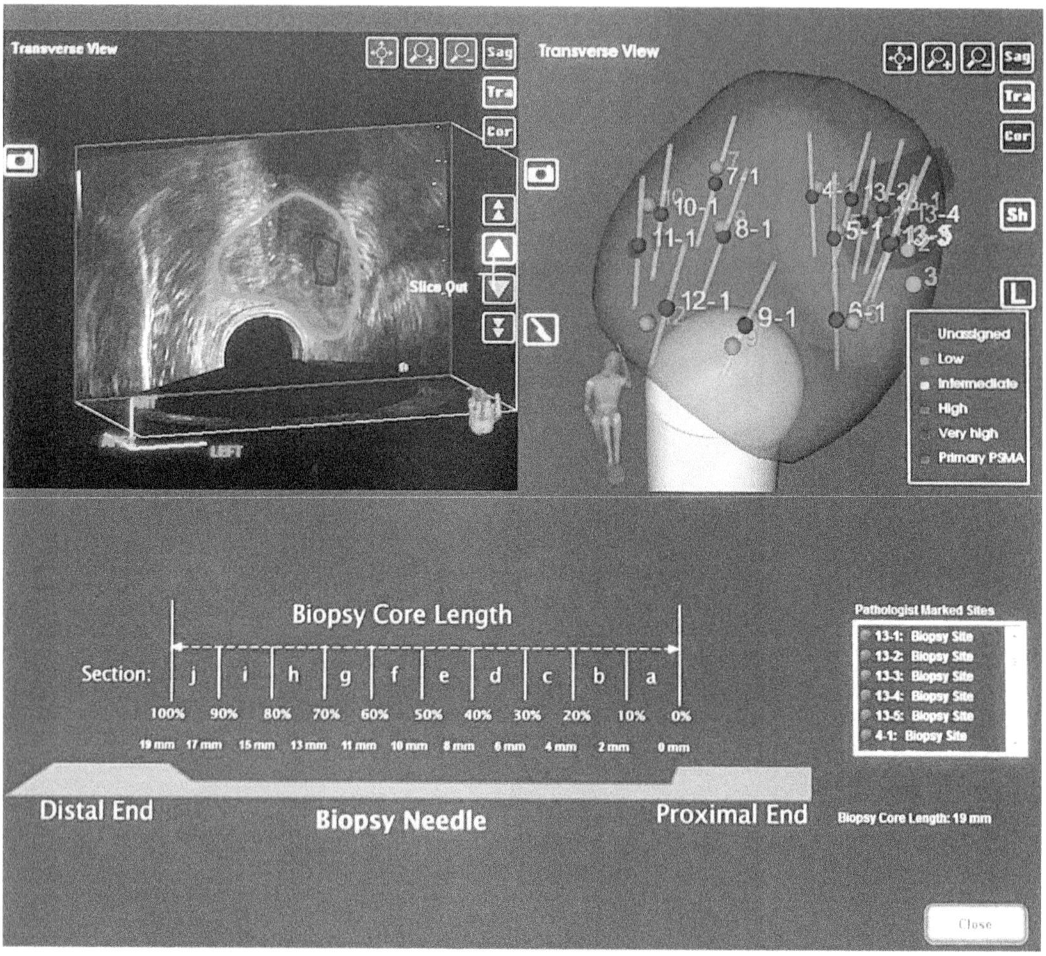

Fig. 10.3 A longitudinal view of the output from Artemis fusion platform. The target lesions are volume-rendered, while the lines show the biopsy needle positions. The center of the biopsy needle where the cores were obtained is indicated by blue and purple dots, while the green dots represent the location of the acquired systematic biopsy sites. (Image courtesy of Leonard S. Marks, MD, Clark Urology Center, UCLA)

technique to register MRI to TRUS images leads to a targeted sampling of the most suspicious PCa foci and thus improves yields for csPCa and risk stratification of PCa. In a head-to-head comparison of TRUS bx and Urostation MRUS-Fbx in 582 men, Siddiqui et al. found that adding MRUS-Fbx to TRUS bx yielded a 67% increase in the detection of high-grade (GS $\geq 4 + 3$) PCa and upgraded GS in 32% of men compared to systematic TRUS bx alone [22]. Wu et al. were the first to perform a meta-analysis on all MRUS-Fbx studies dating prior to August 2015 [29]. In their study of 3105 individuals from 16 paired cohort studies, MRUS fusion biopsy detected more csPCa (RR: 1.19, $P < 0.05$) and less clinically insignificant cancers (RR: 0.68, $P < 0.01$), compared to systematic TRUS bx. In addition, significantly higher core positivity percentage was achieved by MRUS-Fbx compared to TRUS bx (26.6% vs. 10.2%, RR: 2.75, $P < 0.01$).

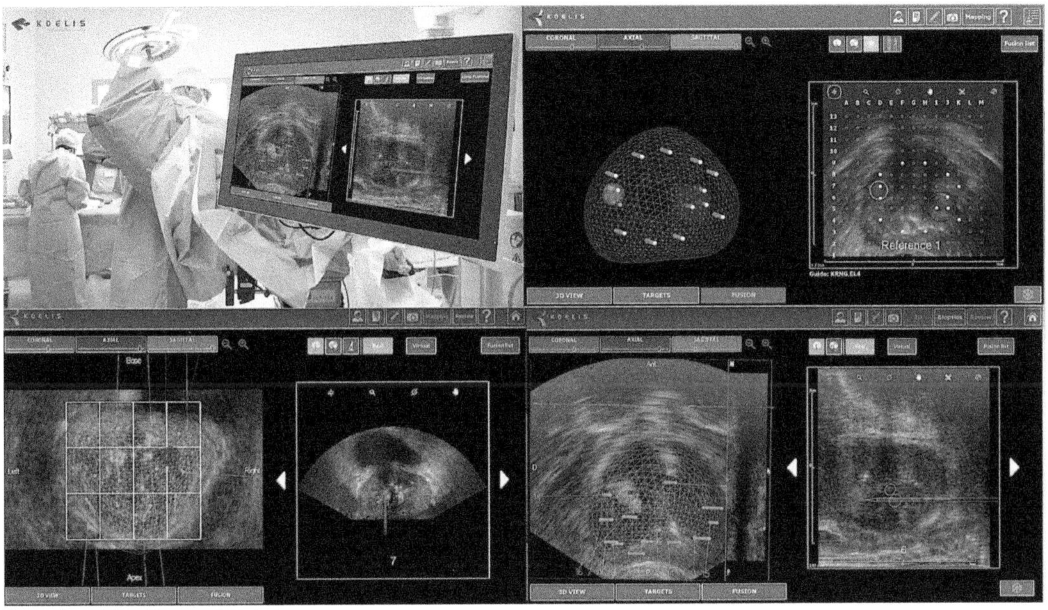

Fig. 10.4 Operator view while performing MRUS fusion biopsy using Urostation (Koelis) platform. The grid planning and the operator view in transrectal and transperineal biopsy approaches are shown. (Adapted and reprinted with permission from Koelis Academy. https://Koelis.Academy [28])

Eliminating the TRUS bx remains somewhat controversial despite the high negative predictive value of multiparametric prostate MRI. Some investigators have suggested combining systematic and targeted biopsies would result in enhanced detection of prostate cancer. PAIREDCAP, a paired cohort study [30], which recruited 300 biopsy-naïve men to undergo three sets of biopsy at the same setting including systematic, MRUS-Fbx (Artemis) and MRUS-Cbx, reported detection of csPCa ranging from 15% in MR-negative to 70% in MR-positive individuals.

MRUS-Fbx has been shown to improve selection of patients for active surveillance (AS). In a study of 113 AS patients, an mpMRI and MRUS-Fbx resulted in reclassification of the disease grade in 36% of patients [31]. As many as 21% of all PCa lesions are found in the anterior region of the prostate gland which are usually more challenging and often missed in physical examination and systematic TRUS bx. Puech et al. found twice as many csPCa detection in anterior of prostate gland by MRUS-Fbx, compared to systematic TRUS bx [32]. Volkin et al. performed 12-core systematic TRUS biopsy and MRUS-FBx in all 241 suspected anterior lesions on prostate mpMRI and found that overall 50.2% (121/241) of targets were positive for PCa, of which 62 (25.7%) were positive on systematic TRUS biopsy, while 97 (40.2%) were positive on MRUS-FBx. (P: 0.001) [3]. Overall, 59 PCa lesions (48.7%) would have been missed on systematic TRUS bx alone, of which 34 were GS $\geq 3 + 4$.

The quality of the MRUS-Fbx of prostate and the final outcome depends on several important steps including optimal MRI acquisition, MRI interpretation by an experienced radiologist, standard sweep ultrasound of the prostate to construct a 3D prostate volume, fusion platform accuracy, and the expertise of the physician performing the fusion biopsy [33]. Structured training of the new users in tertiary centers and courses at international meeting are encouraged to ensure the quality of the procedure.

10.3 Cognitive MR-Guided Biopsy of Prostate

Cognitive or so-called visual MRUS biopsy is the simplest method for targeted biopsy of prostate, as it does not require the sophisticated equipment required for MRUS-FBx and IBMR-Bx. In MRUS-Cbx, the operator reviews the pre-acquired MRI data prior and mentally registers the PIRADS score 3–5 targets to their approximate location on US (apex, midgland or base, anterior or posterior, transitional or peripheral gland). The registered MRUS-Cbx target is usually a hypoechoic nodule or an area with some degree of contrast to the surrounding tissue; however, the visualized target on MRI might not be simply recognized on MRUS-Cbx in some individuals [34]. Current evidence suggest that this visual-targeted technique detects a higher number of PCa lesions, compared to systematic TRUS bx [35]. This technique, however, is highly dependent in the operator expertise, without any tracking or guidance system, making it highly susceptible to human error. Overall, studies have not shown a definite superiority for MRUS-Fbx over MRUS-Cbx for detection of csPCa, although some studies have shown a trend toward improved PCa detection with MRUS-Fbx comparted to MRUS-Cbx. A study of 50 individuals who underwent MRUS-Cbx and MRUS-Fbx showed that the detection rate of csPCa was slightly but not significantly higher for MRUS-Fbx (52% vs. 43% at target level, p: 0.24) [36]. In a cohort of 231 patients who underwent either MRUS-Fbx or MRUS-Cbx, Oberlin et al. showed that MRUS-Fbx detected significantly more lesions (48% vs. 35%, p:0.04), with a nonsignificant increased rate of csPCa (61.5% vs. 48%, p:0.07) [37]. In contrast, in an analysis of a cohort of 391 individuals, both elastic and rigid fusion-targeted techniques were superior to MRUS-Cbx for detection of high-grade PCa [38]. Overall, MRUS cognitive biopsy is the cheapest MR-guided biopsy technique and is the most compatible method for performing prostate biopsy in an office setting. As with other MR-targeted techniques, the quality of communication between the radiologist who interpreted the MRI and the one who performs the biopsy would increase the accuracy of this technique [34].

10.4 In-Bore MR-Guided Biopsy of Prostate

Direct in-bore MR-guided biopsy (IBMR-Bx) of prostate allows within-gantry sampling of prostate. This technique has several advantages. First, MR images are acquired during biopsy with T2- and diffusion-weighted imaging to ensure that the previously noted findings are reproducible. Occasionally sampling may be obviated if MR findings of prostatitis resolve. Second, it is the only technique that ensures MR confirmation of the needle within an MR target. All other techniques are based on approximations. Third, IBMR-Bx usually requires less obtained cores for diagnosis of PCa since oversampling is not required for diagnosis. Finally, IBMR-Bx is versatile and may be performed via TR, TP, or TG routes. Relative drawbacks of the technique include its limited availability relative to MRUS fusion or MRUS cognitive biopsies. Second, the procedure may be more time-consuming at some centers with a median procedure time of 25–68 min. Third, it may be more costly than MRUS-Fbx or MRUS-Cbx.

This technique requires obtaining and interpreting mpMRI images before biopsy planning to identify suspicious targets as with other MR-guided biopsy techniques. IBMR-Bx may be performed with an open- or closed-bore scanner with a commercially available MR-compatible biopsy device (DynaTRIM, Philips-InVivo, Gainesville, Fl). Biopsy localization DynaCAD software is used to identify the target and guide adjustment of the biopsy device in three planes to accurately place the needle within the lesion. On the day of the procedure, patients are placed in prone position in the scanner table, and T2-weighted and DWI sequences are performed to localize the lesion (10–12 min) and transfer this data to the DynaCAD workstation to enable lesion localization for biopsy coordinates (5 min). Individual targets are selected on the workstation with three unique coordinates for each target in anteroposterior, left-to-right, and craniocaudal directions. These coordinates are then adjusted in the biopsy device to keep the proper alignment between the needle guide and the target. After obtaining the appropriate coordinates, the biopsy device with the needle guide is adjusted accordingly, and then a repeat T2-weighted sequence is acquired to confirm appropriate needle guide placement, followed by further manual adjustments of the needle guide as necessary, to allow lesion sampling and sampling of additional targets (15–30 min). During the procedure, patients may move in and out of the gantry several times to confirm needle position within targets and for confirmation of the additional targets. The cycle is repeated to ensure the needle guide orientation toward the desired target (Fig. 10.5). In addition, after obtaining biopsy cores, another confirmatory MR image is acquired. An MR-compatible

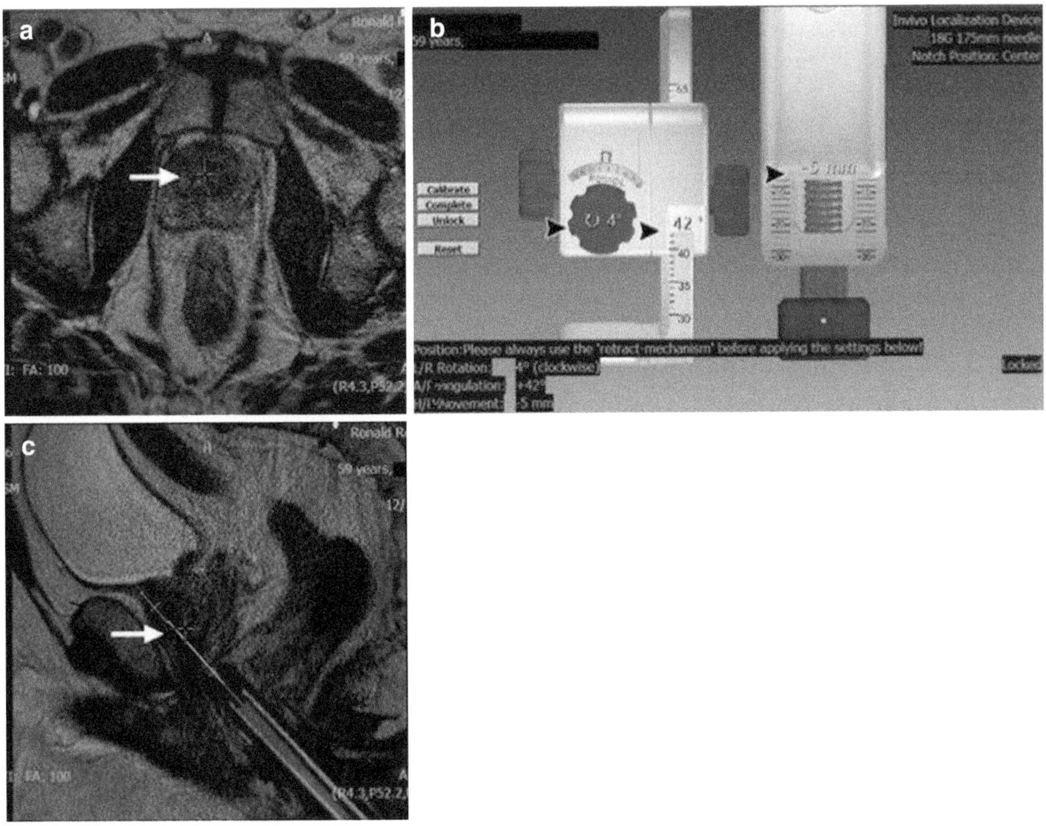

Fig. 10.5 DynaTRIM device (InVivo-Philips, Gainesville, Fl) for performing in-bore MR-guided biopsy of prostate. The workstation allows localization of the target during biopsy procedure (**a**), with target coordinations, adjusted on the dial (arrowhead on **b**) and finally biopsy needle position confirmation within the desired target (Arrow on **c**). (Adapted and reprinted from Tan et al. [41], with permission from Radiological Society of North America (RSNA))

robotic devices have also been be developed and undergone US FDA clearance to assist this procedure [39].

The procedure might be carried out through TR, TP, and TG approaches using intravenous conscious sedation (with midazolam and fentanyl) with the TR route being the most commonly used. The TP route allows a freehand use of the needle and carries a much lower risk of sepsis and rectal bleeding, compared to TR route, as discussed earlier. A TP approach, moreover, is helpful in individuals with history of previous rectal surgery, anal stricture, or perianal disease. A TG route is used in patients with a surgically resected rectum or with anal stricture and may better access to prostate apex.

Overall, in-bore MR-guided biopsy is a safe procedure with rare occurrence of serious complications. Transient hematuria and short-term rectal bleeding may occur in 1–4% of patients. Urinary retention and urosepsis may also occur in up to 2% of patients [40].

10.4.1 Current Opinions on In-Bore MR-Guided Biopsy

In single and multicenter series, IBMR-Bx has detected significantly more csPCa along with a significantly less low-grade PCa compared to systematic TRUS bx with a higher core positivity rate compared to all other targeted techniques. Application of mpMRI and IBMR-Bx of MR-positive lesions can reduce the need for biopsy up to 51% [42]. A systematic review on ten studies dating since 2013 found median PCa and csPCa detection rate of 42% and 81–93%, respectively, for IBMR-Bx [40]. In an update on the review of 23 IBMR-Bx cohorts dated back to mid-2018 [43], csPCa detection rate was 63% among 2632 individuals, much higher than PCa and csPCa detection rates of 30–50% and 10–40% for systematic TRUS bx [44]. In a head-to-head comparative study, van der Leest et al. [45] examined the efficacy of MRI with subsequent MR-guided biopsy against TRUS bx for the diagnosis of prostate cancer in 626 biopsy-naïve men. They found that the MRI pathway leads to avoidance of biopsy in half of individuals, 11% reduction in the number of clinically insignificant PCa and 89% less biopsy cores for diagnosis of PCa. Hambrock et al. also reported that IBMR-Bx cores predicted final Gleason grade at RP in 88% of individuals, much higher than the 55% RP correlation rate of 10-core TRUS bx [46].

The role of IBMR-Bx for the detection of csPCa has been reported in three distinct populations including:

1. Biopsy-naïve individuals with high suspicion of PCa
2. Individuals with high suspicion of csPCa despite a history of prior negative TRUS-guided biopsy
3. Individuals with known low-grade PCa under active surveillance

Current guidelines recommend performing mpMRI when suspicion for PCa remains high after a negative systematic TRUS biopsy, followed by MR-targeted biopsy of the suspicious lesions. A single study of patients with elevated PSA and repeat negative TRUS biopsy found PCa detection rate of 59% by IBMR-Bx. The results showed a significantly better performance for IBMR-Bx over TRUS bx for PCa detection of except in individuals with very high suspicion (PSA > 20 ng/ml, prostate volume > 65 cc, PSAD<0.15, or > 0.5015–0.5 ng/ml/cc), in whom the yield of both techniques was comparable [47]. Pokorny et al. reported the PCa and csPCa detection rate of 60% and 81% in individuals with prior negative prostate biopsy [43]. In one of the largest multicenter IBMR-Bx series of 461 patients to date, Felker et al. [4] reported a PCa and csPCa detection rate of 51% and 65%, suggesting that both biopsy-naïve patients and patients with history of negative TRUS bx can benefit from IBMR-Bx. Felker et al. also found that Gleason

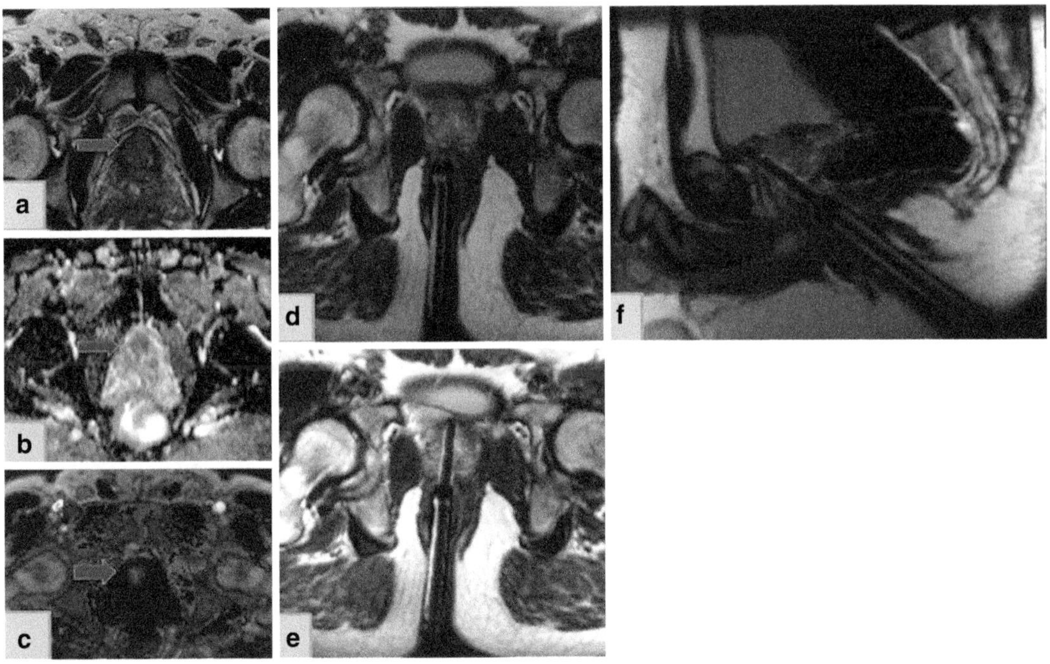

Fig. 10.6 Multiparametric MRI (using a 3-Tesla scanner) of a 65-year-old man with suspicious rise in PSA despite having a negative TRUS bx 6 months ago shows a moderately hypointense lesion on T2-weighted image (**a**) with obscured margins, located in anterior transitional zone. Marked signal hypointensity (407 mic^2/s) is noted on ADC image (**b**). Early and intense focal enhancement and washout was seen on dynamic contrast-enhanced images, shown as increased exchange constant in pharmacokinetic map for K-trans (**c**). Overall PIRADS v2.1 score of 5/5 was assigned. In-bore transrectal MRGB (**d, e, f**) was performed with the specimen showing clinically significant PCa (GS: 4 + 3)

grade was upgraded in 49% of patients under AS. Moreover, they reconfirmed that PIRADS assessment categories of 3, 4, and 5 correlated with csPCa detection rates of 10%, 43%, and 84%, respectively. Another large single-center IBMR-Bx on 475 targets in 379 individuals found an overall PCa of 69.1% and csPCa detection rate of 36.8%, 52.8%, and 50.7% in prior negative TRUS bx patients, biopsy-naïve patients, and active surveillance patients. PIRADSv2.1 score significantly correlated with PCa and csPCa detection (OR: 3.97 and 1.41, respectively) (Figs. 10.6, 10.7, and 10.8).

The yield of IBMR-Bx for PCa and csPCa has been similar in both transition (TZ) and peripheral (PZ) zone targets [41, 48]. This is in contrast with TRUS-bx results, in which 70% of positive lesions come from PZ. The anterior and transitional zones are not sampled in a systematic 12-core TRUS bx, and PCa in these areas is more likely to be undetected on TRUS bx.

10.5 IBMR-Bx vs. MRUS-Fbx

Both IBMR-Bx biopsy and MRUS-Fbx have higher spatial resolution and have the notable advantage of documenting the target location before biopsy, compared to systematic TRUS bx. Both techniques are safe and have similar complication rate to TRUS bx. Both techniques require extra training of the operator (e.g., radiologist, urologist) and staff. Detection rates of PCa and csPCa by targeted techniques have been shown to

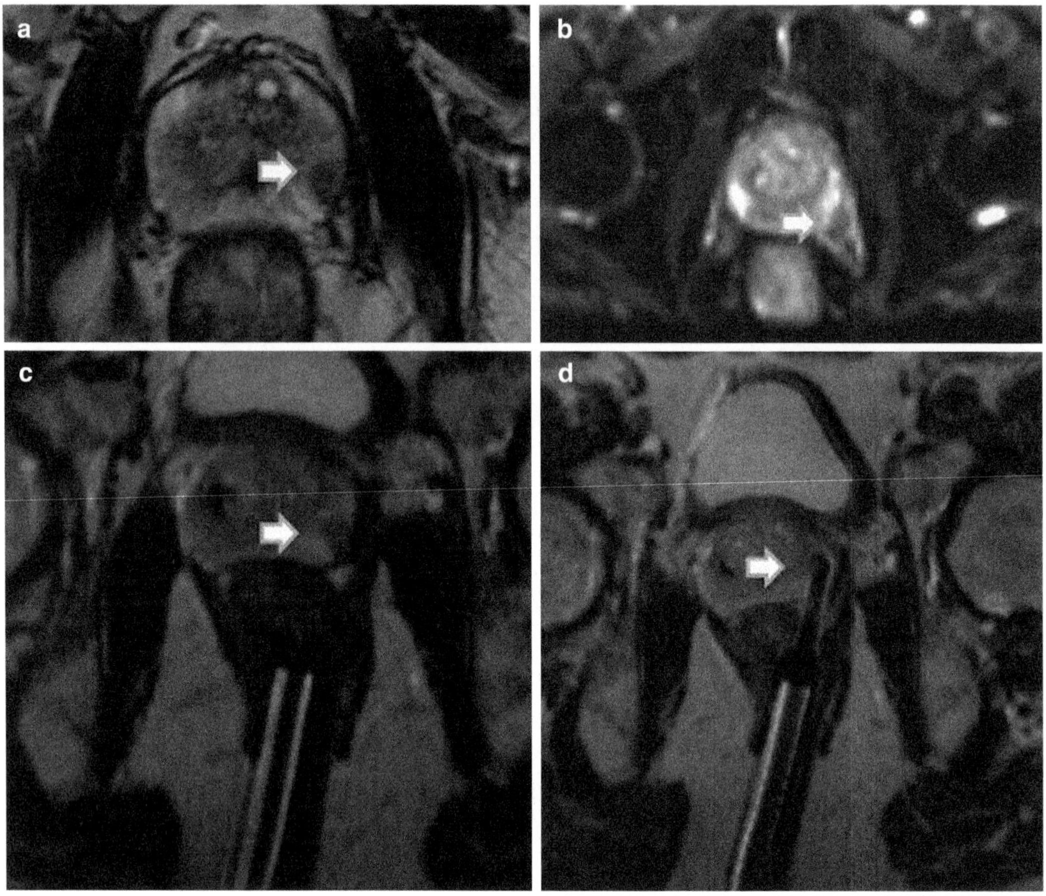

Fig. 10.7 Multiparametric MRI and IBMR-Bx using a 3-Tesla scanner in a 71-year-old biopsy-naïve patient with PSA of 8.2. The arrow points to an oval and markedly hypointense lesion with obscured margins at *TSE* T2-weighted image (**a**) with moderate restricted diffusion (**b**) in left posterolateral peripheral zone in midgland prostate. Overall PIRADS V2.1 score was 4/5. Patient underwent IBMR-Bx (**c, d**), and four core biopsies were obtained. Pathology assessment of the specimen revealed prostate cancer with Gleason score of 3 + 4

be directly influenced by the operator experience. IBMR-Bx, however, is less dependent to operator experience with a small increase in PCa yield and the obtained cancer core length and also a significant decrease in biopsy time from first to second year [49]. In contrast, MRUS-Fbx has a steep learning curve with improved PCa detection rate over time. In a study of 340 individuals who underwent transperineal MRUS-Fbx, the PCa detection rate increased from 27% to 63% over 22 months [50]. IBMR-Bx allows concurrent and direct visualization of the suspicious target and the needle guide in MRI with fewer biopsy cores required for the definite diagnosis. However, drawbacks of IBMR-Bx compared to MRUS-Fbx include its relatively higher expense and time and relatively less widespread availability.

A systematic review of 11 IBMR-Bx, 17 MRUS-Fbx, and 11 MRUS-Cbx and 4 combined MR-targeted biopsy studies showed a significantly higher detection rate of csPCa (RR: 1.16) and a significantly lower detection rate of clinically insignificant cancer (RR:0.47) with MR-targeted methods over TRUS bx. The review did not detect any significant difference between three MR-targeted techniques for the detection of csPCa [10].

In the FUTURE study, a multicenter randomized controlled trial of 665 men with suspected PCa and prior negative systematic biopsy

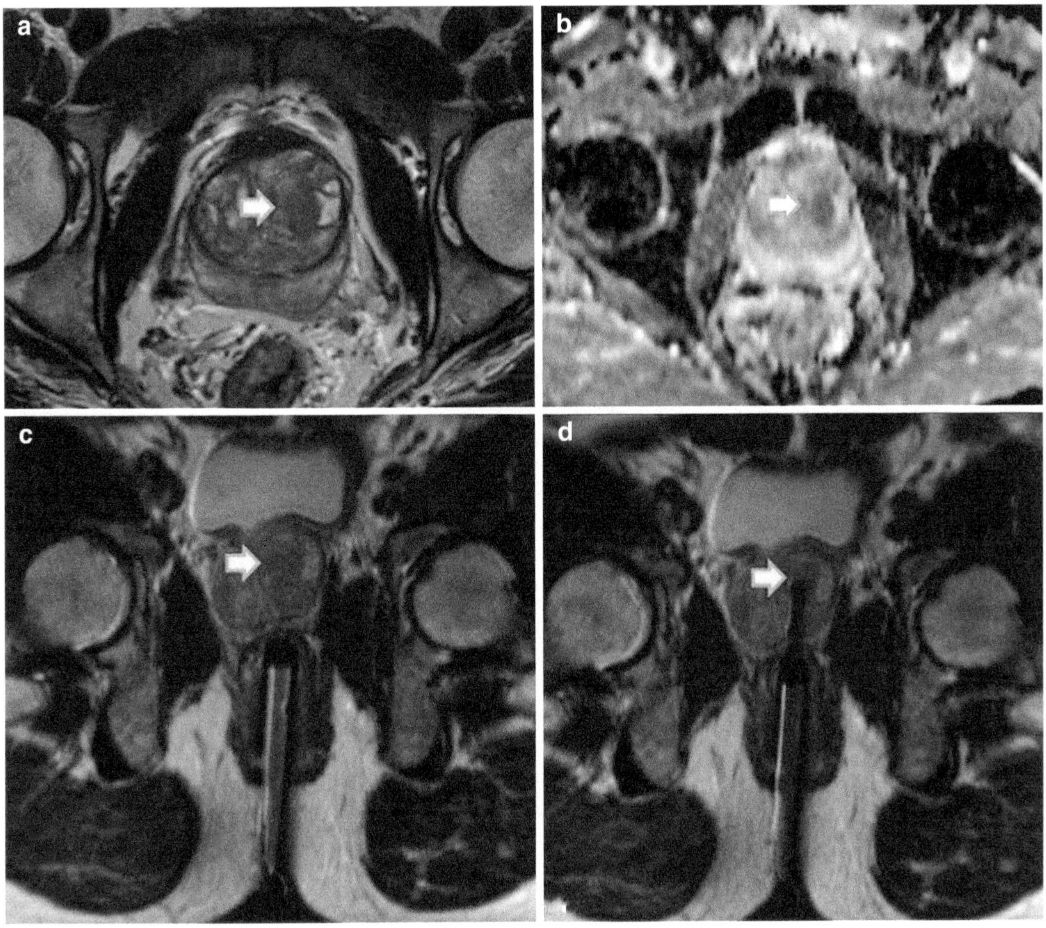

Fig. 10.8 Multiparametric MRI and in-gantry MRGB using a 3-Tesla scanner in a 62-year-old patient with rising PSA and prior negative TRUS bx. Axial TSE T2-weighted image (**a**) showed a suspicious oval, mildly hypointense lesion (arrow) with blurred margins in left anterior transition zone of prostate with moderate restricted diffusion (**b**). PIRADS v2.1 score of 3/5 was assigned, and IBMR-Bx of prostate was performed. An MR-compatible, 18-gauge needle was introduced through a needle guide, and 6-core needle biopsies were obtained from the target (**c, d**). Pathology of the specimen yielded benign lesion

(<4 year) compared three MR-targeted techniques: MRUS-Fbx, MRUS-Cbx, and IBMR-Bx. The study reported no significant difference was found between three subcohorts in the detection rate of prostate cancer (MRUS-Fbx, 49.4%; MRUS-Cbx, 43.6%; IBMR-Bx, 54.5%; p, 0.4) and clinically significant prostate cancer (MRUS-Fbx, 34.2%; MRUS-Cbx, 33.3%; IBMR-Bx, 32.5%; $P > 0.9$); however, core positivity rate was significantly higher by the IBMR bx technique (IBMR-Bx, 47.7%; MRUS-Cbx, 33.3%; MRUS-Fbx, 31.3%) [51]. Another prospective trial also did not find any significant difference in clinically significant prostate cancer detection rate between combined TRUS- MRUS-Fbx and IBMR-Bx [52]. In contrast, a study by Costa et al. [53] found significantly higher detection of csPCa by IBMR-Bx compared to MRUS-Fbx (61% vs. 47%, $p < 0.0001$) and significantly lower detection of insignificant PCa by in-bore technique compared to the fusion technique (11% vs. 18%, P:0.001).

It is noteworthy that systematic reviews of studies on MR-targeted biopsies are usually limited by several factors. First, by heterogeneous population of patients undergoing MR-targeted biopsy, as there are no clear criteria for performing MR-targeted biopsy. The European Association of Urology suggests that in patients with high clinical suspicion of PCa who need a repeat biopsy, mpMRI should be considered with subsequent MR-targeted biopsy if mpMRI is positive (PIRADS category 3 and higher). Second, the definition of clinically significant prostate cancer varies widely between published studies on MR-targeted biopsy. Third, there are variations in the number of obtained cores and the preferred technical aspects.

As there is no general consensus on the preferred MR-targeted method, the optimal biopsy technique should be decided on a per-patient basis and based on the availability of the systems and expertise of the staff.

10.6 Cost-Effectiveness of MR-Targeted Biopsy Strategies

Both MRUS-Fbx and IBMR-Bx have higher initial procedure costs, in comparison with TRUS biopsy; however, both targeted techniques have the beneficial sensitivity of multiparametric MRI to detect clinically significant cancers. Therefore, MR-targeted prostate biopsy methods are cost-effective compared to TRUS bx of prostate, when considering the higher health benefits and the overall lifetime expenses. The use of mpMRI as a screening test before biopsy can avoid the financial burden of unnecessary and repeat biopsies and ultimately unnecessary treatment [20]. In a decision-tree model in biopsy-naïve men in the United States, Pahwa et al. found that the use of mpMRI of prostate followed by MR-guided biopsy of suspicious foci to detect csPCa is cost-effective compared to the standard TRUS bx, when the endpoint was quality-adjusted life-year. IBMR-Bx of MR-positive lesions had the maximum net health benefits compared to systematic TRUS bx and MRUS-Cbx [54]. A study of prostate biopsy cost-effectiveness in a Dutch healthcare setting showed that MRUS-Fbx of MR-positive targets is more cost-effective than systematic TRUS bx. IBMR-Bx may be the most cost-effective method if it has a sensitivity of 89% for detection of csPCa [55].

10.7 Future Directions

When there is suspicion of prostate cancer, systematic TRUS bx remains the standard of care, due to its wide availability, relatively low costs, and ease of use in outpatient setting by urologists. Nevertheless, the future for MR-targeted biopsy is very promising. Several studies have proposed using multiparametric MRI over TRUS bx as the initial screening in patients with abnormal PSA or DRE. Furthermore, there is growing use of multiparametric MRI for the identification of suspicious lesions in patients with negative TRUS bx and in those with known low-grade PCa qualified for active surveillance protocol. Currently, there is little consensus over the preferred method of MR-targeted prostate sampling. Appropriate indications for application of each technique need to be determined. Overall, MRUS-Fbx and IBMR-Bx have been shown to be significantly more effective for detection of clinically significant PCa with each technique having its own advantage and disadvantage; hence the preferred method needs to be chosen per-patient basis, considering the availability, experience of the operators, and patient profile.

References

1. Albertsen PC, Hanley JA, Fine J. 20-year outcomes following conservative management of clinically localized prostate cancer. JAMA. 2005;293(17):2095–101.
2. Popiolek M, Rider JR, Andren O, Andersson SO, Holmberg L, Adami HO, et al. Natural history of early, localized prostate cancer: a final report from three decades of follow-up. Eur Urol. 2013;63(3):428–35.
3. Volkin D, Turkbey B, Hoang AN, Rais-Bahrami S, Yerram N, Walton-Diaz A, et al. Multiparametric magnetic resonance imaging (MRI) and subsequent MRI/ultrasonography fusion-guided biopsy increase the detection of anteriorly located prostate cancers. BJU Int. 2014;114(6b):E43–E9. Pubmed Central PMCID: 5613950.
4. Felker ER, Lee-Felker SA, Feller J, Margolis DJ, Lu DS, Princenthal R, et al. In-bore magnetic resonance-guided transrectal biopsy for the detection of clini-

cally significant prostate cancer. Abdom Radiol. 2016;41(5):954–62.
5. Barentsz JO, Richenberg J, Clements R, Choyke P, Verma S, Villeirs G, et al. ESUR prostate MR guidelines 2012. Eur Radiol. 2012;22(4):746–757. Pubmed Central PMCID: 3297750.
6. Barentsz JO, Weinreb JC, Verma S, Thoeny HC, Tempany CM, Shtern F, et al. Synopsis of the PI-RADS v2 guidelines for multiparametric prostate magnetic resonance imaging and recommendations for use. Eur Urol. 2016;69(1):41–49. Pubmed Central PMCID: 6364687.
7. Padhani AR, Weinreb J, Rosenkrantz AB, Villeirs G, Turkbey B, Barentsz J. Prostate imaging-reporting and data system steering committee: PI-RADS v2 status update and future directions. Eur Urol. 2019;75(3):385–396. Pubmed Central PMCID: 6292742.
8. Venderink W, van Luijtelaar A, van der Leest M, Barentsz JO, Jenniskens SFM, Overduin CG, et al. Multiparametric MRI and follow-up to avoid prostate biopsy in 4259 men. BJU Int. 2019;25:775–84.
9. Ahmed HU, El-Shater Bosaily A, Brown LC, Gabe R, Kaplan R, Parmar MK, et al. Diagnostic accuracy of multi-parametric MRI and TRUS biopsy in prostate cancer (PROMIS): a paired validating confirmatory study. Lancet. 2017;389(10071):815–22.
10. Wegelin O, van Melick HHE, Hooft L, Bosch J, Reitsma HB, Barentsz JO, et al. Comparing three different techniques for magnetic resonance imaging-targeted prostate biopsies: a systematic review of in-bore versus magnetic resonance imaging-transrectal ultrasound fusion versus cognitive registration. Is there a preferred technique? Eur Urol. 2017;71(4):517–31.
11. Smith JB, Popert R, Nuttall MC, Vyas L, Kinsella J, Cahill D. Transperineal sector prostate biopsies: a local anesthetic outpatient technique. Urology. 2014;83(6):1344–9.
12. Rothwax JT, George AK, Wood BJ, Pinto PA. Multiparametric MRI in biopsy guidance for prostate cancer: fusion-guided. BioMed Res Int. 2014;2014:439171. Pubmed Central PMCID: 4122009.
13. Kongnyuy M, George AK, Rastinehad AR, Pinto PA. Magnetic resonance imaging-ultrasound fusion-guided prostate biopsy: review of technology, techniques, and outcomes. Curr Urol Rep. 2016;17(4):32. Pubmed Central PMCID: 4928379.
14. Siddiqui MM, Rais-Bahrami S, Truong H, Stamatakis L, Vourganti S, Nix J, et al. Magnetic resonance imaging/ultrasound-fusion biopsy significantly upgrades prostate cancer versus systematic 12-core transrectal ultrasound biopsy. Eur Urol. 2013;64(5):713–719. Pubmed Central PMCID: 6301057.
15. Venderink W, de Rooij M, Sedelaar JPM, Huisman HJ, Futterer JJ. Elastic versus rigid image registration in magnetic resonance imaging-transrectal ultrasound fusion prostate biopsy: a systematic review and Meta-analysis. Eur Urol Focus. 2018;4(2):219–27.
16. van den Heuvel S, Loeb S, Zhu X, Verhagen PC, Schroder FH, Bangma CH, et al. Complications of initial prostate biopsy in a European randomized screening trial. Am J Clin Exp Urol. 2013;1(1):66–71. Pubmed Central PMCID: 4219277.
17. Grummet JP, Weerakoon M, Huang S, Lawrentschuk N, Frydenberg M, Moon DA, et al. Sepsis and 'superbugs': should we favour the transperineal over the transrectal approach for prostate biopsy? BJU Int. 2014;114(3):384–8.
18. Huang H, Wang W, Lin T, Zhang Q, Zhao X, Lian H, et al. Comparison of the complications of traditional 12 cores transrectal prostate biopsy with image fusion guided transperineal prostate biopsy. BMC Urol. 2016;16(1):68. Pubmed Central PMCID: 5114768.
19. Shoji S. Magnetic resonance imaging-transrectal ultrasound fusion image-guided prostate biopsy: current status of the cancer detection and the prospects of tailor-made medicine of the prostate cancer. Investig Clin Urol. 2019;60(1):4–13. Pubmed Central PMCID: 6318202.
20. Brown AM, Elbuluk O, Mertan F, Sankineni S, Margolis DJ, Wood BJ, et al. Recent advances in image-guided targeted prostate biopsy. Abdom Imaging. 2015;40(6):1788–99.
21. Singh AK, Kruecker J, Xu S, Glossop N, Guion P, Ullman K, et al. Initial clinical experience with real-time transrectal ultrasonography-magnetic resonance imaging fusion-guided prostate biopsy. BJU Int. 2008;101(7):841–845. Pubmed Central PMCID: 2621260.
22. Siddiqui MM, Rais-Bahrami S, Turkbey B, George AK, Rothwax J, Shakir N, et al. Comparison of MR/ultrasound fusion-guided biopsy with ultrasound-guided biopsy for the diagnosis of prostate cancer. JAMA. 2015;313(4):390–397. Pubmed Central PMCID: 4572575.
23. Sonn GA, Natarajan S, Margolis DJ, MacAiran M, Lieu P, Huang J, et al. Targeted biopsy in the detection of prostate cancer using an office based magnetic resonance ultrasound fusion device. J Urol. 2013;189(1):86–91. Pubmed Central PMCID: 3561472.
24. Ukimura O, Desai MM, Palmer S, Valencerina S, Gross M, Abreu AL, et al. 3-dimensional elastic registration system of prostate biopsy location by real-time 3-dimensional transrectal ultrasound guidance with magnetic resonance/transrectal ultrasound image fusion. J Urol. 2012;187(3):1080–6.
25. Mozer P, Roupret M, Le Cossec C, Granger B, Comperat E, de Gorski A, et al. First round of targeted biopsies using magnetic resonance imaging/ultrasonography fusion compared with conventional transrectal ultrasonography-guided biopsies for the diagnosis of localised prostate cancer. BJU Int. 2015;115(1):50–7.
26. Shoji S, Hiraiwa S, Ogawa T, Kawakami M, Nakano M, Hashida K, et al. Accuracy of real-time magnetic resonance imaging-transrectal ultrasound fusion image-guided transperineal target biopsy with needle

tracking with a mechanical position-encoded stepper in detecting significant prostate cancer in biopsy-naive men. Int J Urol. 2017;24(4):288–94.
27. Radtke JP, Schwab C, Wolf MB, Freitag MT, Alt CD, Kesch C, et al. Multiparametric magnetic resonance imaging (MRI) and MRI-Transrectal ultrasound fusion biopsy for index tumor detection: correlation with radical prostatectomy specimen. Eur Urol. 2016;70(5):846–53.
28. Koelis Academy. Available from: https://koelis.academy/. 28 Sep 2019.
29. Wu J, Ji A, Xie B, Wang X, Zhu Y, Wang J, et al. Is magnetic resonance/ultrasound fusion prostate biopsy better than systematic prostate biopsy? An updated meta- and trial sequential analysis. Oncotarget. 2015;6(41):43571–43580. Pubmed Central PMCID: 4791251.
30. Elkhoury FF, Felker ER, Kwan L, Sisk AE, Delfin M, Natarajan S, et al. Comparison of targeted vs systematic prostate biopsy in men who are biopsy naive: the prospective assessment of image registration in the diagnosis of prostate Cancer (PAIREDCAP) study. JAMA Surg. 2019;12. Pubmed Central PMCID: 6563598.
31. Hu JC, Chang E, Natarajan S, Margolis DJ, Macairan M, Lieu P, et al. Targeted prostate biopsy in select men for active surveillance: do the Epstein criteria still apply? J Urol. 2014;192(2):385–390. Pubmed Central PMCID: 4129939.
32. Puech P, Rouviere O, Renard-Penna R, Villers A, Devos P, Colombel M, et al. Prostate cancer diagnosis: multiparametric MR-targeted biopsy with cognitive and transrectal US-MR fusion guidance versus systematic biopsy--prospective multicenter study. Radiology. 2013;268(2):461–9.
33. Valerio M, Donaldson I, Emberton M, Ehdaie B, Hadaschik BA, Marks LS, et al. Detection of clinically significant prostate Cancer using magnetic resonance imaging-ultrasound fusion targeted biopsy: a systematic review. Eur Urol. 2015;68(1):8–19.
34. Puech P, Ouzzane A, Gaillard V, Betrouni N, Renard B, Villers A, et al. Multiparametric MRI-targeted TRUS prostate biopsies using visual registration. BioMed Res Int. 2014;2014:819360. Pubmed Central PMCID: 4266999.
35. Giganti F, Moore CM. A critical comparison of techniques for MRI-targeted biopsy of the prostate. Trans Androl Urol. 2017;6(3):432–443. Pubmed Central PMCID: 5503959.
36. Valerio M, McCartan N, Freeman A, Punwani S, Emberton M, Ahmed HU. Visually directed vs. software-based targeted biopsy compared to transperineal template mapping biopsy in the detection of clinically significant prostate cancer. Urologic Oncol. 2015;33(10):424 e9–16.
37. Oberlin DT, Casalino DD, Miller FH, Matulewicz RS, Perry KT, Nadler RB, et al. Diagnostic value of guided biopsies: fusion and cognitive-registration magnetic resonance imaging versus conventional ultrasound biopsy of the prostate. Urology. 2016;92:75–79. Pubmed Central PMCID: 4882086.
38. Delongchamps NB, Peyromaure M, Schull A, Beuvon F, Bouazza N, Flam T, et al. Prebiopsy magnetic resonance imaging and prostate cancer detection: comparison of random and targeted biopsies. J Urol. 2013;189(2):493–9.
39. Futterer JJ, Barentsz JO. MRI-guided and robotic-assisted prostate biopsy. Curr Opin Urol. 2012;22(4):316–9.
40. Overduin CG, Futterer JJ, Barentsz JO. MRI-guided biopsy for prostate cancer detection: a systematic review of current clinical results. Curr Urol Rep. 2013;14(3):209–13.
41. Tan N, Lin WC, Khoshnoodi P, Asvadi NH, Yoshida J, Margolis DJ, et al. In-bore 3-T MR-guided Transrectal targeted prostate biopsy: prostate imaging reporting and data system version 2-based diagnostic performance for detection of prostate Cancer. Radiology. 2017;283(1):130–139. Pubmed Central PMCID: 5375629.
42. Pokorny MR, de Rooij M, Duncan E, Schroder FH, Parkinson R, Barentsz JO, et al. Prospective study of diagnostic accuracy comparing prostate cancer detection by transrectal ultrasound-guided biopsy versus magnetic resonance (MR) imaging with subsequent MR-guided biopsy in men without previous prostate biopsies. Eur Urol. 2014;66(1):22–9.
43. Pokorny M, Kua B, Esler R, Yaxley J, Samaratunga H, Dunglison N, et al. MRI-guided in-bore biopsy for prostate cancer: what does the evidence say? A case series of 554 patients and a review of the current literature. World J Urol. 2019;37(7):1263–79.
44. Wang Y, Zhu J, Qin Z, Wang Y, Chen C, Wang Y, et al. Optimal biopsy strategy for prostate cancer detection by performing a Bayesian network meta-analysis of randomized controlled trials. J Cancer. 2018;9(13):2237–2248. Pubmed Central PMCID: 6036722.
45. van der Leest M, Cornel E, Israel B, Hendriks R, Padhani AR, Hoogenboom M, et al. Head-to-head comparison of Transrectal ultrasound-guided prostate biopsy versus multiparametric prostate resonance imaging with subsequent magnetic resonance-guided biopsy in biopsy-naive men with elevated prostate-specific antigen: a large prospective Multicenter clinical study. Eur Urol. 2019;75(4):570–8.
46. Hambrock T, Hoeks C, Hulsbergen-van de Kaa C, Scheenen T, Futterer J, Bouwense S, et al. Prospective assessment of prostate cancer aggressiveness using 3-T diffusion-weighted magnetic resonance imaging-guided biopsies versus a systematic 10-core transrectal ultrasound prostate biopsy cohort. Eur Urol. 2012;61(1):177–84.
47. Hambrock T, Somford DM, Hoeks C, Bouwense SA, Huisman H, Yakar D, et al. Magnetic resonance imaging guided prostate biopsy in men with repeat negative biopsies and increased prostate specific antigen. J Urol. 2010;183(2):520–7.

48. Quentin M, Blondin D, Arsov C, Schimmoller L, Hiester A, Godehardt E, et al. Prospective evaluation of magnetic resonance imaging guided in-bore prostate biopsy versus systematic transrectal ultrasound guided prostate biopsy in biopsy naive men with elevated prostate specific antigen. J Urol. 2014;192(5):1374–9.
49. Friedl A, Schneeweiss J, Sevcenco S, Eredics K, Kunit T, Susani M, et al. In-bore 3.0-T Magnetic Resonance Imaging-guided Transrectal Targeted Prostate Biopsy in a Repeat Biopsy Population: Diagnostic Performance, Complications, and Learning Curve. Urology. 2018;114:139–46.
50. Gaziev G, Wadhwa K, Barrett T, Koo BC, Gallagher FA, Serrao E, et al. Defining the learning curve for multiparametric magnetic resonance imaging (MRI) of the prostate using MRI-transrectal ultrasonography (TRUS) fusion-guided transperineal prostate biopsies as a validation tool. BJU Int. 2016;117(1):80–6.
51. Wegelin O, Exterkate L, van der Leest M, Kummer JA, Vreuls W, de Bruin PC, et al. The FUTURE trial: a Multicenter randomised controlled trial on target biopsy techniques based on magnetic resonance imaging in the diagnosis of prostate Cancer in patients with prior negative biopsies. Eur Urol. 2019;75(4):582–90.
52. Arsov C, Rabenalt R, Blondin D, Quentin M, Hiester A, Godehardt E, et al. Prospective randomized trial comparing magnetic resonance imaging (MRI)-guided in-bore biopsy to MRI-ultrasound fusion and transrectal ultrasound-guided prostate biopsy in patients with prior negative biopsies. Eur Urol. 2015;68(4):713–20.
53. Costa DN, Goldberg K, Leon AD, Lotan Y, Xi Y, Aziz M, et al. Magnetic resonance imaging-guided in-bore and magnetic resonance imaging-transrectal ultrasound fusion targeted prostate biopsies: an adjusted comparison of clinically significant prostate Cancer detection rate. Eur Urol Oncol. 2019;2(4):397–404.
54. Pahwa S, Schiltz NK, Ponsky LE, Lu Z, Griswold MA, Gulani V. Cost-effectiveness of MR imaging-guided strategies for detection of prostate Cancer in biopsy-naive men. Radiology. 2017;285(1):157–166. Pubmed Central PMCID: 5621719.
55. Venderink W, Govers TM, de Rooij M, Futterer JJ, Sedelaar JPM. Cost-effectiveness comparison of imaging-guided prostate biopsy techniques: systematic Transrectal ultrasound, direct in-bore MRI, and image fusion. AJR Am J Roentgenol. 2017;208(5):1058–63.

11 Prostate MRI from Radiation Oncology Perspective

Gordon Guo

11.1 Introduction

Multiparametric MRI (mp-MRI), compared with computed tomography (CT), significantly improves diagnostic accuracy in extraprostatic extension (EPE) and seminal vesicle invasion (SVI). The latest prostate cancer staging combines anatomical (TMN staging), Gleason score, and prostate-specific antigen (PSA) level.

While the optimal treatment for high-risk prostate cancer is debatable between surgery and radiation, contemporary studies prefer multi-modality treatment, and the decision is generally made based upon staging and patient preference.

Anatomic staging plays a central role in treatment decision-making. Clinical T3 disease by digital rectal exam has been challenging for urological surgeons due to higher risk of positive surgical margins and increased morbidity from aggressive prostate resections. MRI-visible T3 disease has an intermediate prognosis between organ-confined disease and palpable T3 disease [1].

There are multiple radiation-based treatment modalities for prostate cancer across virtually all stages. For low and favorable intermediate risk disease (NCCN guideline), radiation alone is sufficient. Endorectal coil MRI and combined endorectal MRI-MR spectroscopy can contribute significant incremental value to staging nomograms in predicting organ-confined prostate cancer [2]. For unfavorable intermediate-risk and high-risk disease, addition of androgen deprivation therapy (ADT) improves all prostate cancer-associated clinical end points. Mp-MRI can change local tumor staging (T stage) in 20–25% of cases [3, 4]. MRI-visible EPE and/or SVI represent clinical T3 disease, which is high risk by definition. Patients with such unfavorable features have aggressive tumor biology and significant risk of regional nodal metastases. Conventionally dosed radiation alone is associated with 50–60% clinical failure in 8–10 years. Radiation dose escalation and hormonal therapy have been shown to improve outcome [5–7].

There are three types of radiation dose escalation to primary disease in prostate gland and seminal vesicle. External beam radiation therapy (EBRT) by intensity-modulated radiotherapy (IMRT) modern delivery technique can safely raise radiation dose to 78–80 Gy. Brachytherapy is the ultimate dose escalation whereby either a low-dose-rate source such as iodine-125 or a high-dose-rate source such as iridium-192 is placed surgically inside the prostate gland. Prostate brachytherapy can help deliver over 90 Gy in 2 Gy equivalent to the prostate gland and even higher doses to the intraprostatic gross disease. Stereotactic body

G. Guo (✉)
Indiana University Simon Cancer Center, Department of Radiation Oncology, Indianapolis, IN, USA

T. Tirkes (ed.), *Prostate MRI Essentials*, https://doi.org/10.1007/978-3-030-45935-2_11

radiotherapy (SBRT) is a form of highly precise radiation treatment that can deliver much high doses per fraction than IMRT. SBRT as monotherapy has been shown to achieve similar results to IMRT. SBRT as a boost to prostate is actively being investigated, and preliminary results are promising.

11.2 Radiation Dose Painting via IMRT, Brachytherapy, or SBRT

Multiparametric MRI has excellent sensitivity and specificity in identifying extracapsular extension (EPE) and seminal vesicle invasion (SVI). Therefore a pre-treatment MRI improves staging accuracy and helps radiation oncologists make the optimal treatment recommendations to patients. MR imaging combines anatomical (T2W) with functional and physiological assessment such as DCE, DWI, and ADC. Value of these imaging techniques has been discussed at other chapters and will not be discussed here.

Dominant intraprostatic lesion (DIL) is defined by the mp-MRI. There is linear dose-response relationship between dose to DIL and biochemical relapse-free survival [8]. Dose escalation to DIL can be achieved with brachytherapy [9], SBRT [10], or intensity-modulated radiotherapy with simultaneously integrated boost (SIB) [11]. While most reported acceptable toxicity profile using different types of dose escalation, brachytherapy techniques, especially HDR, were superior in terms of normal tissues sparing [12]. A 74-year-old man with unfavorable intermediate risk prostate cancer, Gleason score 4 + 3 disease from left posterior mid gland. MRI revealed DIL in the left posterior lateral gland with broad contact against capsule. Patient underwent Palladium 103 seeds implant and supplemental EBRT to the pelvis. DIL received higher dose from seeds as shown in post-implant CT scan (Fig. 11.1).

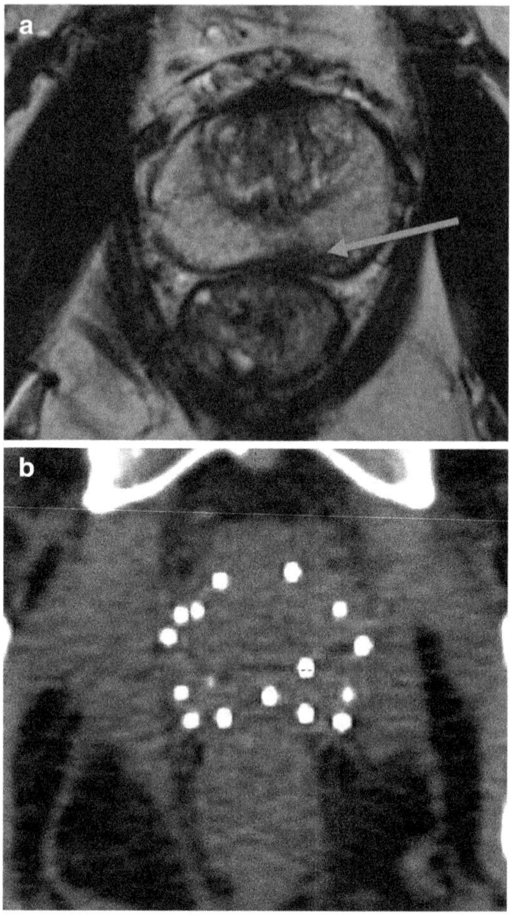

Fig. 11.1 A 74-year-old man was diagnosed with low-volume Gleason 7 prostate cancer on biopsy. (**a**) MRI revealed a left posterior lesion in broad contact with prostatic capsule (arrow). Given risk of microscopic extraprostatic disease, he was treated with Pd-103 seed implant plus complementary EBRT. (**b**) PIRADS 4 lesion in the same patient received focal boost with radiotherapy seeds

11.3 MRI-Guided Focal Dose Painting with Brachytherapy and IMRT/SBRT

Dose optimization by inverse planning can create dose heterogeneity. Radiation oncologists need to accurately delineate location of intraprostatic tumor location to fully take advantage of this dose painting capability. PIRADS 4 and 5 lesions on mp-MRI correlate strongly with clinically significant cancer. In EBRT, T2W MR images are fused with CT simulation images to allow radiation oncologists to contour tumor foci. In brachytherapy, radiation plans are usually based on transrectal ultrasound images. MR images are overlaid with live ultrasound images through deformable registration to guide focal dose escalation.

11.4 MRI-Fusion Biopsy in Radio-Recurrent Prostate Cancer and MRI-Guided Salvage HDR Brachytherapy

After definitive EBRT, 20–30% of patients will experience local recurrence. Many of these patients have systemic disease at the time of biochemical failure, but some have true local treatment failure. PSA < 10, PSA doubling time > 6 months, and Gleason score ≤ 7 generally suggest local only radio-recurrent disease [13]. With proper patient selection, salvage HDR brachytherapy can achieve excellent biochemical control and clinical progression-free survival.

Patients who are suspected of radio-recurrent disease should have MRI-fusion-targeted biopsy to have pathological confirmation and restaging CT scans, whole body bone scans, and, if available, PET/CT or PET/MRI scans utilizing prostate-specific isotopes such as choline, fluclovine, or PSMA to rule out metastases. Mp-MRI can help delineate intraprostatic tumor foci, which can be boosted to higher dose during HDR brachytherapy. Whole gland HDR salvage brachytherapy has shown excellent biochemical progression-free survival and metastases-free survival with acceptable urinary and bowel toxicities [14]. In order to further reduce morbidity, focal HDR salvage therapy has been tested in a prospective Phase II trial, and early results are promising.

Deformable registration between MRI and ultrasound images can help radiation oncologists identify intraprostatic foci that most likely contain gross tumor. Such areas can be focally boosted with HDR or LDR brachytherapy.

Mp-MRI can be a useful tool for tumor localization in focal salvage therapy. However, postradiation changes complicate image interpretation. A recent study suggested that quantitative analysis of certain mp-MRI sequences together with location information resulted in optimal distinction between tumor and benign voxels [15].

Local recurrences after radiotherapy are dose-dependent and predominantly occur in the DIL [16]. Clinically significant tumor foci can be reliably detected on both pre-RT and post-RT MRI. They displayed strikingly similar appearances between pre-RT, post-RT, and step-section pathology. Ratios between tumor volume on pathology and post-RT MRI can range between 0.52 and 2.8; therefore post-RT MRI may underestimate the extent of radio-recurrent prostate cancer [16].

A 66-year-old man received EBRT only for a low-volume Gleason score 3 + 4, favorable intermediate-risk prostate cancer 5 years ago. PSA increased to 8; restaging CT and bone scans did not show evidence of metastases. MRI-fusion biopsy revealed Gleason score 4 + 5 radio-recurrent tumor in the left apex. He was treated with HDR brachytherapy which was local salvage therapy, 21 Gy in 2 fractions to the whole gland, and 27 Gy in 2 fractions to MRI-avid DIL as shown in Fig. (11.2). PSA declined to 0.1 2 years after treatment.

11.5 T2-Weighted MRI and CT Image Fusion in Treatment Planning and Posttreatment Dosimetric Evaluation

The four common indications of T2W/CT image fusion are:

- SpaceOAR rectal spacer
- Pre-radiation planning to improve target delineation
- Post-radioactive seed implant dosimetry
- MRI-LINAC

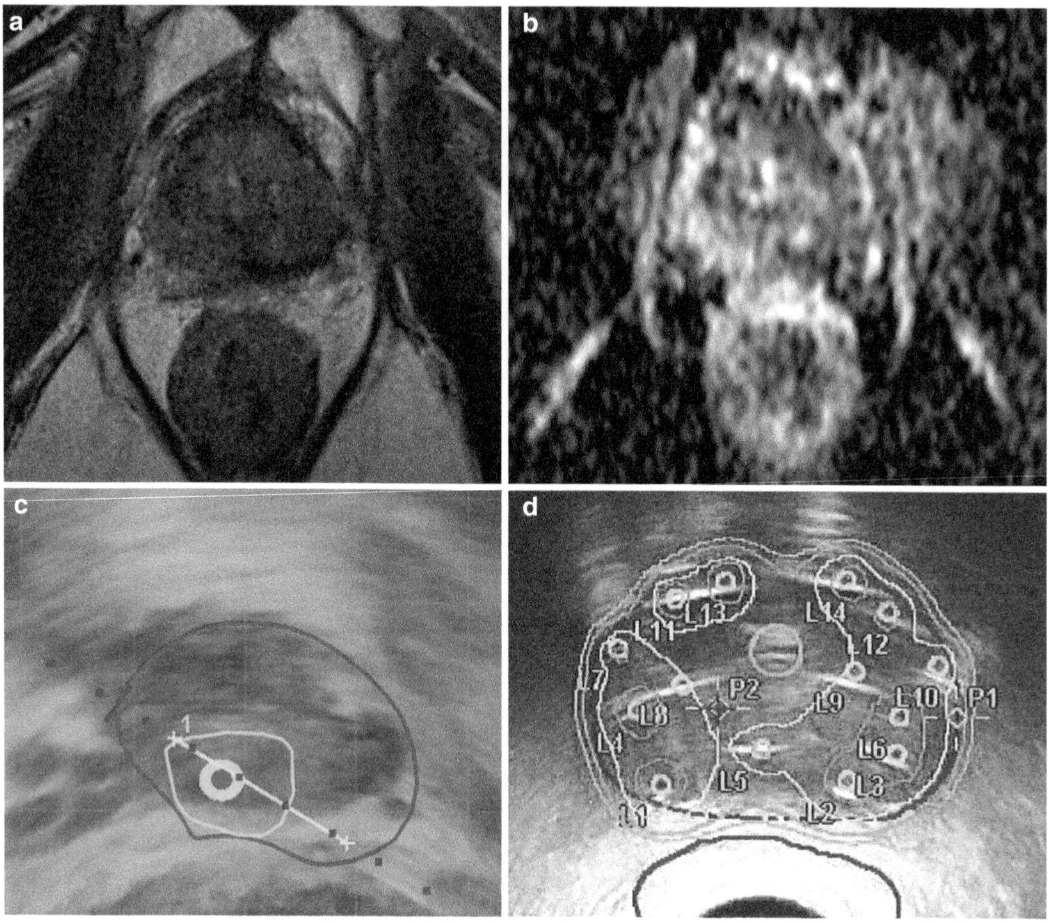

Fig. 11.2 A 66-year-old man received EBRT for low-volume Gleason 7, favorable intermediate risk prostate cancer 5 years ago. PSA subsequently increased to 8. Patient underwent MRI evaluation. (**a**) Loss of T2 signal abnormalities after radiation. (**b**) DCE and ADC images localized a PRIADS 4 left posterior lesion. (**c**) Targeted biopsy revealed Gleason 4 + 5 prostate adenocarcinoma. (**d**) MRI-guided HDR focal boost to left posterior lesion

11.5.1 SpaceOAR Rectal Spacer

The SpaceOAR system is a FDA-approved hydrogel indicated to create separation between prostate and anterior rectal wall. The hydrogel is injected through the perineum under ultrasound guidance, as shown in the schematic diagram (Fig. 11.3).

Spacer application is well tolerated with a 99% technical success rate. The mean additional space created by SpaceOAR hydrogel is just over 1 cm. The hydrogel material remains stable for at least 3 months to allow radiotherapy delivery, then liquefies, absorbed and clears by renal filtration. Multiple phase 2 and 3 clinical trials have demonstrated that spacer application significantly reduces rectal radiation dose and results in significantly lower late rectal toxicity and improvements in bowel, urinary, and sexual QOL (Fig. 11.4).

The hydrogel material appears hyperintense on T2-weighted images. A non-contrast MRI is typically performed at least 1 week after injection to allow trapped air to dissipate. The MRI images are then fused with CT simulation images for treatment planning (Fig. 11.5).

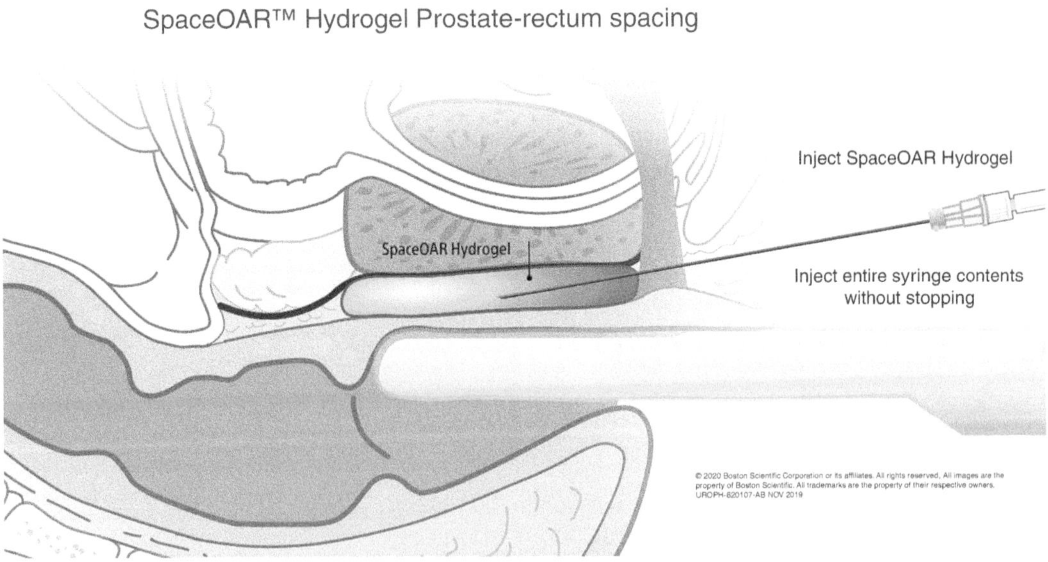

Fig. 11.3 Transperineal placement of biodegradable SpaceOAR hydrogel under ultrasound guidance. Image used with permission from Boston Scientific Corporation

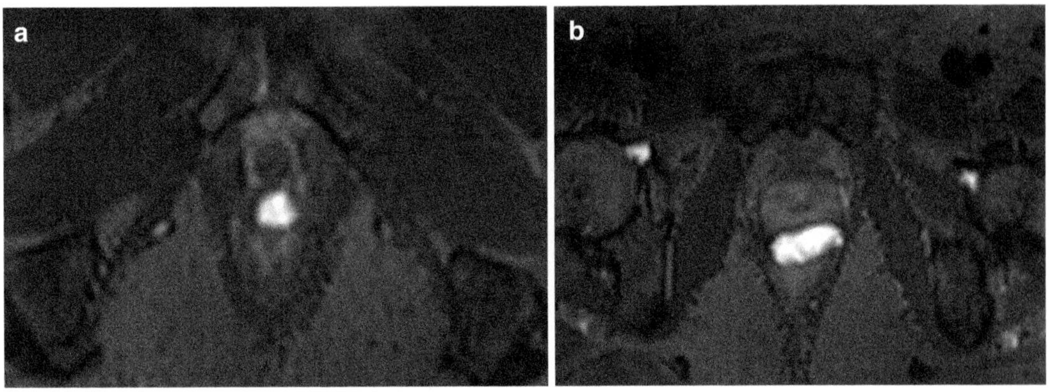

Fig. 11.4 T2W images show SpaceOAR hydrogel (bright signal) placed to create separate between prostate and anterior rectum (**a**) at the level of prostate apex and (**b**) at the level of mid gland

11.5.2 Pre-radiation Planning Improves Target Delineation

MRI-based prostate radiotherapy planning is superior to CT-based planning because important landmarks such as bladder neck and prostate apex can be readily delineated on MRI images. Radiation can be more precisely focused on prostate while minimizing dose to important organs at risk such as bladder and penile bulb (Fig. 11.6).

11.5.3 Post-radioactive Seed Implant Dosimetry

After permanent radioactive seed implant, T2-weighted MRI images can be fused with CT

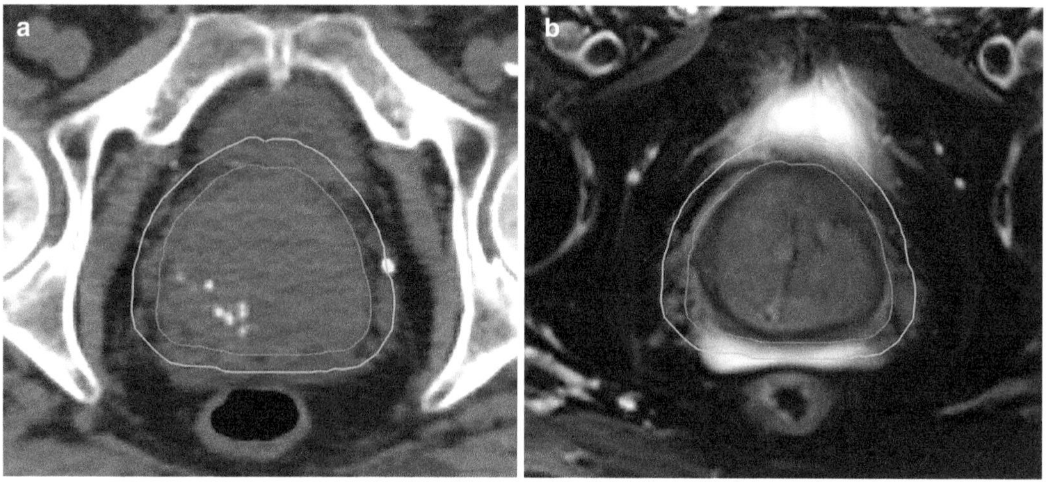

Fig. 11.5 SpaceOAR hydrogel reduces radiation to rectum by creating separation between prostate and rectum. (**a**) Hydrogel has similar density to soft tissue on simulation CT image. (**b**) Hydrogel is hyperintense on T2W images. CT simulation and T2W MR images are fused to help radiation oncologist contour target (orange). After a 5 mm posterior expansion to account for set up uncertainty, the planned target volume (PTV) does not spill over into the rectum

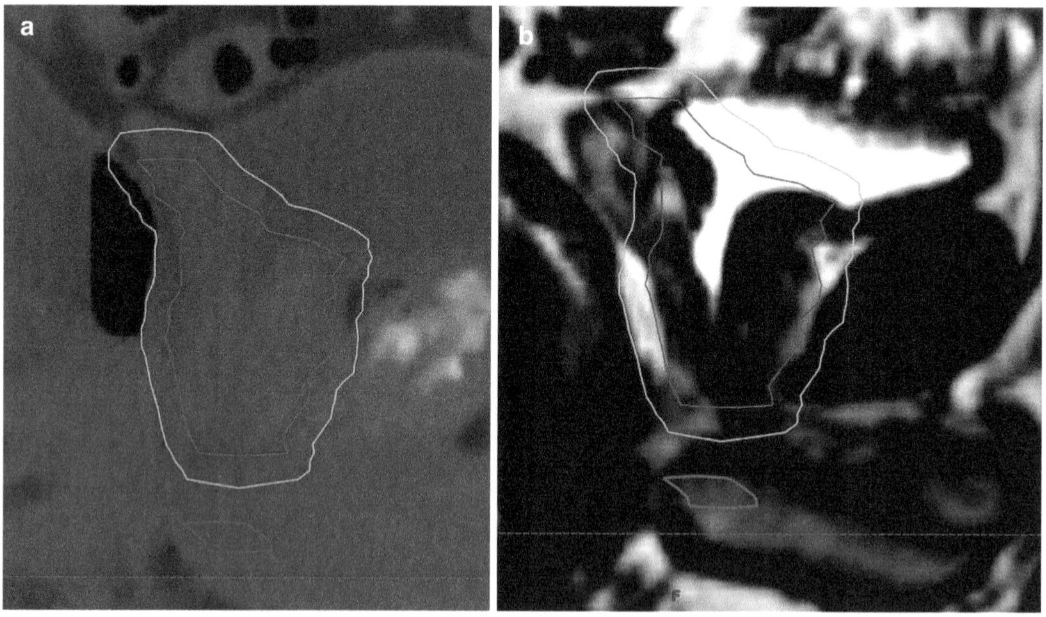

Fig. 11.6 Target delineation on CT-MRI fusion technique. (**a**) Prostate and proximal seminal vesicles are contoured on CT. (**b**) Prostate apex and penile bulb are visualized on sagittal T2W MR image

images to better delineate prostate gland, seminal vesicles, urethra, and rectum. Organs of interest are contoured on T2W images; dose map is generated on CT images; CT/MRI fusion creates accurate dosimetry and allows the radiation oncologist to review quality of implant. EBRT or additional seeds can make up for areas that were not adequately covered by initial implant (Fig. 11.7).

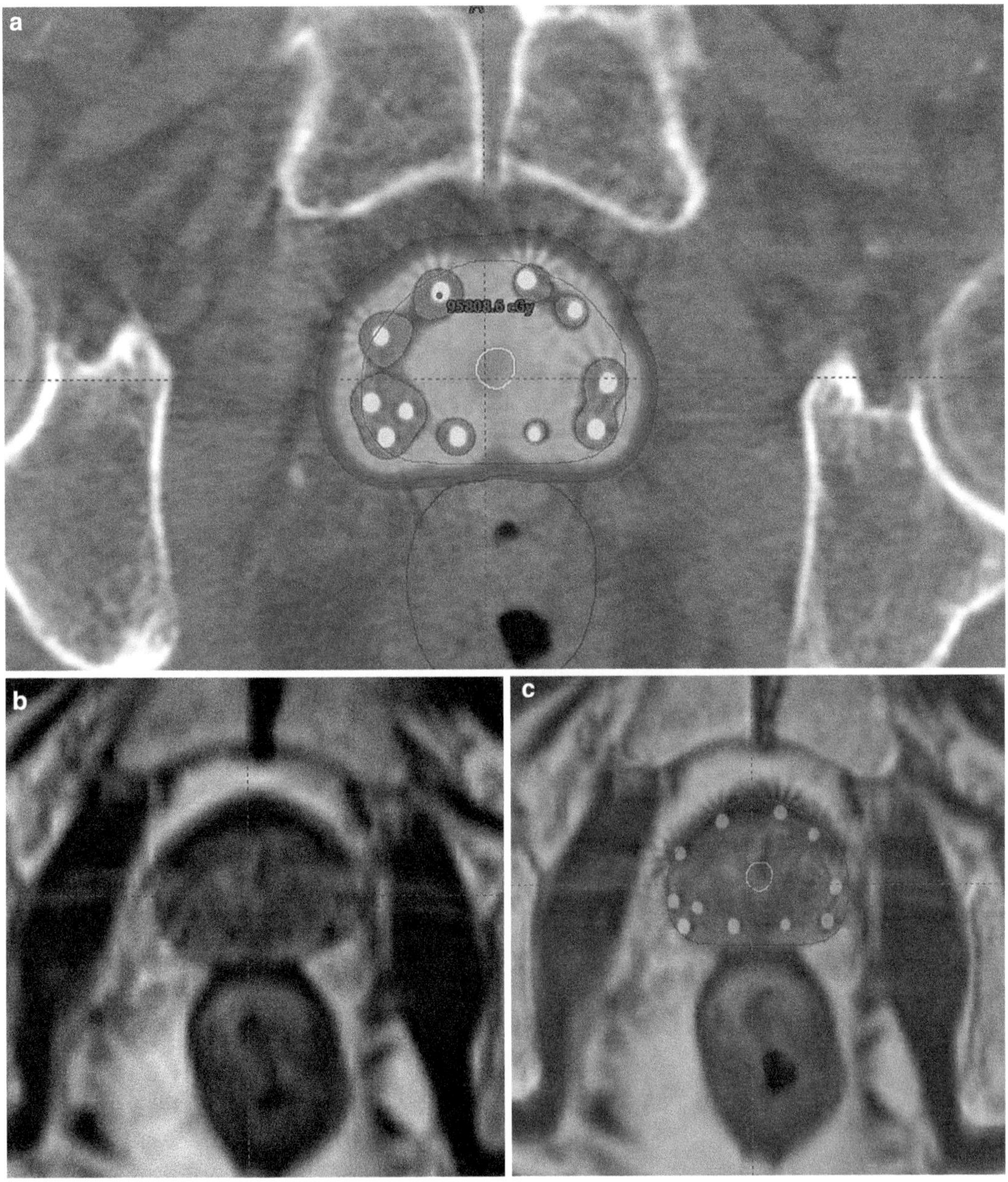

Fig. 11.7 CT and T2W MR images overlaid to create post-implant dosimetry. (**a**) Dose color wash. Seeds have metal coating that makes them radiopaque. (**b**) MRI provides better soft tissue differentiation. (**c**) CT/T2W fusion

11.5.4 MRI-LINAC

More recently, newer generation of linear accelerator (LINAC) is equipped with MR unit named MRI-LINAC which is being used for radiation treatment guidance. Compared to X-ray image guidance, MR-LINAC reduces uncertainty in target delineation and minimizes dose to normal organs at risk. When MR images demonstrate anatomic deviation, radiation plan can be adapted based on real-time soft tissue anatomy, allowing the most precise dose delivery.

The "Unity" MR-LINAC by Elekta uses a 1.5 T magnet. It has the ability to react to change in target shape and/or location, giving physician the ability to adapt radiation plan to patient's real-time anatomy. A handful of radiation centers in the USA and Europe have started using MR-LINAC, and it is expected to become more common in the near future.

References

1. Muralidhar V, Dinh KT, Mahal BA, et al. Differential post-prostatectomy cancer-specific survival of occult t3 vs. Clinical t3 prostate cancer: Implications for managing patients upstaged on prostate magnetic resonance imaging. Urol Oncol. 2015;33(7):330.e19–25. https://doi.org/10.1016/j.urolonc.2015.03.010.
2. Wang L, Hricak H, Kattan MW, et al. Prediction of organ-confined prostate cancer: incremental value of MR imaging and MR spectroscopic imaging to staging nomograms. Radiology. 2006;238:597–603.
3. D'Amico AV, Schnall M, Whittington R, et al. Endorectal coil magnetic resonance imaging identifies locally advanced prostate cancer in select patients with clinically localized disease. Urology. 1998;51:449–54.
4. Hegde JV, Chen MH, Mulkern RV, et al. Preoperative 3-tesla multiparametric endorectal magnetic resonance imaging findings and the odds of upgrading and upstaging at radical prostatectomy in men with clinically localized prostate cancer. Int J Radiat Oncol Biol Phys. 2013;85(2):e101–7. https://doi.org/10.1016/j.ijrobp.2012.08.032.
5. Bolla M, Collette L, Blank L, et al. Long-term results with immediate androgen suppression and external irradiation in patients with locally advanced prostate cancer (an eortc study): a phase iii randomised trial. Lancet. 2002;360(9327):103–6.
6. Stock RG, Cahlon O, Cesaretti JA, et al. Combined modality treatment in the management of high-risk prostate cancer. Int J Radiat Oncol Biol Phys. 2004;59:1352–9.
7. Kuban DA, Tucker SL, Dong L, et al. Long-term results of the m. D. Anderson randomized dose-escalation trial for prostate cancer. Int J Radiat Oncol Biol Phys. 2008;70:67–74.
8. Cellini N, Morganti AG, Mattiucci GC, et al. Analysis of intraprostatic failures in patients treated with hormonal therapy and radiotherapy: implications for conformal therapy planning. Int J Radiat Oncol Biol Phys. 2002;53:595–9.
9. Gomez-Iturriaga A, Casquero F, Urresola A, et al. Dose escalation to dominant intraprostatic lesions with MRI-transrectal ultrasound fusion high-dose-rate prostate brachytherapy. Prospective phase ii trial. Radiother Oncol. 2016;119(1):91–6. https://doi.org/10.1016/j.radonc.2016.02.004.
10. Miralbell R, Molla M, Rouzaud M, et al. Hypofractionated boost to the dominant tumor region with intensity modulated stereotactic radiotherapy for prostate cancer: a sequential dose escalation pilot study. Int J Radiat Oncol Biol Phys. 2010;78(1):50–7. https://doi.org/10.1016/j.ijrobp.2009.07.1689.
11. Sundahl N, De Meerleer G, Villeirs G, et al. Combining high dose external beam radiotherapy with a simultaneous integrated boost to the dominant intraprostatic lesion: analysis of genito-urinary and rectal toxicity. Radiother Oncol. 2016;119(3):398–404. https://doi.org/10.1016/j.radonc.2016.04.031.
12. Georg D, Hopfgartner J, Gora J, et al. Dosimetric considerations to determine the optimal technique for localized prostate cancer among external photon, proton, or carbon-ion therapy and high-dose-rate or low-dose-rate brachytherapy. Int J Radiat Oncol Biol Phys. 2014;88(3):715–22. https://doi.org/10.1016/j.ijrobp.2013.11.241.
13. Nguyen PL, D'Amico AV, Lee AK, et al. Patient selection, cancer control, and complications after salvage local therapy for postradiation prostate-specific antigen failure: a systematic review of the literature. Cancer. 2007;110(7):1417–28.
14. Yamada Y, Kollmeier MA, Pei X, et al. A phase ii study of salvage high-dose-rate brachytherapy for the treatment of locally recurrent prostate cancer after definitive external beam radiotherapy. Brachytherapy. 2014;13(2):111–6. https://doi.org/10.1016/j.brachy.2013.11.005.
15. Dinis Fernandes C, van Houdt PJ, Heijmink S, et al. Quantitative 3t multiparametric MRI of benign and malignant prostatic tissue in patients with and without local recurrent prostate cancer after external-beam radiation therapy. J Magn Reson Imaging. 2019;50(1):269–78. https://doi.org/10.1002/jmri.26581.
16. Pucar D, Hricak H, Shukla-Dave A, et al. Clinically significant prostate cancer local recurrence after radiation therapy occurs at the site of primary tumor: magnetic resonance imaging and step-section pathology evidence. Int J Radiat Oncol Biol Phys. 2007;69:62–9.

Post-Treatment MR Imaging of Prostate

12

Annemarijke van Luijtelaar, Joyce G. R. Bomers, and Jurgen J. Fütterer

12.1 Introduction

Multi-parametric magnetic resonance imaging (mpMRI) is the preferred technique for detection and staging of prostate cancer due to its multiplanar anatomical imaging and excellent soft tissue contrast [1, 2]. Prostate mpMRI plays an important role in evaluation and follow-up after prostate cancer therapy. Traditional prostate cancer treatments include radical prostatectomy (RP) or radiation therapy (RT), which incorporates brachytherapy or external beam radiation therapy (EBRT). In men with localized prostate cancer, RP is the preferred technique; RT is favored in elder patients or patients that are not eligible for surgery with low- to high-risk prostate cancer [3, 4]. After prostate cancer treatment, mpMRI is being used to differentiate between the failure of therapy and post-treatment changes [5]. Despite improved management approaches, the disease still recurs in up to 40% of the patients that underwent definitive treatment [6, 7]. The location of recurrent disease may vary depending on the kind of treatment that was used. Patients who underwent whole gland prostate cancer treatment are followed closely based on serum prostate-specific antigen (PSA) levels, as it is a sensitive marker for disease recurrence. The most important role of post-treatment MR imaging is to localize potential recurrent or residual disease so that active surveillance, salvage therapy, or systemic therapy can be promptly instituted. As minimally invasive treatment methods and novel management approaches emerge, the use of mpMRI in prostate cancer therapy is increasing [8]. These treatment options include cryotherapy, focal laser ablation (FLA), high-intensity focused ultrasound (HIFU), and irreversible electroporation (IRE). An understanding of the various treatment options available and the MR imaging features used for assessment of the prostate and pelvic region is essential for accurate post-treatment mpMRI evaluation and follow-up.

12.2 Radical Prostatectomy

The most used surgical prostate cancer treatment remains radical prostatectomy (RP), which is typically performed in cancers that are limited to the prostate gland (stage T1 or T2) [9]. Certain surgical approaches for RP include open, laparoscopic, and robot-assisted procedures. However, there is still no consensus favoring one technique over another in specific situations [10]. A successful radical prostatectomy includes total removal of the prostate gland and, if necessary, along with the seminal vesicles and a varying

A. van Luijtelaar (✉) · J. G. R. Bomers
J. J. Fütterer
Radboud University Medical Center, Department of Radiology and Nuclear Medicine, Nijmegen, The Netherlands
e-mail: annemarijke.vanLuijtelaar@radboudumc.nl; joyce.bomers@radboudumc.nl; jurgen.futterer@radboudumc.nl

T. Tirkes (ed.), *Prostate MRI Essentials*, https://doi.org/10.1007/978-3-030-45935-2_12

extended dissection of the pelvic lymph nodes for evaluation of potential metastasis [11].

12.2.1 MR Imaging Findings After Radical Prostatectomy

Prostate mpMRI may help distinguish between local prostate cancer recurrence and distant metastatic disease. The functional components of a post-treatment mpMRI contribute to differentiation between recurrent disease, residual tissue, inflammatory tissue, and normal postoperative fibrosis and therefore play an important role in evaluating the postsurgical bed. T2-weighted (T2W) imaging is used for the anatomical orientation and evaluation of signal patterns. Diffusion-weighted imaging (DWI) may be useful for distinguishing tumor from inflammation or benign prostate tissue. The DWI can be degraded by artifacts if metallic clips were used during surgery. DCE imaging can be used for detecting recurrent disease. In a normal postoperative DCE imaging, there should not be an early enhancement in the arterial phase; however, there should be some low-level enhancement of the surgical bed during the venous phase (Fig. 12.1).

MR images following prostatectomy show a descended bladder and levator sling into the prostatectomy fossa [12]. The vesicourethral anastomosis is located inferior to the bladder neck and should appear as low-signal intensity on all sequences, which corresponds to postoperative fibrosis [11]. Secondary to edema, a hyperintense signal may be present at the prostatic fossa on the T2W images during the 6-week follow-up images. If the seminal vesicles can be preserved (in 20% of the patients), the MR imaging shows their characteristic tubular structure at its original location on T1W or T2W imaging. The retained seminal vesicles exhibit as intermediate to high intensity on T2W imaging, depending on the degree of postoperative fibrosis, with a restricted diffusion on DWI and early enhancement on

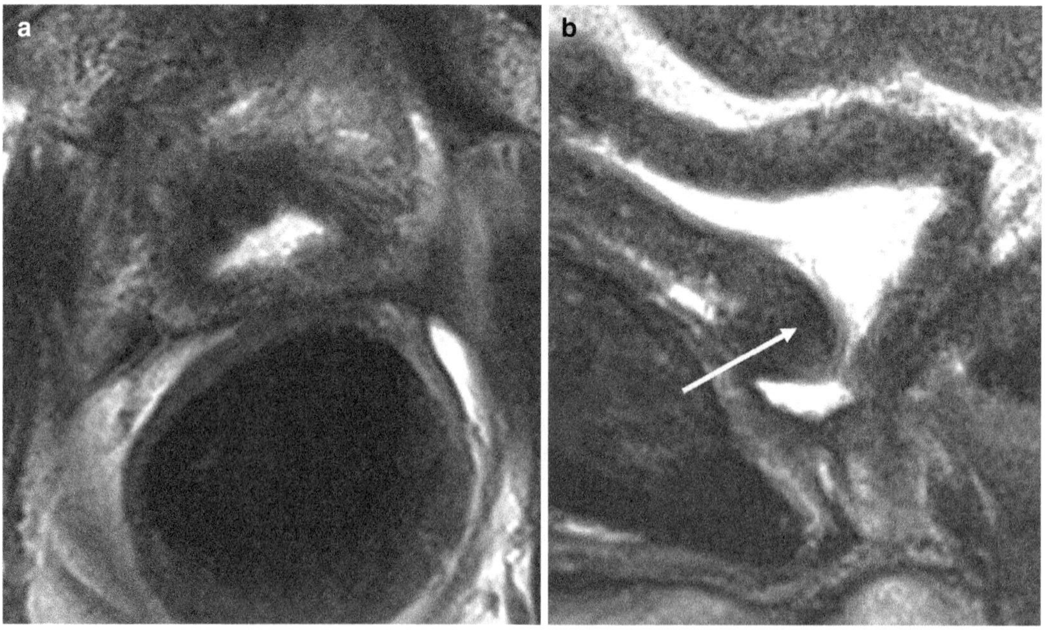

Fig. 12.1 Image findings after radical prostatectomy. Multi-parametric MRI of a 66-year-old male with a serum PSA of 1.8 ng/mL. Patient underwent a radical prostatectomy in 2018 as treatment for a Gleason score 4 + 3 = 7 prostate cancer. Eight months after the radical prostatectomy, the axial (**a**) and sagittal (**b**) T2W images show absence of the prostate and the descended bladder and levator sling into the prostatic fossa (white arrow)

DCE [13]. The signal patterns of fibrosis may differ between patients, depending on the surgical approach that was used. Typical postsurgical fibrosis is characterized by minimal to no enhancement on DCE images during the venous phase and displays a low-signal intensity in all sequences [11]. Additionally, lymphoceles may appear 3–8 weeks after surgery at the locations of former lymph nodes. Lymphoceles show a low T1W and high T2W signal intensity and demonstrate no enhancement on DCE [12].

12.2.2 Features of Recurrence After Radical Prostatectomy

Certain pre-surgical tumor characteristics, such as seminal vesicle invasion, extraprostatic extension, lymph node invasion, increased tumor volume, and positive surgical margins, increase the risk of recurrent disease. Normally, with a total removal of the prostate gland, serum PSA levels should be undetectable within 2–3 weeks after a successful RP. Any detectable serum PSA might indicate persistent or recurrent disease. Local recurrence of prostate cancer in patients that underwent RP may occur anywhere at the prostatic fossa; however, the most common site is the vesicourethral anastomosis [14]. Overall, the signal patterns of recurrent prostate cancer on mpMRI are very similar to de novo prostate cancer. It tends to occur as a soft tissue nodule with a hyperintense signal on T2W imaging and is isointense to the muscle on T1W imaging (Fig. 12.2). The recurrent disease will exhibit as hypointense on the ADC map and hyperintense on high b-value images. Prompt enhancement during the arterial phase followed by a quick washout during the venous phase on DCE images is highly suspicious for recurrence [15, 16]. However, it is often readily confused with a prominent periprostatic venous plexus. In contrast, local recurrent disease appears as a rounded area with enhancement. DCE enhancement contrasts sharply with the normal postsurgical low-level venous enhancement at the vesicourethral anastomosis and therefore is the most important sequence in detection of recurrent disease after prostate cancer treatment [17].

12.3 Radiation Therapy

Radiation therapy is the second most common radical treatment for stage 1 or 2 cancers that are limited to the prostate gland [18]. It is generally used in (elderly) men that are not eligible to surgery. To maximize the treatment efficacy, RT may be combined with neoadjuvant or adjuvant systemic (hormonal) therapy [19]. Normally, there remains benign prostate tissue after RT which complicates the interpretation of elevated serum PSA levels. Undetectable levels of serum PSA after treatment with RT are not achieved as quickly as with RP since it takes around 18 months to achieve PSA nadir [20].

12.3.1 External Beam Radiation Therapy

External beam radiation therapy (EBRT) involves the direction of external radiation through focused beams in order to destroy cancerous cells. It can be performed by delivering either photons or protons (proton beam therapy). Using advanced computer-based planning systems, EBRT allows precise targeted radiation therapy with a subsequently reduced dose exposed to healthy tissue. Ultrasound-guided placement of intraprostatic fiducials allows accurate treatment accuracy and is a standard of care in EBRT [21]. It is generally offered to patients with early diagnosed prostate cancer.

12.3.1.1 MR Imaging Findings After EBRT

Both the prostate and seminal vesicles show a reduced volume and hypointense signal on TW2 imaging after EBRT. Differentiation between peripheral, transition, and central zone is more difficult due to destruction of the normal cells

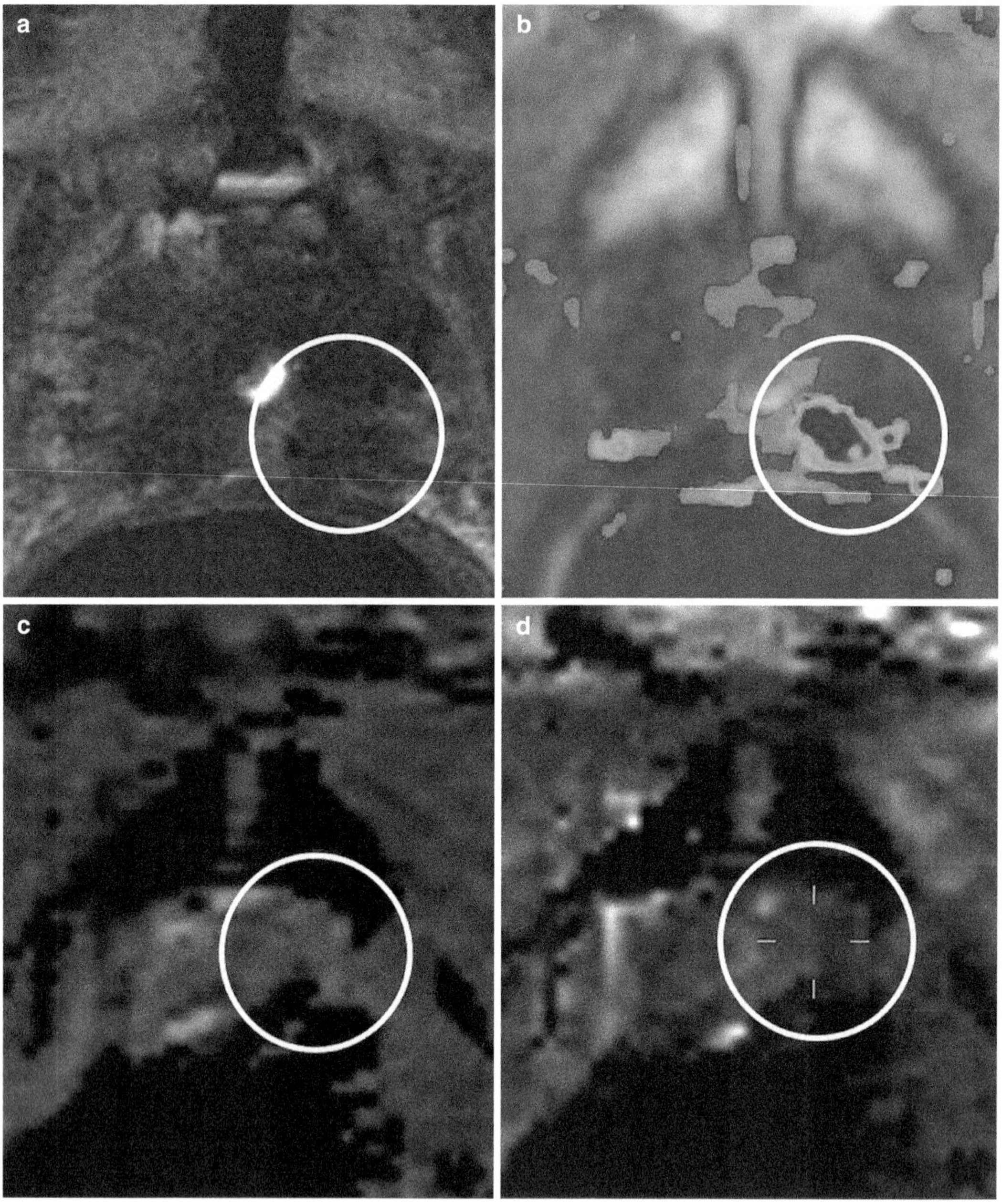

Fig. 12.2 Recurrence after radical prostatectomy. Multiparametric MRI of a 71-year-old male who underwent a radical prostatectomy in 2011 as treatment for a de novo lesion (Gleason score 3 + 4 = 7) at the left peripheral zone. After the radical prostatectomy, the serum PSA has dropped to 1.2 ng/mL but then risen to 4.3 ng/mL. Follow-up imaging demonstrated a lesion in the left prostatic fossa that is highly suspicious for residual disease. It exhibits as a hyperintense signal on T2W imaging with diffusion restriction on DWI and focal enhancement on DCE-MRI (white circles). Pathology results showed a Gleason score 4 + 3 = 7 in 2 cores. (**a**) Axial T2W imaging; (**b**) axial DCE-MRI with minimal to no enhancement; (**c**) axial ADC map; (**d**) axial DWI with $b = 1400$ (calculated)

and subsequent fibrosis (Fig. 12.3) [22]. As a result, the prostate is less cellular and lacking vascularity, and therefore DWI and DCE characteristics are altered as well. The surrounding structures appear different on post-EBRT imaging. The pelvic sidewall muscles may show increased signal intensity on T2W images, and bone marrow may appear relatively hypointense

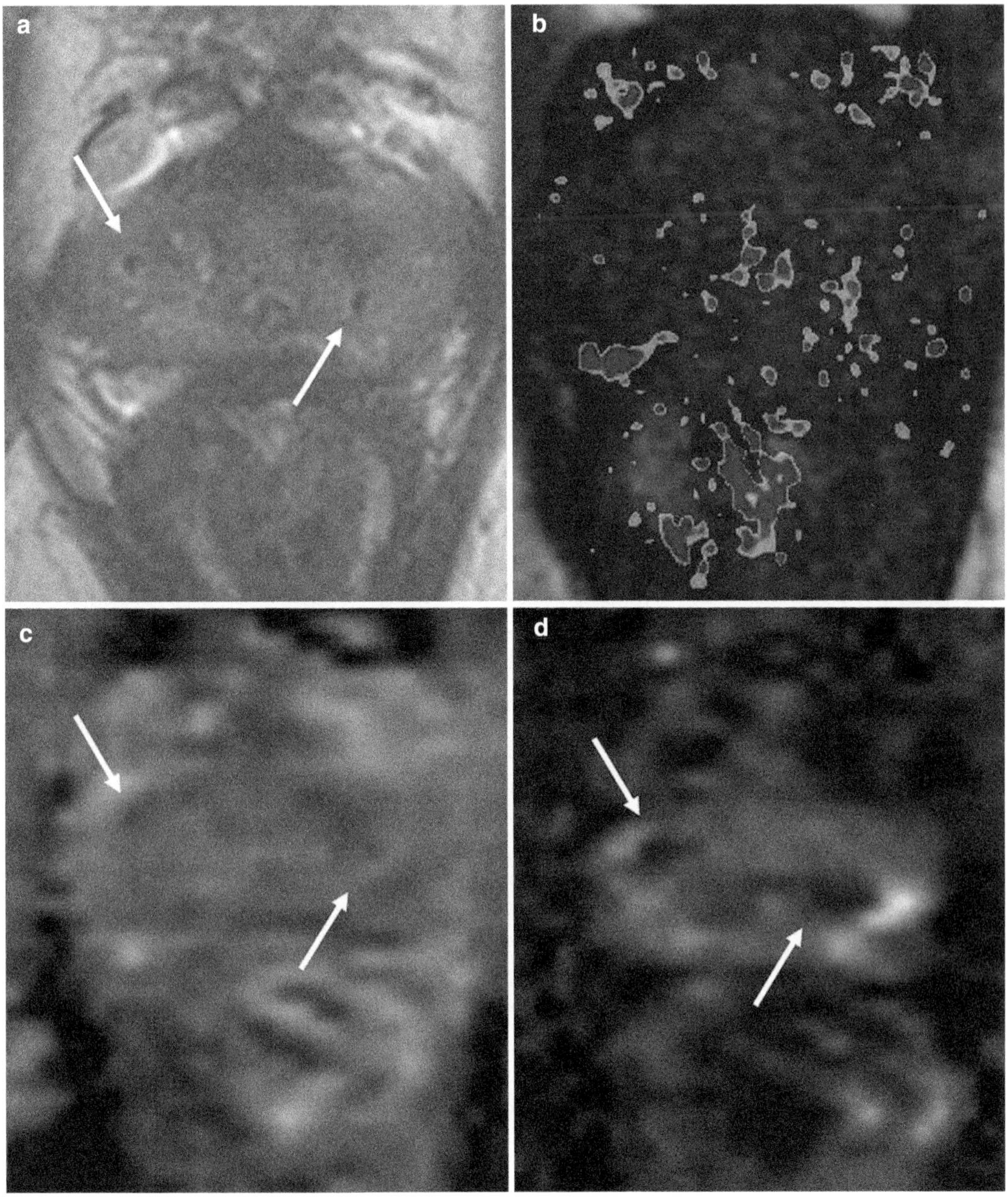

Fig. 12.3 Imaging findings after external beam radiation therapy. Multi-parametric MRI of a 66-year-old male with an initial serum PSA of 6.9 ng/mL. Patient underwent EBRT in 2013 as treatment for a Gleason score 3 + 4 = 7 lesion at the left peripheral zone. Follow-up imaging in 2018 shows characteristic findings of post-radiation change, including gold markers (white arrows). (**a**) Axial T2W image shows the altered background signal of the prostate, with a diffuse low-signal intensity and loss of zonal distinction. (**b**) Axial DCE-MRI with minimal to no enhancement; (**c**) axial ADC map; (**d**) axial DWI with $b = 1400$ (calculated)

on fat-saturated T1W images due fatty replacement [23]. Other effects of EBRT may include prominence of the perirectal fascia and increased signal intensity of the bladder and rectal wall.

12.3.1.2 Features of Recurrence After EBRT

Recurrence of prostate cancer after treatment with EBRT usually occurs at the original tumor site [24]. It commonly emerges as a hypointense T2W signal nodule and often demonstrates capsular bulging as a result of increased growth relative to the atrophic benign prostate gland [25]. Detection of recurrent disease after EBRT may be challenging on T2W imaging as it has notable limitations due to post-radiation changes, i.e., decreased background signal intensity [26]. The distinction between benign and tumor tissue is more difficult due to atrophy and fibrosis of the prostate gland. Therefore, the apparent diffusion coefficient (ADC) map and early enhancement on DCE images play a more dominant role in the detection of recurrent disease (Fig. 12.4). Normal post-treatment changes on DWI and DCE images are not as comprehensive as seen on T2W imaging, making these functional sequences more suitable for detection of recurrent disease after EBRT. Characteristics of recurrence on DWI are very similar to those of the original tumor, with a low-signal intensity on the ADC map and hyper-

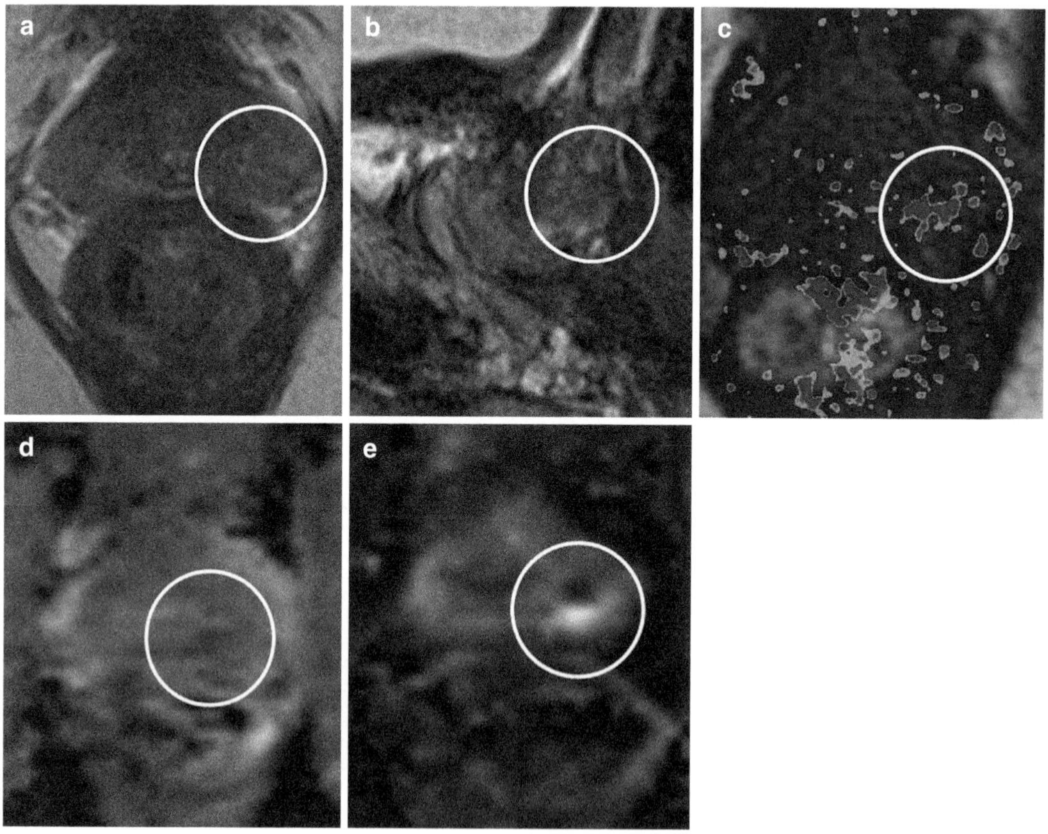

Fig. 12.4 Recurrence after EBRT. Multi-parametric MRI of a 66-year-old male with an initial serum PSA of 6.9 ng/mL. Patient underwent EBRT in 2013 as treatment for a de novo lesion (Gleason score 3 + 4 = 7) at the left peripheral zone. During follow-up, the serum PSA has risen from 1.2 to 4.5 ng/mL, and MRI demonstrated a residual tumor at the left peripheral zone (white circles) and left seminal vesicle. (**a**) Axial T2W imaging of the prostate base with a hyposignal intensity at the left peripheral zone; (**b**) sagittal T2W imaging with a low-signal intensity near the left prostate base; (**c**) axial DCE-MRI with focal enhancement; (**d**) axial ADC image shows a low-signal intensity with diffusion restriction and a minimal ADC value of 940; (**e**) axial DWI with b = 1400 (calculated). Pathology results revealed a Gleason 4 + 3 = 7 cancer in 3 cores

intensity on high b-value DWI that correlates with a nodule seen on T2W images [27]. Early hyperenhancement on DCE has been proven to be useful in detection of recurrent disease as the cancerous cells are expected to retain vascular supply due to neovascularization [28]. In contrast, a normal irradiated prostate is lacking normal vascularization as a result of glandular atrophy and will exhibit no to minimal enhancement on DCE.

12.3.2 Brachytherapy

Brachytherapy uses radioactive seeds that are implanted within the prostate under image guidance and sometimes referred to as internal radiation. Brachytherapy allows specific distribution of high doses of radiation in order to treat a prostate tumor with fewer side effects than EBRT. It can be given as high-dose rate therapy (HDR) in a brief treatment session delivered by temporary implanted radioactive pellets, or alternatively it is performed as low-dose rate therapy (LDR) where tiny radioactive titanium seeds are implanted and left in place. The main advantage of HDR is higher precision in dosimetry as the source dwell time and position can be modulated [29]. However, LDR brachytherapy is more commonly used as it is most suitable for indolent prostate cancer in patients with a small prostate volume [30]. To improve prostate cancer treatment, brachytherapy may be combined with EBRT [31].

12.3.2.1 MR Imaging Findings After Brachytherapy

Overall, MRI post-treatment changes of the brachytherapy and EBRT are very similar [23]. The prostate gland shows lower-signal intensity compared to pre-treatment imaging. Similar to EBRT, the zonal and tissue distinction may be very difficult due to the altered background signal of the prostate (Fig. 12.5) [22]. The metallic seeds may cause artifacts, making interpretation more challenging. After completion of the brachytherapy, the prostate will progressively shrink in size

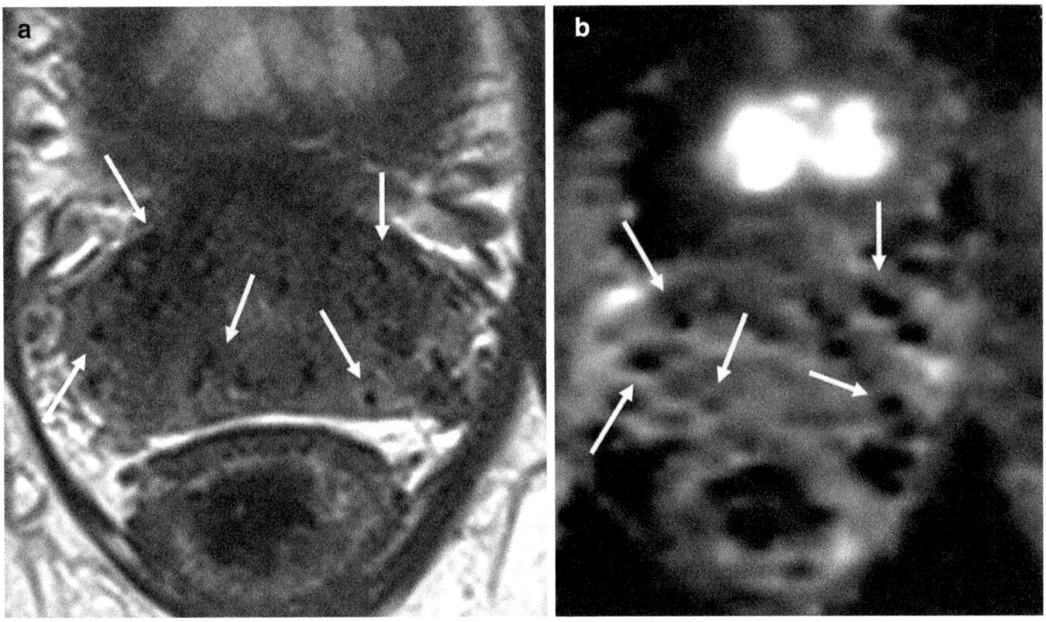

Fig. 12.5 Imaging findings after brachytherapy. Multiparametric MRI of a 68-year-old male with an initial PSA of 7.4 ng/mL who underwent brachytherapy in 2012 as treatment for a Gleason score 3 + 4 = 7 prostate cancer at the left peripheral zone. Follow-up imaging shows ellipsoid brachytherapy seeds (white arrows). (**a**) Axial T2W imaging demonstrates a diffuse hypointense signal and loss of differentiation between the transition zone and peripheral zone. (**b**) Axial ADC map

due to atrophy, allowing the seeds to be seen more peripherally within the gland [32]. The seeds appear as small ellipsoid T2W hypointense foci scattered throughout the gland. Interpretation of the DWI sequence is difficult due to artifacts caused by the metallic seeds [33]. In case of a HDR brachytherapy, the post-treatment imaging differs since the seeds are removed from the body. The use of MR imaging to evaluate HDR brachytherapy has yet to be validated.

12.3.2.2 Features of Recurrence After Brachytherapy

The general signal characteristics of recurrent disease after brachytherapy remain similar to EBRT. Recurrence is most often seen at the site of original cancer and will appear as a nodular structure with low T2W signal intensity [34]. Interpretation of the T2W imaging may be challenging, just as with EBRT, due to glandular atrophy and fibrosis [26, 35]. On DWI, it appears as a hypointense signal on the ADC map and hyperintense on high b-value images [36]. However, the DWI sequence is limited after treatment with LDR brachytherapy due to artifacts caused by metallic seeds. Overall, DCE imaging is more reliable compared to other sequences with an early hyperenhancement strongly suggestive of recurrence.

12.4 Minimally Invasive Therapies

Minimally invasive (or nonsurgical) therapies are a novel strategy for organ-confined prostate cancer. It offers targeted treatment of the index lesion, while preserving the benign tissue. The principle of most techniques is based on local destruction of cancerous cells in the prostate gland while using various energy sources [37]. An advantage to preservation of healthy prostatic tissue is to reduce treatment-related complications and morbidity [38]. The serum PSA levels are not very reliable for follow-up after focal ablation treatment as there is still prostatic tissue left behind [37].

It is recommended to perform a baseline prostate MRI before treatment in order to establish any post-treatment changes [39]. Evaluation of a post-treatment mpMRI may be challenging as normal post-treatment changes induced by minimally invasive treatment have similar signal characteristics as the prostate cancer [40]. To make interpretation more difficult, the treated area changes dynamically during the first year following treatment due to recovery and phagocytosis. Regardless of the energy source that was used, all techniques should result in atrophy at the location of the targeted area. This exhibits as a hypointense signal on T2W imaging along with a low-signal intensity on DWI and little to no enhancement on DCE images [41]. Since T2W image characteristics of recurrent disease after all minimal invasive treatment forms are very similar to prostate cancer, functional sequences of much more value for detection of any recurrences [25]. It is important to pay attention to the anterior rectum as it is most sensitive for injury and more carefully ablated, hence might find residual disease after minimal invasive treatment. Other locations at risk include the periurethral tissue, neurovascular bundle, and pubic bone marrow. Recurrent disease shows hypointense signal on T2W imaging with diffusion restriction on the ADC maps and early hyperenhancement on DCE images [41]. The DCE imaging tends to be the most reliable sequences in this context, due to its higher sensitivity and specificity [42].

12.4.1 Cryoablation

Cryoablation is based on the in situ destruction of prostate tissue by application of alternating freeze and thaw cycles to induce cell death. Tissue injury mainly occurs by lowering the temperature of extracellular water. This results in an osmotic gradient and cellular dehydration, followed by coagulative necrosis, thrombosis, and tissue hypoxia. The process is enhanced by intracellular ice formation causing a complete cell disruption. Traditionally, cryoablation is applied to whole gland for localized prostate cancer or as local recurrence after RT. Efforts have been made to apply cryoablation as focal or targeted treatment, especially as alternative salvage treatment option in patients with local recurrence after RT.

12.4.1.1 MR Imaging Findings After Cryoablation

The effects of cryoablation are overestimated on MR imaging as the visible area is often larger than the actual treated area. Normal post-treatment changes demonstrate a distorted prostate architecture with a low-signal intensity on T2W imaging (Fig. 12.6) [43]. T1W imaging

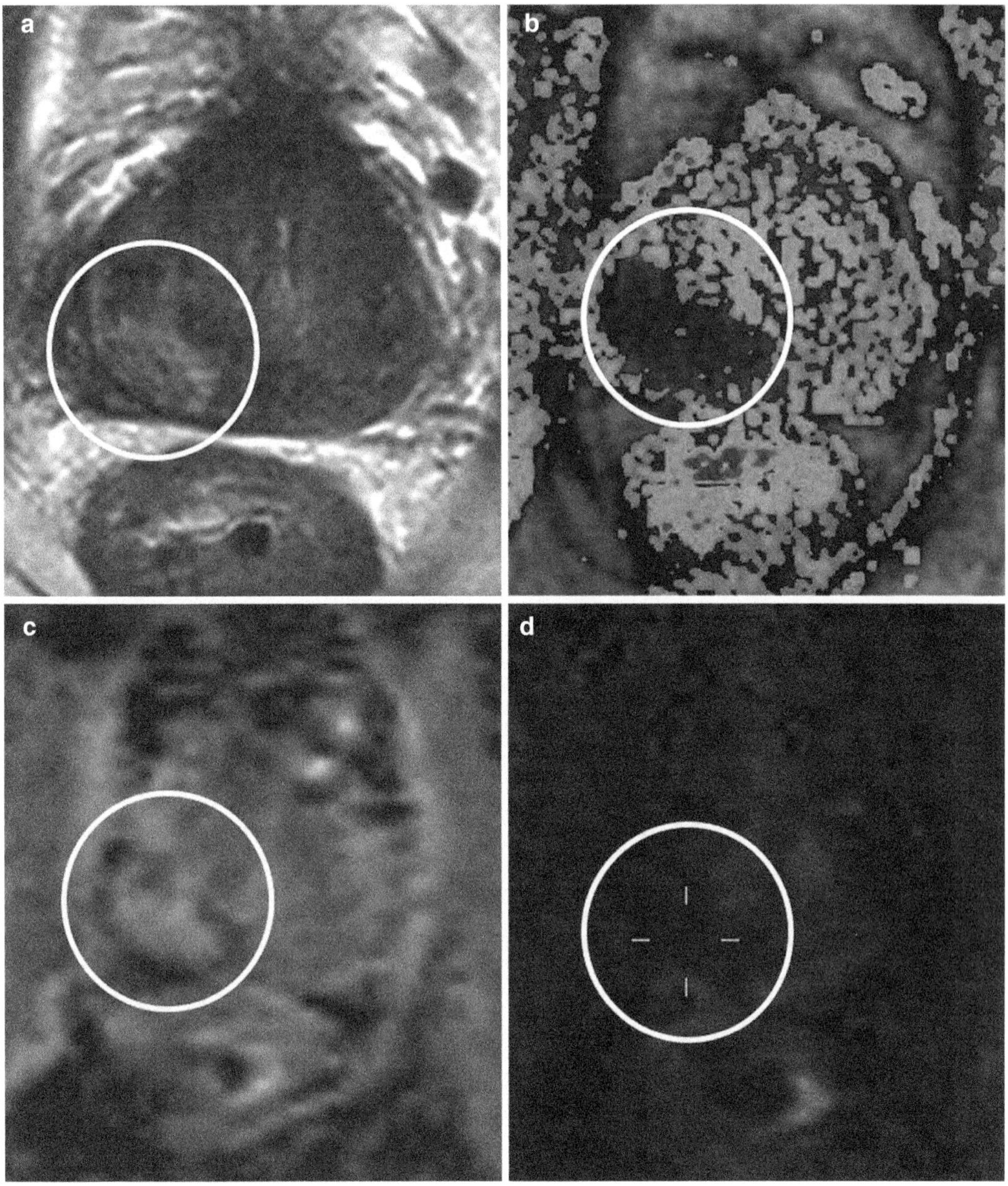

Fig. 12.6 Imaging findings after cryoablation. Multiparametric MRI of a 77-year-old male with an initial PSA of 11.4 ng/mL. Patient underwent EBRT in 2012 as treatment for a de novo lesion (Gleason score 4 + 4 = 8) at the right peripheral zone. During follow-up, serum PSA has risen from 1.1 to 2.7 ng/mL, and imaging showed a recurrent lesion at the right peripheral zone. Pathology showed a Gleason score 4 + 5 = 9 in two cores, and patient underwent cryotherapy. During the 3-month follow-up, mpMRI shows areas of heterogeneous signal, mingled with necrosis along with a rim of hypointense T2W signal and enhancement on DCE-MRI (white circles). (**a**) Axial T2W imaging; (**b**) axial DCE-MRI with an enhanced peripheral rim; (**c**) axial ADC map; (**d**) axial DWI with $b = 1400$ (calculated)

shows areas of heterogeneous enhancement mingled with necrosis along with a thickened capsule, urethra, and rectal wall. DCE imaging is more useful, especially when performed immediately after treatment. The treated area can be delineated as it exhibits no enhancement and is surrounded by an enhanced peripheral rim of prostatic tissue [44]. The urethral wall, neurovascular bundle, rectal wall, and pelvic bone marrow may not demonstrate enhancement on the DCE images directly after treatment; however, enhancement may be seen on follow-up examinations.

12.4.2 Focal Laser Ablation

Focal laser ablation (FLA) is a novel technique as the laser fiber is applied within the index lesion under image guidance. This technique is based on thermal energy ablation by raising the temperature within targeted area using the energy of the laser. When the temperature reaches more than 60 °C, cell necrosis is accomplished. The number of ablations needed depends on the volume of the intended lesion and the type of the laser fiber. MR-based temperature mapping allows real-time feedback of the thermal distribution in the prostate during treatment increasing efficacy. Therefore, FLA has become a more targeted and predictable approach compared to other treatment options and has a wide potential for use as it is safe and feasible for low- and intermediate-risk prostate cancer as well as salvage therapy.

12.4.2.1 MR Imaging Findings After Focal Laser Ablation

After FLA, MR imaging is mainly used to evaluate the degree and distribution of the expected necrosis in the targeted region. Directly after FLA, T2W imaging is not helpful in due to signal changes from hemorrhage and coagulative necrosis. Post-treatment DCE images demonstrate a focal defect with no enhancement in the treated area. The targeted lesion is oftentimes no longer visible on the 6-month follow-up imaging. After 6 months, mpMRI shows reduced prostate volume due to glandular atrophy [45]. The FLA treatment zone may show heterogeneous low-signal intensity on T2W imaging along with a restricted diffusion on DWI (Fig. 12.7).

12.4.2.2 High-Intensity Focused Ultrasound (HIFU)

During treatment with HIFU, energy from high-frequency ultrasound is used to heat and destroy the targeted tissue. HIFU is applied to the prostate either via an endorectal or transurethral probe. The ultrasound beam is focused on tumor tissue to rise to certain temperature. This results in thermal tissue coagulation and necrosis. It is suitable as treatment of localized prostate cancer or local recurrence after RT [46].

12.4.2.3 MR Imaging Findings After HIFU

Post-treatment imaging after HIFU demonstrates a heterogeneous and diffuse low-signal intensity on T2W imaging [47]. The targeted area appears as hypointense signal surrounded by a peripheral rim of enhancement which corresponds to necrosis and surrounding rim of inflammatory response. Directly after whole gland HIFU, a complete loss of the prostate zonal anatomy occurs with a separation of the central gland from the peripheral zone. Further distinction between benign and malign prostate tissue may be challenging due to the decreased background signal intensity. Hemorrhage and necrosis of the surrounding fatty tissue cause more difficulties in evaluation of the post-treatment images. On DCE images, the ablated area should exhibit no enhancement, but there might be a rim of residual enhancement surrounding the treatment area [48]. There may also be residual enhancement of the prostatic tissue near the apex and rectum wall since these areas are usually spared.

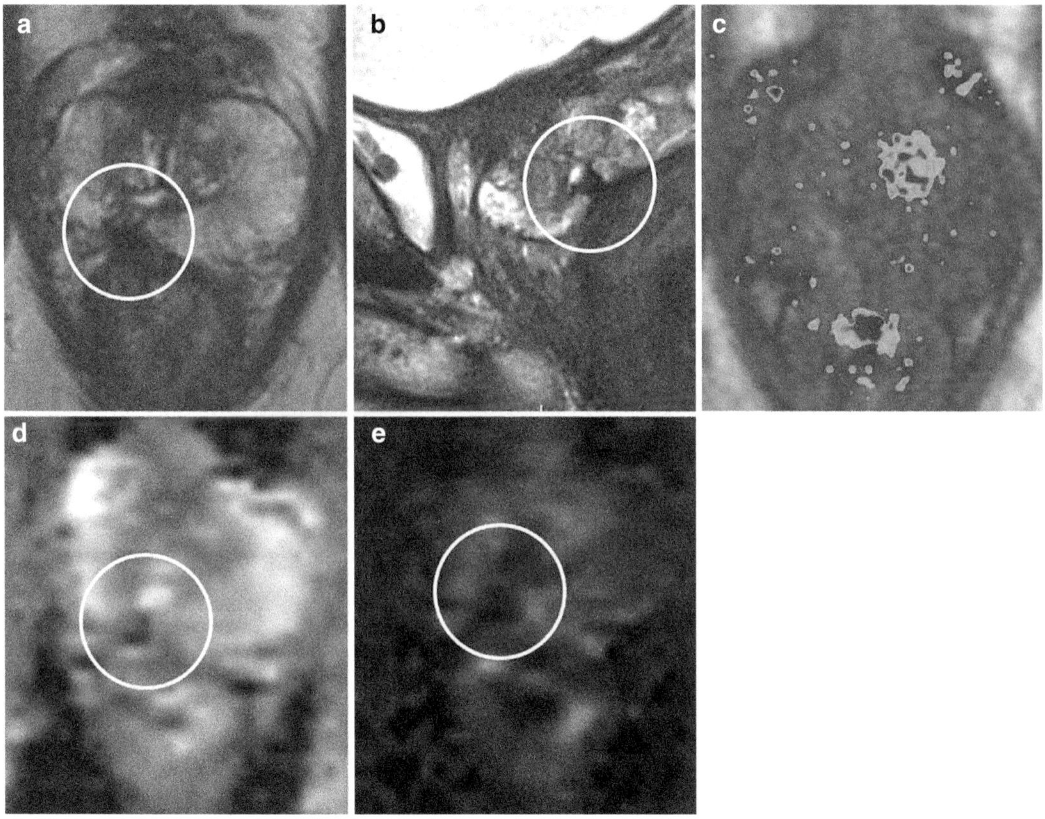

Fig. 12.7 Imaging findings after focal laser ablation. Multi-parametric MRI of a 61-year-old male with an initial PSA of 6.8 ng/mL who underwent focal laser ablation (FLA) as treatment for a de novo lesion (Gleason score 3 + 4 = 7) at the right peripheral zone (PI-RADS 4). On the 6-month follow-up MRI, ablated area exhibits as a heterogeneous low T2W signal intensity along with a restricted diffusion on DWI and demonstrates no enhancement in the treated area (white circles). (**a**) Axial T2W imaging of the mid prostate base with the ablation zone at the right peripheral zone; (**b**) sagittal T2W imaging with the ablation zone in the peripheral zone; (**c**) axial DCE MRI shows no enhancement; (**d**) axial ADC map; (**e**) axial DWI with $b = 1400$ (calculated)

12.4.2.4 Transurethral Ultrasound Ablation (TULSA)

TULSA is a novel technology that combines MR-based treatment planning and real-time monitoring with ablating prostate tissue using transurethral ultrasound [49]. This technique induces thermal coagulation of the prostate and is able to deliver accurate whole gland or focal ablation. The ablation volume can be prescribed precisely by using axial T2W images obtained at the time of the treatment. In addition, real-time temperature feedback control algorithm provided by the MRI results in reduced risk of damage to vital structures [50]. Normal post-treatment changes after TULSA demonstrate a total absence of the prostate with fibrotic tissue in the prostatic fossa on T2W imaging. The urethra and rectal wall are spared due to active water-based cooling (Fig. 12.8).

12.4.3 Irreversible Electroporation

Irreversible electroporation (IRE) is a relatively new type of treatment method for prostate cancer. It uses a surgical ablation technique where

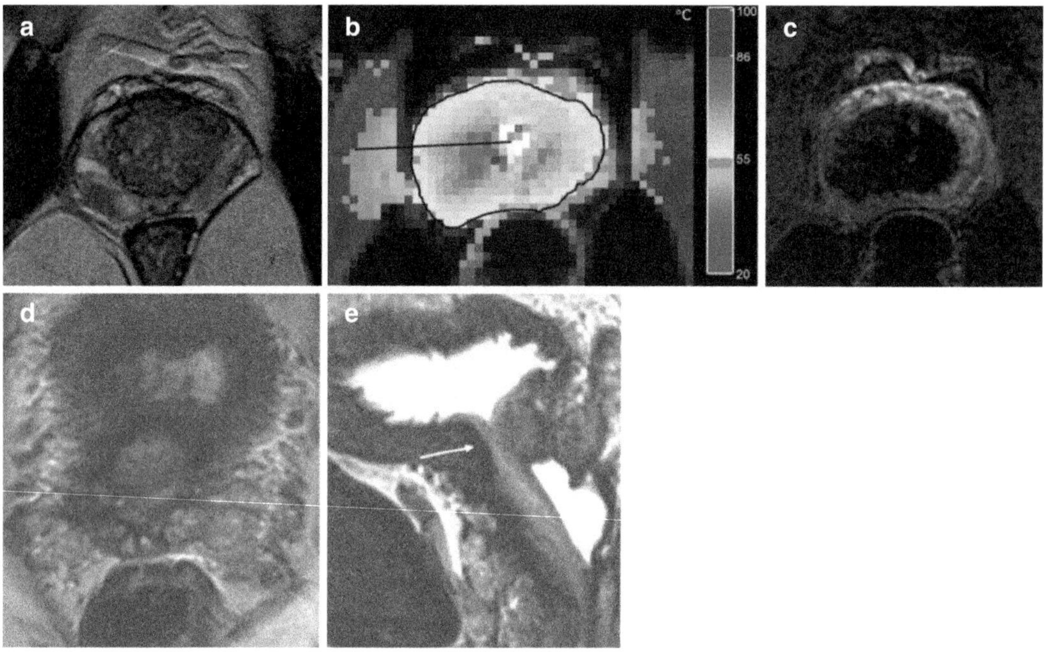

Fig. 12.8 Imaging findings after transurethral ultrasound ablation (TULSA). Multi-parametric MRI of a 65-year-old male with an initial PSA of 6.0 ng/mL. This patient underwent TULSA as treatment for a Gleason score 3 + 4 = 7 lesion at the left peripheral zone (PI-RADS 5). (**a**) Pre-treatment axial T2W imaging; (**b**) axial real-time temperature image during the treatment. (**c**) Axial post-treatment post-contrast T1-weighted image showing no internal enhancement. Eight months after the ablation, axial (**d**) and sagittal (**e**) T2W images demonstrate no residual prostate tissue, while the urethra is still visible (white arrow)

electrical pulses travel between electrodes inserted transperineally [51]. The electrical pulses induce an increased permeability of the cell membranes which result in apoptosis of the cancerous cells.

12.4.3.1 MR Imaging Findings After IRE

MR imaging findings after treatment with IRE are often very similar to other prostate cancer treatments. It includes heterogeneous signal intensity in the treated area on T2W imaging along with no enhancement on DCE images after administration of contrast agent [52].

12.5 Systemic Therapy

Prostate cancer occurs when normal cells become abnormal and start to grow and/or reproduce with no self-regulation. As it grows, it requires androgens as fuel by receptor activation. This is especially true during the early stages of prostate cancer development. Therefore, stopping the androgen production is one of the backbones of prostate cancer treatment. This can be accomplished surgically by a bilateral orchiectomy or using systemic drugs, better known as androgen deprivation therapy (ADT) [53].

12.5.1 Androgen Deprivation Therapy (ADT)

Systemic therapy is traditionally used as treatment for metastatic prostate cancer. However, ADT is commonly used as a supplementary regimen, in patients with rising PSA levels after local treatment, or as additional therapy in RT candidates [54]. Commonly used drugs are androgen receptor antagonists, antiandrogen drugs, gonadotropin-releasing hormone agonists, gonadotropin-releasing hormone antagonists, or 5a-reductase inhibitors [55]. Unfortunately, resistance to systemic drugs is relatively common with prolonged use.

12.5.1.1 MR Imaging Findings After ADT

None of the biochemical markers are reliable for distinction between local and distant tumor recurrence; therefore, a mpMRI is very valuable when monitoring for recurrent disease. The prostate volume decreases following ADT, with a greater extent in the peripheral zone compared to the transitional zone (Fig. 12.9). Depending on the type and duration of the therapy, patients demonstrate fluctuating responses to ADT on mpMRI, varying from no changes to reduced signal intensity on T2W imaging. The ADC value of the tumor is significantly increased after ADT compared to normal appearing peripheral and transitional zones. Additionally, the seminal vesicles shrink and show a hypointense signal on T2W images [56]. ADT reduces the tumor volume but does not necessarily result in downgrading of the staging of prostate cancer.

12.5.1.2 Features of Recurrence After ADT

An elevated serum PSA after treatment with ADT is an indication for persistent or recurrent disease. Typically, prostate cancer recurrence after ADT has the same imaging features as seen after RT. In most cases, tumor is readily identified on T2WI. Differentiation between tumor and normal post-treatment effect may be challenging due to the varying degrees of decreased signal intensity in the peripheral zone, resulting in overestimation of the recurrent or residual disease [56]. These inherent variabilities of changes to the prostate limit the clinical relevance of MR imaging after ADT.

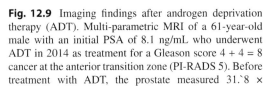

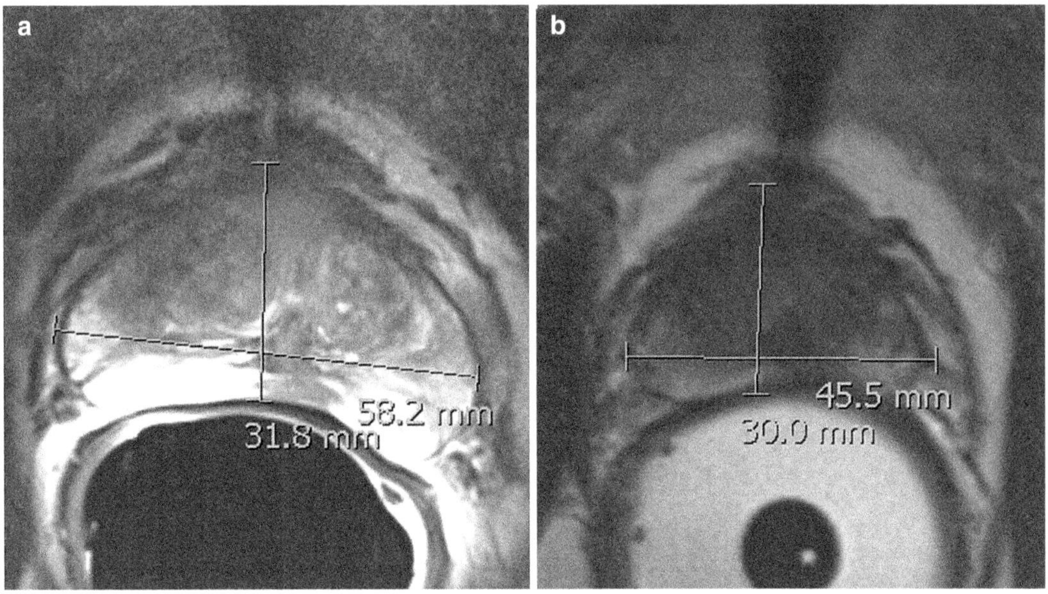

Fig. 12.9 Imaging findings after androgen deprivation therapy (ADT). Multi-parametric MRI of a 61-year-old male with an initial PSA of 8.1 ng/mL who underwent ADT in 2014 as treatment for a Gleason score 4 + 4 = 8 cancer at the anterior transition zone (PI-RADS 5). Before treatment with ADT, the prostate measured 31.`8 × 58.2 mm using the axial dimensions. Six months after treatment with ADT, the mpMRI prostate measured 30.0 mm x 45.5 mm. (**a**) Axial T2W imaging before treatment with ADT; (**b**) axial T2W imaging after treatment with ADT

References

1. Rosenkrantz AB, Verma S, Choyke P, Eberhardt SC, Eggener SE, Gaitonde K, et al. Prostate magnetic resonance imaging and magnetic resonance imaging targeted biopsy in patients with a prior negative biopsy: a consensus statement by AUA and SAR. J Urol. 2016;196(6):1613–8.
2. European Association U. European Association of Urology guidelines. 2018 Edition. Arnhem: European Association of Urology Guidelines Office; 2018.
3. Siegel R, DeSantis C, Virgo K, Stein K, Mariotto A, Smith T, et al. Cancer treatment and survivorship statistics, 2012. CA Cancer J Clin. 2012;62(4):220–41.
4. Mottet N, Bellmunt J, Bolla M, Briers E, Cumberbatch MG, De Santis M, et al. EAU-ESTRO-SIOG guidelines on prostate Cancer. Part 1: screening, diagnosis, and local treatment with curative intent. Eur Urol. 2017;71(4):618–29.
5. Mertan FV, Greer MD, Borofsky S, Kabakus IM, Merino MJ, Wood BJ, et al. Multiparametric magnetic resonance imaging of recurrent prostate Cancer. Top Magn Reson Imaging. 2016;25(3):139–47.
6. Hull GW, Rabbani F, Abbas F, Wheeler TM, Kattan MW, Scardino PT. Cancer control with radical prostatectomy alone in 1,000 consecutive patients. J Urol. 2002;167(2 Pt 1):528–34.
7. Stephenson AJ, Scardino PT, Eastham JA, Bianco FJ Jr, Dotan ZA, Fearn PA, et al. Preoperative nomogram predicting the 10-year probability of prostate cancer recurrence after radical prostatectomy. J Natl Cancer Inst. 2006;98(10):715–7.
8. Valerio M, Cerantola Y, Eggener SE, Lepor H, Polascik TJ, Villers A, et al. New and established Technology in Focal Ablation of the prostate: a systematic review. Eur Urol. 2017;71(1):17–34.
9. Bill-Axelson A, Holmberg L, Ruutu M, Garmo H, Stark JR, Busch C, et al. Radical prostatectomy versus watchful waiting in early prostate cancer. N Engl J Med. 2011;364(18):1708–17.
10. Tewari A, Sooriakumaran P, Bloch DA, Seshadri-Kreaden U, Hebert AE, Wiklund P. Positive surgical margin and perioperative complication rates of primary surgical treatments for prostate cancer: a systematic review and meta-analysis comparing retropubic, laparoscopic, and robotic prostatectomy. Eur Urol. 2012;62(1):1–15.
11. Allen SD, Thompson A, Sohaib SA. The normal post-surgical anatomy of the male pelvis following radical prostatectomy as assessed by magnetic resonance imaging. Eur Radiol. 2008;18(6):1281–91.
12. Hricak H, Williams RD, Spring DB, Moon KL Jr, Hedgcock MW, Watson RA, et al. Anatomy and pathology of the male pelvis by magnetic resonance imaging. AJR Am J Roentgenol. 1983;141(6):1101–10.
13. Sella T, Schwartz LH, Hricak H. Retained seminal vesicles after radical prostatectomy: frequency, MRI characteristics, and clinical relevance. AJR Am J Roentgenol. 2006;186(2):539–46.
14. Cirillo S, Petracchini M, Scotti L, Gallo T, Macera A, Bona MC, et al. Endorectal magnetic resonance imaging at 1.5 T to assess local recurrence following radical prostatectomy using T2-weighted and contrast-enhanced imaging. Eur Radiol. 2009;19(3):761–9.
15. Vargas HA, Wassberg C, Akin O, Hricak H. MR imaging of treated prostate cancer. Radiology. 2012;262(1):26–42.
16. Sella T, Schwartz LH, Swindle PW, Onyebuchi CN, Scardino PT, Scher HI, et al. Suspected local recurrence after radical prostatectomy: endorectal coil MR imaging. Radiology. 2004;231(2):379–85.
17. Notley M, Yu J, Fulcher AS, Turner MA, Cockrell CH, Nguyen D. Pictorial review. Diagnosis of recurrent prostate cancer and its mimics at multiparametric prostate MRI. Br J Radiol. 2015;88(1054):20150362.
18. Cooperberg MR, Broering JM, Carroll PR. Time trends and local variation in primary treatment of localized prostate cancer. J Clin Oncol. 2010;28(7):1117–23.
19. Bolla M, Van Tienhoven G, Warde P, Dubois JB, Mirimanoff RO, Storme G, et al. External irradiation with or without long-term androgen suppression for prostate cancer with high metastatic risk: 10-year results of an EORTC randomised study. Lancet Oncol. 2010;11(11):1066–73.
20. Pickles T. Prostate-specific antigen (PSA) bounce and other fluctuations: which biochemical relapse definition is least prone to PSA false calls? An analysis of 2030 men treated for prostate cancer with external beam or brachytherapy with or without adjuvant androgen deprivation therapy. Int J Radiat Oncol Biol Phys. 2006;64(5):1355–9.
21. Ng M, Brown E, Williams A, Chao M, Lawrentschuk N, Chee R. Fiducial markers and spacers in prostate radiotherapy: current applications. BJU Int. 2014;113(Suppl 2):13–20.
22. Sugimura K, Carrington BM, Quivey JM, Hricak H. Postirradiation changes in the pelvis: assessment with MR imaging. Radiology. 1990;175(3):805–13.
23. Chan TW, Kressel HY. Prostate and seminal vesicles after irradiation: MR appearance. J Magn Reson Imaging. 1991;1(5):503–11.
24. Zumsteg ZS, Spratt DE, Romesser PB, Pei X, Zhang Z, Kollmeier M, et al. Anatomical patterns of recurrence following biochemical relapse in the dose escalation era of external beam radiotherapy for prostate Cancer. J Urol. 2015;194(6):1624–30.
25. McCammack KC, Raman SS, Margolis DJ. Imaging of local recurrence in prostate cancers. Future Oncol (London, England). 2016;12(21):2401–15.
26. Sala E, Eberhardt SC, Akin O, Moskowitz CS, Onyebuchi CN, Kuroiwa K, et al. Endorectal MR imaging before salvage prostatectomy: tumor localization and staging. Radiology. 2006;238(1):176–83.

27. Barchetti F, Panebianco V. Multiparametric MRI for recurrent prostate cancer post radical prostatectomy and postradiation therapy. Biomed Res Int. 2014;2014:316272.
28. Rouviere O, Valette O, Grivolat S, Colin-Pangaud C, Bouvier R, Chapelon JY, et al. Recurrent prostate cancer after external beam radiotherapy: value of contrast-enhanced dynamic MRI in localizing intraprostatic tumor–correlation with biopsy findings. Urology. 2004;63(5):922–7.
29. Tamada T, Sone T, Jo Y, Hiratsuka J, Higaki A, Higashi H, et al. Locally recurrent prostate cancer after high-dose-rate brachytherapy: the value of diffusion-weighted imaging, dynamic contrast-enhanced MRI, and T2-weighted imaging in localizing tumors. AJR Am J Roentgenol. 2011;197(2):408–14.
30. Koukourakis G, Kelekis N, Armonis V, Kouloulias V. Brachytherapy for prostate cancer: a systematic review. Ther Adv Urol. 2009;2009:327945.
31. Sylvester JE, Blasko JC, Grimm PD, Meier R, Malmgren JA. Ten-year biochemical relapse-free survival after external beam radiation and brachytherapy for localized prostate cancer: the Seattle experience. Int J Radiat Oncol Biol Phys. 2003;57(4):944–52.
32. Coakley FV, Hricak H, Wefer AE, Speight JL, Kurhanewicz J, Roach M. Brachytherapy for prostate cancer: endorectal MR imaging of local treatment-related changes. Radiology. 2001;219(3):817–21.
33. Rouviere O, Vitry T, Lyonnet D. Imaging of prostate cancer local recurrences: why and how? Eur Radiol. 2010;20(5):1254–66.
34. Pucar D, Hricak H, Shukla-Dave A, Kuroiwa K, Drobnjak M, Eastham J, et al. Clinically significant prostate cancer local recurrence after radiation therapy occurs at the site of primary tumor: magnetic resonance imaging and step-section pathology evidence. Int J Radiat Oncol Biol Phys. 2007;69(1):62–9.
35. Westphalen AC, Coakley FV, Roach M 3rd, McCulloch CE, Kurhanewicz J. Locally recurrent prostate cancer after external beam radiation therapy: diagnostic performance of 1.5-T endorectal MR imaging and MR spectroscopic imaging for detection. Radiology. 2010;256(2):485–92.
36. Yu J, Fulcher AS, Turner MA, Cockrell CH, Cote EP, Wallace TJ. Prostate cancer and its mimics at multiparametric prostate MRI. Br J Radiol. 2014;87(1037):20130659.
37. Bozzini G, Colin P, Nevoux P, Villers A, Mordon S, Betrouni N. Focal therapy of prostate cancer: energies and procedures. Urol Oncol. 2013;31(2):155–67.
38. Eggener S, Salomon G, Scardino PT, De la Rosette J, Polascik TJ, Brewster S. Focal therapy for prostate cancer: possibilities and limitations. Eur Urol. 2010;58(1):57–64.
39. Muller BG, van den Bos W, Brausi M, Cornud F, Gontero P, Kirkham A, et al. Role of multiparametric magnetic resonance imaging (MRI) in focal therapy for prostate cancer: a Delphi consensus project. BJU Int. 2014;114(5):698–707.
40. Ahmed HU, Moore C, Lecornet E, Emberton M. Focal therapy in prostate cancer: determinants of success and failure. J Endourol. 2010;24(5):819–25.
41. De Visschere PJ, De Meerleer GO, Futterer JJ, Villeirs GM. Role of MRI in follow-up after focal therapy for prostate carcinoma. AJR Am J Roentgenol. 2010;194(6):1427–33.
42. Verma S, Turkbey B, Muradyan N, Rajesh A, Cornud F, Haider MA, et al. Overview of dynamic contrast-enhanced MRI in prostate cancer diagnosis and management. AJR Am J Roentgenol. 2012;198(6):1277–88.
43. Martino P, Scattoni V, Galosi AB, Consonni P, Trombetta C, Palazzo S, et al. Role of imaging and biopsy to assess local recurrence after definitive treatment for prostate carcinoma (surgery, radiotherapy, cryotherapy, HIFU). World J Urol. 2011;29(5):595–605.
44. Rosenkrantz AB, Scionti SM, Mendrinos S, Taneja SS. Role of MRI in minimally invasive focal ablative therapy for prostate cancer. AJR Am J Roentgenol. 2011;197(1):W90–6.
45. Felker ER, Raman SS, Lu DSK, Tuttle M, Margolis DJ, ElKhoury FF, et al. Utility of multiparametric MRI for predicting residual clinically significant prostate cancer after focal laser ablation. AJR Am J Roentgenol. 2019;213:1–6.
46. Blana A, Murat FJ, Walter B, Thuroff S, Wieland WF, Chaussy C, et al. First analysis of the long-term results with transrectal HIFU in patients with localised prostate cancer. Eur Urol. 2008;53(6):1194–201.
47. Rouviere O, Lyonnet D, Raudrant A, Colin-Pangaud C, Chapelon JY, Bouvier R, et al. MRI appearance of prostate following transrectal HIFU ablation of localized cancer. Eur Urol. 2001;40(3):265–74.
48. Kirkham AP, Emberton M, Hoh IM, Illing RO, Freeman AA, Allen C. MR imaging of prostate after treatment with high-intensity focused ultrasound. Radiology. 2008;246(3):833–44.
49. Chopra R, Colquhoun A, Burtnyk M, N'Djin WA, Kobelevskiy I, Boyes A, et al. MR imaging-controlled transurethral ultrasound therapy for conformal treatment of prostate tissue: initial feasibility in humans. Radiology. 2012;265(1):303–13.
50. Chin JL, Billia M, Relle J, Roethke MC, Popeneciu IV, Kuru TH, et al. Magnetic resonance imaging-guided transurethral ultrasound ablation of prostate tissue in patients with localized prostate Cancer: a prospective phase 1 clinical trial. Eur Urol. 2016;70(3):447–55.
51. Rubinsky B, Onik G, Mikus P. Irreversible electroporation: a new ablation modality--clinical implications. Technol Cancer Res Treat. 2007;6(1):37–48.

52. Scheltema MJ, Postema AW, de Bruin DM, Buijs M, Engelbrecht MR, Laguna MP, et al. Irreversible electroporation for the treatment of localized prostate cancer: a summary of imaging findings and treatment feedback. Diagn Intervent Radiol (Ankara, Turkey). 2017;23(5):365–70.
53. Massard C, Fizazi K. Targeting continued androgen receptor signaling in prostate cancer. Clin Cancer Res. 2011;17(12):3876–83.
54. Bolla M, de Reijke TM, Van Tienhoven G, Van den Bergh AC, Oddens J, Poortmans PM, et al. Duration of androgen suppression in the treatment of prostate cancer. N Engl J Med. 2009;360(24):2516–27.
55. Sharifi N, Gulley JL, Dahut WL. Androgen deprivation therapy for prostate cancer. JAMA. 2005;294(2):238–44.
56. Chen M, Hricak H, Kalbhen CL, Kurhanewicz J, Vigneron DB, Weiss JM, et al. Hormonal ablation of prostatic cancer: effects on prostate morphology, tumor detection, and staging by endorectal coil MR imaging. AJR Am J Roentgenol. 1996;166(5):1157–63.

Molecular Imaging of Prostate Cancer

13

Moozhan Nikpanah, Esther Mena, Peter L. Choyke, and Baris Turkbey

13.1 Introduction

With 174,650 new cases and 31,620 deaths per year, prostate cancer (PCa) is the most commonly diagnosed non-cutaneous cancer and the second cause of cancer-associated mortality in men in the USA [1]. The biological behavior and clinical course of PCa show a broad spectrum from indolent intraprostatic tumors to aggressive metastatic disease [2–4].

Imaging is a crucial aspect of prostate cancer management [5]. In spite of considerable advances, currently used diagnostic imaging modalities for primary tumor diagnosis, evaluation of metastatic disease, and detecting sites of biochemical recurrence (BCR) seem to be suboptimal [6]. Transrectal ultrasonography (TRUS)-guided biopsy subsequent to prostate-specific antigen (PSA) screening has been the primary tool for assessment of PCa [7]. Multiparametric MRI (mpMRI) has been utilized to further identification of clinically aggressive prostate tumors, underdiagnosed with screening-driven TRUS-guided biopsies. Even though mpMRI has proven its utility in detection and local staging of the untreated prostatic tumors, evaluating invasion, and detecting recurrences, its success rate is still limited [3, 8, 9]. Hence, molecular imaging with positron emission tomography (PET) has been increasingly taken into consideration in prostate cancer as this noninvasive imaging method targets certain biological aspects of tumors [3, 10]. PET is often merged with computed tomography (CT) or magnetic resonance imaging (MRI) for better anatomical localization of increased metabolic avidity in addition to differentiation of physiologic activity from pathologic uptake [11]. The landscape of available PET radiotracers for PCa imaging includes probes interrogating tumor metabolism (^{18}F-FDG), fatty acids metabolism (^{11}C acetate), the biology of choline (^{11}C/^{18}F Choline), amino acid transport upregulation (^{18}F FACBC), those targeting prostate-specific membrane antigen (PSMA) receptors (^{68}Ga-PSMA, ^{18}F-DCFBC, ^{18}F-DCFPyl, ^{18}F-PSMA-1007), and other agents targeting hormone receptors or gastrin-releasing peptide receptor [3]. In this chapter, we review some of these clinically available tracers in the setting of primary disease diagnosis, staging, and biochemical recurrence prostate cancer.

M. Nikpanah
NIH, Clinical Center, Radiology and Imaging Sciences, Bethesda, MD, USA
e-mail: seyedehmoozhan.nikpanah@nih.gov

E. Mena · P. L. Choyke · B. Turkbey (✉)
NCI, NIH, Molecular Imaging Program, Bethesda, MD, USA
e-mail: esther.menagonzalez@nih.gov; pchoyke@mail.nih.gov; turkbeyi@mail.nih.gov

T. Tirkes (ed.), *Prostate MRI Essentials*, https://doi.org/10.1007/978-3-030-45935-2_13

13.2 ^{18}F-FDG

^{18}F-FDG-PET/CT has become the basis of molecular imaging in detection, staging, and monitoring of a vast majority of malignancies [12]. The amount of FDG avidity is mainly associated with the rate of glucose metabolism by tumor cells comparing to non-cancer cells, originally known as the Warburg effect [13]. Increased glucose uptake by tumor cells is mainly caused by overexpression of membrane glucose transporters (GLUTs) and increased hexokinase activity [14]. Beyond the routine standard of care ^{18}F-FDG-PET/CT imaging in many malignant tumors, it has demonstrated limited value for imaging the typically indolent PCa [3, 15, 16], mostly as a result of low glucose metabolism in prostate cancer cells [17–19]. Previous studies have demonstrated insufficient results in the use of FDG in primary diagnosis, initial staging, or evaluation of biochemical recurrence [20–23]. Recent studies have shown higher FDG avidity in more aggressive PCa tumors [24–26] (Fig. 13.1). In fact, the phase of the disease seems to be the determinant factor for the utility of ^{18}F-FDG PET in prostate cancer [27].

13.2.1 Primary Disease

Overlap between FDG uptake of PCa tumors, benign prostatic hyperplasia (BPH), and normal

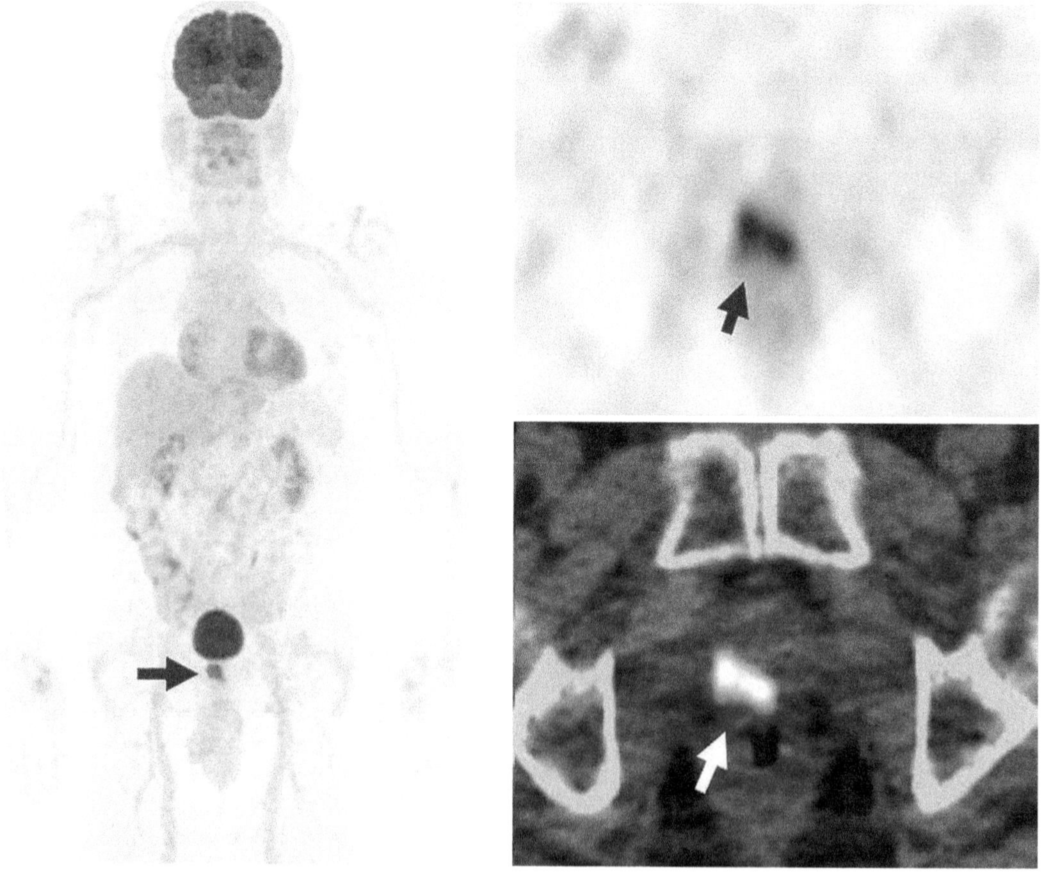

Fig. 13.1 77-year-old patient with history of high-risk cT3b, Gleason 10 (5 + 5) prostate cancer, treated with external beam radiation and neoadjuvant, concomitant and long-term ADT for 2 years. Patient had biochemical recurrence 9 years after treatment, with PSA of 0.15 ng/mL (patient currently on ADT). 18F-FDG PET/CT imaging, including maximal intensity projection, and axial PET and PET/CT fused images demonstrate a large hypermetabolic focus at the right mid-to-base peripheral zone of the prostate gland consistent with disease recurrence (arrows)

prostate tissue, which are frequently present in the same gland, has been previously reported [19, 27]. Minamimoto et al. [28] evaluated the role of ^{18}F-FDG PET/CT prior to biopsy in 50 patients with elevated PSA levels, reporting sensitivity and specificity within the prostate of 51.9% and 75.7%, respectively. In particular, the sensitivity and specificity were 22.7% and 85.9% in the central zone and 73.3% and 64.3% in the peripheral zone, respectively [28]. Other studies have reported even lower sensitivities for primary tumor detection [29, 30]. However, biopsy-proven malignant prostate lesions that showed higher ^{18}F-FDG uptake were reported to be more aggressive tumors. Minamimoto et al. [28] reported a positive predictive value (PPV) of 87% and sensitivity of 80% for ^{18}F-FDG PET/CT in detecting lesions with Gleason score ≥7 [28]. These studies highlight the fact that while ^{18}F-FDG PET/CT detects more advanced prostate cancers with higher Gleason scores, it is not the method of choice for prostate cancer detection since it misses the majority of typically indolent, less aggressive prostate cancers.

Previous studies have assessed the role of incidental high ^{18}F-FDG avidity in primary prostate cancer detection. Bertagna et al. evaluated the risk of malignancy and prevalence of incidental ^{18}F-FDG uptake detected by ^{18}FDG-PET/CT in a meta-analysis and systematic review of 6 studies, including 444 patients [31]. For high incidental FDG uptake, a poor prevalence of 1.8% was observed. The overall pooled risk of malignancy in cases with high FDG avidity was 17% (95%CI, 12–23%) and increased to 62% in the biopsy-proven cohort (n = 121). They found a trend of higher maximum standardized uptake value (SUV_{max}) in malignant tumors with high incidental uptake; however, there was no statistically significant difference when compared to benign lesions with high incidental FDG avidity [31]. In another study by Kang et al., higher SUV_{max} was reported in prostate cancer tumors than benign lesions. However, no significant association was found between SUV_{max} and serum PSA, Gleason score, and prostate tumor volume [32]. ^{18}F-FDG-PET/CT was not able to differentiate cancerous from benign lesions. Therefore, it was concluded that prostatic biopsy was not suggested in cases with incidental high FDG avidity. However, further clinical investigations such as PSA were recommended in patients with high incidental uptake on ^{18}F-FDG PET/CT scans [32]. Consistent with prior studies, in a study by Reesink et al., incidental FDG uptake on PET/CT images showed a low positive predictive value for prostate cancer [33]. Sahin et al. observed incidental FDG avidity in 1.3% of patients who underwent PET/CT scans. Furthermore, SUV_{max} was not able to differentiate benign from cancerous lesions, and no association was observed between serum PSA and SUV_{max} [34]. Brown et al. recommended that high incidental FDG avidity with SUV_{max} >6 needed to be further evaluated by mpMRI [35]. In a study by Kwon et al., further evaluation, for instance, PSA measurement, was suggested to be performed in patients with higher SUV_{max}, and prostate biopsy was recommended in those with high PSA levels [36].

13.2.2 Staging

^{18}F-FDG PET/CT has shown unsatisfactory results in primary staging of PCa. Therefore, limited number of studies has focused on this subject in the past years. Beauregard et al. studied 54 patients with primary tumors Gleason score ≥8 whose FDG PET/CT was performed prior to biopsy. Surgical lymphadenectomy was performed on 41 out of 54 patients. Based on histopathology reports, 11/41 (27%) of patients had lymph node metastases, among whom only 3 (3/11, 27%) were positive on FDG scans [26]. Liu et al. retrospectively assessed nine prostate cancer patients with ^{18}F-FDG PET/CT at the time of initial staging; despite showing a low sensitivity (33%) in detection of primary malignant tumors, ^{18}F-FDG PET/CT demonstrated nodal or bone metastases in six out of nine cases [29]. It could be concluded that ^{18}FDG PET/CT has a higher sensitivity in localizing metastases than detection of primary PCa tumors [29]. However, in general, ^{18}FDG PET/CT is limited for primary staging of PCa.

13.2.3 Biochemical Recurrence

Localizing the site of recurrence has a high clinical significance in patients with BCR, as it is beneficial for planning the proper management. Same as the primary diagnosis and initial staging, ^{18}F-FDG PET/CT has a limited value in evaluation of biochemical recurrence in PCa patients. In a retrospective study by Schöder et al. that was performed on 91 patients with BCR, it was reported that FDG PET was able to detect localized or systemic disease in 31% of cases. In addition, the likelihood of disease detection showed an increase with a rise in PSA levels [37]. However, in a different study, Chang et al. investigated the FDG avidity in 24 patients with biochemical recurrence that had undergone FDG PET/CT scan prior to pelvic nodal dissection [38]. They reported sensitivity, specificity, accuracy, negative predictive value, and positive predictive of 75%, 100%, 83.3%, 67.7%, and 100%, respectively, for localizing lymph node metastases [38]. In another study assessing the efficacy of ^{11}C-choline and ^{18}F-FDG in BCR PCa patients, ^{18}F-FDG and ^{11}C-choline showed sensitivity of 31% and 60.6%, respectively [39]. When PSA levels were >1.9 ng/mL, sensitivities increased up to 40% and 80%, respectively [39]. Öztürk et al. retrospectively investigated the use of ^{18}F-FDG PET/CT in detection of recurrence in 28 patients, who had received external beam radiation therapy or undergone radical prostatectomy [40]. They reported sensitivity of 61.6% and specificity of 75.0% for ^{18}F-FDG PET/CT [40]. In the retrospective study by Liu et al., assessing 16 patients with biochemical recurrence, ^{18}FDG PET/CT detected metastatic disease in 12 cases [29]. It was also able to identify recurrent tumors within the prostate gland in two patients. Moreover, there was a statistically significant difference in PSA values between patients with negative vs. those with positive results on ^{18}FDG PET/CT [29]. In another study that prospectively evaluated the role of ^{18}F-FDG PET/CT and ^{18}F-NaF PET/CT in identifying occult metastases in 37 patients with BCR, ^{18}FDG PET/CT demonstrated overall detection rate of 8.1% [41]. Present findings suggest that ^{18}FDG PET/CT has a limited utility in the assessment of BCR PCa patients, with more value in those with higher PSA levels.

13.3 ^{11}C/^{18}F-Acetate

Acetate is converted to fatty acids that are incorporated in the cell membrane in a two-step mechanism (acetate to acetyl-CoA via acetyl-CoA synthase and acetyl-CoA to fatty acids via fatty acid synthase) [3]. Enhanced fatty acid synthase activity causes increased acetate uptake in PCa lesions, which has been indicated to be associated with the aggressiveness of these tumors [42]. Both ^{11}C- and ^{18}F-labeled acetate tracers have been developed; however, ^{11}C-acetate is significantly less practical [3]; since it has a short half-life (20 min), that makes its utility limited to centers with an on-site cyclotron [5, 43]. However, its negligible urinary tract excretion makes it a desirable tracer for evaluation of local prostate disease recurrence [15, 44].

13.3.1 Primary Disease

Even though ^{11}C-acetate has shown success in detection of advanced PCa, it has not been reported to be helpful in assessing localized disease [5]. Mena et al. investigated 39 cases of localized PCa who underwent ^{11}C-acetate PET/CT and mpMRI before prostatectomy [45]. SUVs derived from ^{11}acetate PET were compared with findings from mpMRI and histopathology reports. Despite showing a significantly higher ^{11}C-acetate uptake by tumor cells compared to normal prostate tissue, considerable overlap in tracer uptake was found between malignant tumors and benign prostatic hyperplasia. In comparison with histopathology, ^{11}acetate PET/CT showed sensitivity of 61.6% and specificity of 80% for tumors >0.5 cm. Multiparametric MRI demonstrated sensitivity of 82.3% and specificity of 95.1%. Comparable results were revealed for ^{11}acetate PET/CT and mpMRI in lesions >0.9 cm [45]. In a study by Jabor et al. on 36 patients with untreated, nonmetastatic PCa, a sensitivity and specificity of 88% and 41%, respectively, were reported for ^{11}C-acetate PET/CT in detection of primary tumors [46]. In a meta-analysis by Mohsen et al. including 23 studies, a pooled sensitivity of 75.1% and specificity of 75.8% were reported for ^{11}C-acetate PET regarding primary tumor detection [47]. Furthermore, they reported that ^{11}C-acetate PET not only showed high uptake in benign prostatic hyperplasia but also was not able to detect small lesions [47]. In general, despite showing higher sensitivity than ^{18}F-FDG reported by previous studies [48, 49], the use of ^{11}C-acetate PET/CT is not justified over conventional imaging methods such as mpMRI for primary prostate cancer detection [15].

13.3.2 Staging

Haseebuddin et al. performed ^{11}C-acetate PET/CT on 107 patients with intermediate- or high-risk prostate cancer, who had no lymph node involvement on conventional imaging [50]. ^{11}C-acetate PET/CT demonstrated positive findings for pelvic lymph node involvement or distant metastases in 36 out of 107 (33.6%) patients. Based on histopathology reports, lymph node metastasis was present in 25 cases (23.4%). ^{11}C-acetate PET/CT demonstrated sensitivity, specificity, negative predictive value, and positive predictive value of 68%, 78.1%, 88.9%, and 48.6%, respectively, for identification of nodal metastasis. ^{11}C-acetate PET/CT was suggested as an useful asset in staging of pelvic lymph nodes and therapeutic decision-making [50]. In a study by Schumacher et al., 19 PCa patients underwent extended pelvic lymph node dissection subsequent to ^{11}C-acetate PET/CT scan [51]. In the patient-based analysis, ^{11}C-acetate PET/CT demonstrated high sensitivity (90%) but low sensitivity (67%). However, nodal region-based analysis revealed low sensitivity (62%) and high specificity (89%). Furthermore, ^{11}C-acetate PET/CT was reported to have limitations in detecting small lesions and the exact nodal disease location, which caused false-positive and false-negative results in more than one-third of the patients [51].

13.3.3 Biochemical Recurrence

In the meta-analysis of 23 studies by Mohsen et al., ^{11}C-acetate PET showed pooled sensitivity and specificity of 64% and 93%, respectively, for evaluation of BCR PCa patients [47]. A retrospective study by Leisser et al. evaluated 123 patients with suspected local recurrence using ^{11}C-acetate PET/CT, which demonstrated positive uptake in 82 patients [52]. PSA velocity was shown to be notably higher in patients with positive PET findings. In addition, a positive association between higher SUV_{max} and the initial primary tumor Gleason score was observed. Hence, they proposed that ^{11}C-acetate PET could be a prognostic tool for recurrent prostate cancers [52]. In a retrospective study on 120 patients by Dusing et al., higher positive results were observed on ^{11}C-acetate PET/CT for PSA >1.24 ng/mL or PSA velocity >W1.32 ng/mL/year [53]. Therefore, it can be concluded that in biochemical recurrence, ^{11}C-acetate might be useful as an indicator of tumor aggressiveness [5]. In a recent study by Almeida et al., the performance of ^{11}C-acetate PET/CT in detecting biochemical recurrence and its correlation with PSA value was evaluated [54]. ^{11}C-acetate PET/CT scans showed positive results in localizing the site of recurrence or metastasis in 637 out of 721 (88%) patients with biochemical recurrence [54]. In addition, it was reported that with optimal threshold values of PSA >1.09 ng/mL, or PSA doubling time of <3.8 months, ^{11}C-acetate PET/CT scans had the highest likelihood of showing positive results [54]. The role of ^{11}C-acetate PET/CT as a predictor of survival in patients with BCR was investigated by Regula et al. [55]. Five-year prostate cancer-specific survival was reported as 100% and 80% in cases with negative and positive ^{11}C-acetate PET/CT results, respectively. It was suggested that ^{11}C-acetate PET/CT might be useful in determining high-risk cases among patients with biochemical recurrence [55].

13.4 $^{11}C/^{18}F$-Choline

Choline is a precursor for phosphatidylcholine, which is the main phospholipid in cell membrane. Through choline transporters, choline is internalized into cells and metabolized by choline kinase, which has a pivotal role in cellular membrane synthesis. Increased choline uptake by prostate tumor cells has been reported to be due to overexpression of choline kinase [56]. Analogs of choline tracer are different in excretion patterns and half-life. Short half-life of ^{11}C-labeled choline (20 min) needs the presence of an on-site cyclotron [57], whereas ^{18}F analog with a longer half-life of 110 min has the viability for transport and application in multicenter settings [57]. Excretion of ^{11}C-choline is mainly through the hepatobiliary system, which is desired for prostate assessment [5, 58]. ^{18}F-choline, however, has urinary excretion, which may interfere with the interpretation of pelvic findings [5, 57].

13.4.1 Primary Disease

The utility of choline radiotracers in the primary diagnosis of prostate cancer has been widely investigated. Overlap in ^{11}C or ^{18}F-Choline avidity between PCa tumors and BPH or even prostatitis has been reported, which limits the diagnostic performance of this tracer [5, 57]. Bundschuh et al. assessed 20 patients using ^{11}C-choline PET/CT prior to prostatectomy, reporting that ^{11}C-choline PET/CT could localize less than 50% of the pathologically proven prostate cancers [59]. Grosu et al. in a study with 28 patients with PCa demonstrated that preoperative ^{11}C-choline PET/CT was not useful in differentiating cancerous from normal prostate tissue [60]. Interestingly, some of the non-neoplastic prostate tissues demonstrated higher uptake [60]. Pinaquy and collaborators prospectively compared the diagnostic performance of diffusion-weighted MRI (DWI) and ^{18}F-choline in 47 patients before surgery. The accuracy of ^{18}F-choline PET/CT in tumor localization and evaluation of extra-prostatic invasion did not show any superiority over mpMRI [61]. To summarize, the utility of ^{11}C- or ^{18}F-choline PET/CT for detection of primary PCa is not justified.

13.4.2 Staging

Several studies have evaluated the performance of choline PET/CT in initial PCa staging. In a meta-analysis, Evangelista et al. evaluated the role of ^{18}F- and ^{11}C-choline PET and PET/CT in initial staging of PCa and reported a pooled sensitivity of as low as 49.2% and pooled specificity of 95% [62]. In another large meta-analysis by von Eyben et al. assessing the diagnostic accuracy of ^{11}C- and ^{18}F-choline PET/CT in PCa patients, choline PET/CT demonstrated pooled sensitivity and pooled specificity of 62% and 92%, respectively, in localization of metastatic lymph nodes [63]. A retrospective study on 48 cases with intermediate- to high-risk PCa compared bone scan and abdominopelvic CT with ^{18}F-choline PET/CT for initial staging [64]. The overall accuracy for detection of lymph node involvement was 83.3% with ^{18}F-choline PET/CT. ^{18}F-choline PET/CT showed a similar specificity (92.3% vs. 92.3%) but a higher sensitivity (46.2% vs. 69.2%) comparing to the CT scan. In addition, both specificity (86.4% vs. 77.2%) and sensitivity (100% vs. 90%) were higher in ^{18}F-choline PET/CT than bone scans. Moreover in 33% of prostate cancer patients, the findings of ^{18}F-choline PET/CT altered the staging of PCa [64]. In a prospective study, Van Den Bergh et al. utilized DWMRI and ^{11}C-choline PET/CT to assess nodal staging in 75 high-risk PCa patients with N0 lesions on contrast-enhanced CT [65]. Thirty-seven out of 75 patients showed positive results on histology. For ^{11}C-choline PET/CT, the PPV and sensitivity were 63.6% and 18.9%, respectively. DWI demonstrated a PPV of 86.7% and a sensitivity of 36.1%. On a region-based analysis, PPV of ^{11}C-choline PET/CT was 50.0% and a sensitivity of 8.2% while for DWI showed PPV of 40.0% and sensitivity of 9.5%. It was concluded that these imaging modalities were not useful for pretreatment evaluation of nodal staging in PCa patients with negative results on CT scan [65].

13.4.3 Biochemical Recurrence

The utility of choline tracers in evaluating BCR PCa has been widely studied. Based on the location of biochemical recurrence and PSA levels, choline PET/CT has shown a wide range of detection rate [66]. Evangelista et al. reported a detection rate of 11%–75% for prostate gland recurrences, 30% for lymph nodes metastases, and 20%–50% for skeletal metastases in a meta-analysis [66]. Furthermore, as a function of PSA, for both ^{11}C- and ^{18}F-choline, the detection rate was reported as <30% for PSA level <1 ng/mL and >50% for PSA level >2 ng/mL [66]. It was also shown that the detection rate was higher in PSA velocity of >5 ng/mL/year and PSA doubling time of less than 2 or 3 months [66]. A study by Cimitan et al. on 1,000 patients with biochemical relapse demonstrated that a high primary tumor Gleason score (>8) at the time of diagnosis was a strong predictive factor for ^{18}F-choline PET/CT positivity, even at low PSA levels [67].

A principal approach to evaluate the role of a PET tracer is to consider its impact on patient survival and therapeutic management. In a study by Garcia et al., prognostic value of therapeutic response by ^{11}C-choline PET/CT was evaluated in 37 patients with BCR [68]. ^{11}C-choline PET/CT demonstrated high ability in detecting infra-diaphragmatic nodal metastases that helped in distinguishing patients who might benefit from salvage radiotherapy and planning further therapeutic approach. In another study, Goldstein et al. investigated the use of ^{11}C-choline PET/CT in biochemically recurrent PCa management [69]. Increased ^{11}C-choline uptake in prostate, prostate fossa, or pelvic lymph node was shown in 17 patients, and distant metastases were observed in 9 cases, whereas ^{11}C-choline PET failed to localize recurrence in 7 patients. In 55% (18/33) of patients, ^{11}C-choline PET/CT changed the therapeutic approach ($p = 0.05$). It was concluded that in patients with biochemical recurrence PCa, ^{11}C-choline PET/CT might have a role in improving care by targeting appropriate patients for salvage radiotherapy, by developing a better radiation treatment plan, and by postponing or avoiding androgen deprivation therapy [69]. Incerti et al. retrospectively investigated the predictive value of ^{11}C-choline PET/CT on survival outcomes in 68 patients, who underwent helical tomotherapy following a positive ^{11}C-choline PET scan [70]. PET-derived parameters, including SUV_{max}, mean standardized uptake value (SUV_{mean}), and metabolic tumor volume (MTV) with a threshold of 40%, 50%, and 60% was determined. There was no significant correlation between SUV_{max}, SUV_{mean}, and the survival outcomes. However, using the receiver operating characteristic (ROC) curve, metabolic tumor volume (MTV) showed to be the best predictor for relapse-free survival. Notably, MTV and the presence of extra-pelvic choline-avid lymph nodes were reported as independent prognostic factors, which might be used to select therapeutic strategy [70]. In another retrospective study by the same group on 302 hormone-naïve BCR PCa patients following radical prostatectomy, ^{11}C-choline PET/CT was able to predict survival with 15-year prostate cancer-specific survival being 42.4% in patients with ^{11}C-choline PET positivity and 95.5% in patients with a negative ^{11}C-choline PET scan [71]. The same group evaluated the role of ^{11}C-choline PET/CT in predicting prostate cancer-specific survival in 195 cases treated with radical prostatectomy in whom ^{11}C-choline PET/CT was performed due to BCR while patients were on androgen deprivation therapy [72]. The results showed prostate cancer-specific survival of 11.2 and 16.4 years in patients with ^{11}C-choline PET/CT positivity and negativity, respectively ($p < 0.001$) [72].

In conclusion, choline PET tracer has shown a promising performance in evaluating BCR at high PSA levels. It has also shown to be helpful in differentiating local and regional relapse from distant metastases, which directs to the appropriate clinical management [73]. In 2012, the Food and Drug Administration (FDA) approved ^{11}C-choline PET/CT for evaluation of BCR in PCa patients with rising PSA values following definitive treatment [74]. However, concerns exist that sensitivity of choline tracers might be unsatisfactory at low PSA levels (~0.5 ng/mL) that question the value of this probe in decision toward salvage radiotherapy [43].

13.5 ^{18}F-FACBC (Fluciclovine)

^{18}F-FACBC (anti-1-amino-3-^{18}F-fluorocyclobuate-1-carboxylic acid), recently renamed as ^{18}F-fluciclovine or Axumin™ (brand name), is a synthetic analog of the amino acid L-leucine that targets amino acid transport [2]. Same as many other cancers, upregulation of transport and metabolism of amino acids is present in prostate cancer which highlights the role of amino acid analogs as PET tracers [57]. Delayed renal excretion and favorable biodistribution have made ^{18}F-FACBC a desirable tracer for prostate cancer imaging [75]. Moreover, the long half-life of ^{18}F-FACBC allows its use without the need for on-site cyclotron [76].

13.5.1 Primary Disease

^{18}F-FACBC has shown a poor performance in detection of primary PCa tumors. In a study by Schuster et al. in 10 patients who underwent ^{18}F-FACBC PET/CT imaging prior to radical prostatectomy, the highest combined sensitivity of 81.3% and specificity of 50% were reported [77]. Even though the highest SUV_{max} was observed in malignant sextants, overlap was reported between cancerous and benign prostate tissue [77]. In a prospective study by Turkbey et al., the ^{18}F-FACBC PET/CT uptake in cases with localized PCa, BPH, and normal prostate was investigated. In addition, the utility of ^{18}F-FACBC PET/CT in localizing pathologically confirmed PCa was evaluated and compared with the results from mpMRI [78]. PCa demonstrated a significantly higher mean SUV_{max} compared to normal prostate tissue ($p < 0.001$). However, they did not indicate a statistically significant difference compared to BPH nodules ($p = 0.27$). Sector-based analysis revealed a lower sensitivity (67% vs. 73%) and specificity (66% vs. 79%) for ^{18}F-FACBC PET/CT compared to T2-weighted MRI. The PPV of combined ^{18}F-FACBC PET/CT and mpMRI for primary tumor localization was reported as 82%, which was significantly higher ($p < 0.001$) than the PPV of each of the modalities alone (50% for ^{18}F-FACBC PET/CT and 76% for mpMRI). It was concluded that although ^{18}F-FACBC PET/CT had low specificity in detection of primary PCa tumors independently, its conjoint utility with conventional imaging modalities such as mpMRI might be helpful in detection of primary cancerous lesions [78]. In another study by Jambor et al., the role of ^{18}F-FACBC PET/CT, PET/MRI, and mpMRI was investigated in 26 patients [79]. Results showed high sensitivity (87%) and a low specificity (56%) for ^{18}F-FACBC PET/CT in identification of primary PCa lesions. Moreover, both PET/MRI and mpMRI performed better than ^{18}F-FACBC PET/CT in PCa detection [79]. Kairemo et al. retrospectively assessed 26 patients with ^{18}F-FACBC PET/CT and correlated with PSA levels and PSA doubling times [80]. No statistically significant difference was found between patients who showed positive and negative results on ^{18}F-FACBC PET/CT with regard to PSA levels. However, significantly shorter PSA doubling time was observed in patients who had positive ^{18}F-FACBC uptake leading to the conclusion that ^{18}F-FACBC uptake might be an indicator of PCa aggressiveness [80]. To conclude, same as previous tracers, due to low specificity and overlaps in uptake, ^{18}F-FACBC PET/CT has a limited value in detection of primary disease.

13.5.2 Staging

Currently, limited data exists on the role of ^{18}F-FACBC PET/CT in primary PCa staging. Suzuki et al. in a multicenter Phase IIb clinical trial on 68 patients compared the diagnostic performance of NMK36 (trans-1-amino-3-[18F] fluorocyclobutanecarboxylic acid)-PET/CT with conventional imaging methods including whole-body contrast-enhanced CT for assessing involvement of regional lymph nodes and combination of bone scintigraphy and contrast-enhanced CT for detection of bone metastasis [81]. Comparable diagnostic accuracy was reported for conventional imaging methods and ^{18}F-fluciclocine PET/CT. However, though not confirmed by reference standard, some sub-centimeter lymph nodes (5–9 mm short axis) and bone metastases were only identified on ^{18}F-fluciclocine PET/

CT, which needed further investigations to confirm the utility of ^{18}F-FACBC PET/CT in PCa staging [81].

13.5.3 Biochemical Recurrence

^{18}F-FACBC PET/CT has demonstrated to be most beneficial in localization of BCR than for evaluation of primary disease. Based on the data gathered from more than 700 PCa patients from the USA and Europe, FDA approved ^{18}F-fluciclocine in 2016, under the trade name Axumin™, for evaluation of prostate cancer recurrence in cases with increasing PSA levels after previous treatment [82].

In a multicenter study including 596 patients with BCR by Bach-Gansmo et al., an overall detection rate of 67.7% was reported for ^{18}F-fluciclocine PET/CT [83]. In addition ^{18}F-fluciclocine PET/CT could identify local and distant PCa recurrence within a broad range of PSA levels [83]. Odewole et al. in a study of 53 BCR PCa patients with negative bone scans, ^{18}F-FACBC PET/CT was compared to CT with regard to lesion detection. Results demonstrated that the diagnostic performance of ^{18}F-FACBC PET/CT was far better than CT [84]. Nanni et al. compared accuracy of ^{11}C-choline PET/CT with ^{18}F-FACBC PET/CT in patients with biochemical relapse after radical prostatectomy; overall similar performance was reported for both of these tracers. However, by classifying patients by PSA values, ^{18}F-FACBC PET/CT showed higher sensitivity in nearly all PSA ranges [85]. Therefore, it was suggested that in the evaluation of BCR patients following radical prostatectomy, ^{18}F-FACBC PET/CT might be a better alternate than ^{11}C-choline PET/CT [85]. Overall, ^{18}F-FACBC has demonstrated high sensitivity but low specificity in localizing BCR. Schuster et al. compared ^{18}F-FACBC PET/CT to ProstaScint (PMSA-targeted ^{111}In-capromab pendetide) in detecting prostate cancer relapse [86]. In the evaluation of the prostatic bed, ^{18}F-FACBC PET/CT showed sensitivity of 90.2% and specificity of 40%, whereas PMSA-targeted ^{111}In-capromab pendetide demonstrated far lower numbers [86]. In a meta-analysis including six studies, Rem et al. investigated the utility of ^{18}F-FACBC PET/CT in BCR PCa patients, reporting a pooled sensitivity and specificity of 87% and 66%, respectively. Moreover, an area under the receiver operating characteristic curve (AUC) of 0.93 was reported [87]. Despite showing high sensitivity, ^{18}F-FACBC has the disadvantage of having a high false-positive rate in detecting tumor recurrence, which makes its utility questionable considering the development of newer tracers.

13.6 PSMA-Targeting Tracers

Prostate-specific membrane antigen (PSMA) is a transmembrane protein highly upregulated in prostate cancer and weakly expressed in normal prostate tissue [88]. PSMA expression is correlated with both grade and stage of the lesions representing disease aggressiveness [89]. PSMA has shown increased uptake in some other malignancies, in addition to physiologic uptake in the proximal renal tubules, bladder, salivary/lacrimal glands, small intestine, liver, and spleen [90, 91].

The extracellular domain of PSMA with catalytic activity is used for tumor targeting [92]. Several PSMA PET radioligands, with minor differences, have been developed; however, none of them are currently approved by FDA. The only PSMA radiotracer that is approved by FDA is ^{111}In-capromab pendetide (ProstaScint), which is a radiolabeled PSMA antibody. However, its use has been limited due to disadvantages such as slow clearance and binding to intracellular component of PSMA which leads to low uptake and high background ratio [93]. Nearly all of these PSMA PET agents excrete through urinary tract excluding ^{18}F-PSMA-1007 which has a higher hepatobiliary excretion [89]. Some of the PSMA PET tracers including ^{68}Ga-PSMA-HBED-CC (PSMA-11), ^{18}F-DCFBC, ^{18}F-DCFPyL, and ^{18}F-PSMA-1007 will be reviewed.

^{68}Ga-PSMA-11

^{68}Ga-PSMA-11 (also known as ^{68}Ga-HBED-CC-PSMA) was first described by Eder et al. for

PET imaging [94]. Ever since, it has been widely utilized and investigated in all stages of prostate cancer disease [95, 96].

13.6.1 Primary Disease

In a study including 53 biopsy-proven PCa patients, Eiber et al. evaluated the diagnostic performance of ^{68}Ga-PSMA-11 PET/MRI against mpMRI for the detection of primary PCa [97]. Combined ^{68}Ga-PSMA-11 PET/MRI showed better performance in localizing primary prostate cancer than mpMRI (AUC: 0.88 vs. 0.73; $p < 0.001$) and PET alone (AUC: 0.88 vs. 0.83; $p = 0.002$). ^{68}Ga-PSMA-11 PET/MR showed higher sensitivity (76%) and specificity (97%), compared to mpMRI (58% and 82%, respectively) and PET alone (64% and 94%). This study also suggested the possible use of ^{68}Ga-PSMA-11 PET/MR for image-guided biopsy [97].

13.6.2 Staging

There have been some debates regarding the utility of ^{68}Ga-PSMA-11 PET/CT in initial staging of PCa tumors. Herlemann et al. evaluated the accuracy of ^{68}Ga-PSMA-11 PET/CT for preoperative nodal staging in 71 lymph node regions from 34 patients with intermediate- or high-risk prostate cancer [98]. The reference standard was histopathology reports from surgery. It was reported that with a higher sensitivity and specificity, ^{68}Ga-PSMA-11 PET/CT showed higher performance than CT, particularly in lymph nodes that did not meet the CT size criteria [98]. Budaus et al., in another study, compared baseline ^{68}Ga-PSMA-11 PET/CT with postoperative histopathology reports in terms of evaluating lymph node metastases [99]. ^{68}Ga-PSMA-11 PET/CT showed overall sensitivity of 33.3% and overall specificity of 100% in localization of lymph nodes [99]. The considerable number of false positives (67.7%) reported was mainly attributed to the size of metastatic lymph nodes [99]. In general, the performance of ^{68}Ga-PSMA in lymph node staging seems to outperform conventional imaging methods.

13.6.3 Biochemical Recurrence

Regarding evaluation of BCR, PSMA PET/CT has demonstrated the highest value compared to other imaging methods. Numerous studies have reported promising results for the utility of ^{68}Ga-PSMA-11 PET/CT in recurrent PCa. In a large retrospective study of 319 patients with BCR by Afshar-Oromieh et al., 82.8% of patients showed 1 or more lesions representing disease recurrence. For ^{68}Ga-PSMA-11 PET/CT, lesion-based analysis showed sensitivity and specificity of 76.6% and 100%, respectively, demonstrating that this radiotracer was highly specific for prostate cancer [100]. Moreover, tumor detection was found to be positively correlated with PSA values; however, no association was reported between ^{68}Ga-PSMA-11 PET/CT positivity and Gleason score or faster PSA doubling time [100]. Perera et al. in a meta-analysis reported an association between pre-scan PSA values and positive results on ^{68}Ga-PSMA-11 PET/CT [101]. By stratifying PSA into 4 groups, 0–0.2, 0.2–1, 1–2, and >2 ng/ml, ^{68}Ga-PSMA-11 PET/CT demonstrated positive findings in 42%, 58%, 76%, and 95% of scans, respectively [101]. Moreover, shorter PSA doubling time was reported to show more positive findings on ^{68}Ga-PSMA-11 PET/CT [101]. In another study, Verburg et al. retrospectively evaluated the correlation between PSA values, PSA doubling time, Gleason score, and ^{68}Ga-PSMA-11 PET/CT results in 155 patients with BCR [102]. ^{68}Ga-PSMA-11 PET/CT showed positive findings in 44% of cases with PSA values ≤ 1 ng/mL, 79% with PSA levels 1–2 ng/mL, and 89% with PSA ≥ 2 ng/ml. In addition, shorter PSA doubling times and higher PSA values were reported to be independent factors for positivity of ^{68}Ga-PSMA-11 PET/CT scans and extra-pelvic metastatic disease. However, there was not association between Gleason score and the extent of the disease on imaging studies [102]. In another study, Eiber et al. investigated the detection rate of ^{68}Ga-PSMA-11 PET/CT in patients with BCR. In total, the detection rate was reported as 89.5%. Among patients with PSA values of ≥ 2, 1–2, 0.5–1, and 0.2–0.5, the detection rates were 96.8%, 93.0%, 72.7%, and

57.9%, respectively [103]. This highlights the fact that ^{68}Ga-PSMA-11 PET/CT is beneficial in identification of BCR, even at low PSA levels. In a retrospective study on a larger cohort of 1007 patients, Afshar-Oromieh et al. reported that ^{68}Ga-PSMA-11 PET/CT was able to detect at least one lesion indicative of recurrent prostate cancer in 79.5% of patients [104]. While lower than the number reported in previous studies [100, 103], the detection rate of ^{68}Ga-PSMA-11 PET/CT was still high. Moreover, tumor detection rate was associated with PSA values and ongoing androgen deprivation therapy [104]. Morigi et al. compared the detection rate of ^{18}F-choline PET/CT and ^{68}Ga-PSMA-11 in patients with BCR [105]. Even though a better detection rate was reported for ^{68}Ga-PSMA-11 PET/CT rather than ^{18}F-choline PET/CT at all PSA levels, the main benefit was seen at low PSA values. At PSA levels <0.5, the detection rate was 12.5% for ^{18}F-choline PET/CT and 50% for ^{68}Ga-PSMA-11 PET/CT. At PSA levels 0.5–2.0 ng/mL, ^{18}F-choline showed detection rate of 31% compared to 69% for ^{68}Ga-PSMA-11 [105]. In a recent single-arm prospective trial with 635 patients, Fendler et al. evaluated ^{68}Ga-PSMA-11 PET in identifying BCR [106]. The scans were reviewed by three blinded readers, among whom the inter-reader reliability was considerable. The PPV was reported as 84–92% with overall detection rate of 75% that showed a significant increase with PSA levels: 38% for PSA <0.5 ng/mL, 57% for PSA 0.5 to −<1 ng/mL, 84% for PSA 1 to <2 ng/mL, 86% for PSA 2 to <5 ng/mL, and 97% for PSA ≥5 ng/mL [106].

To conclude, in the evaluation of recurrent PCa, ^{68}Ga-PSMA-11 PET/CT has shown promise even at low PSA values that many other tracers are not able to identify metastatic disease.

Fluorinated PSMA-Targeted Radiotracers

Beside the gallium-labeled tracers, the group of fluorinated agents have been developed that same as gallium-based ones are urea-based small molecules which attach to extracellular part of PSMA [89]. ^{18}F-labeled PSMA inhibitors have shown several benefits over ^{68}Ga-PSMA tracers. These radiotracers have a longer half-life compared to ^{68}Ga-labeled ones (109 vs. 68 min) which makes mass production in a central location and delivery to distant sites possible [107]. Moreover, a better image resolution, improved lesion detection rate, and higher mean tumor-to-background ratio have been reported for these ^{18}F-based compounds compared to gallium-labeled ones [108, 109].

To date, three fluorine-based radiotracers have been described including ^{18}F-DCFBC, ^{18}F-DCFPyL, and the latest one ^{18}F-PSMA-1007, which will be further explained.

^{18}F-DCFBC and ^{18}F-DCFPyL

^{18}F-DCFBC was developed as the first generation of ^{18}F-labeled PSMA radiotracers. However, ^{18}F-DCFBC has a long clearance time from blood because of being bound to serum proteins, which limits the efficiency of this tracer for evaluating lymph nodes close to blood vessels [89]. ^{18}F-DCFPyL, on the other hand, has the advantage of considerably faster blood clearance and superior tumor-to-background ratio [89, 110]. Moreover, in comparison with-DCFBC, ^{18}F-DCFPyL has shown significantly higher affinity to PSMA, which leads to improved detection of primary and metastatic PCa lesions [89, 110]. Therefore, ^{18}F-DCFPyL has become available as the second generation of ^{18}F-labeled PSMA agents, and its use has received more attention in the past years.

13.6.4 Primary Disease

Rowe et al. compared ^{18}F-DCFBC PET/CT with mpMRI regarding primary prostate cancer detection [111]. Even though ^{18}F-DCFBC PET/CT showed lower sensitivity for localization of primary PCa than mpMRI, it demonstrated higher specificity in detecting tumors with high Gleason scores (≥8) and size of ≥1 mL. Moreover, ^{18}F-DCFBC avidity was reported to be negligible in BPH comparing to PCa tumors. This lead to the conclusion that ^{18}F-DCFBC PET/CT in combination with mpMRI, in addition to distinguishing indolent from aggressive disease, could make detection and biopsy of the most clinically significant high-grade tumors possible [111]. In a study by Turkbey et al., the performance of

^{18}F-DCFBC PET/CT to identify localized PCa was evaluated in association with mpMRI and histopathology [112]. For detection of PCa, lower sensitivity was reported for ^{18}F-DCFBC PET/CT compared to mpMRI. In addition, ^{18}F-DCFBC PET/CT showed a higher SUV_{max} in primary PCa tumors compared to BPH or normal prostate tissue. Moreover, a moderate correlation was found between ^{18}F-DCFBC uptake and Gleason score. It was concluded that in order to achieve high sensitivity in detecting primary PCa, it is crucial to utilize the combination of mpMRI and ^{18}F-DCFBC PET/CT [112].

13.6.5 Staging

The viability of ^{18}F-DCFBC PET/CT in PCa staging was studied by Rowe et al., reporting that the detection rate of metastatic lesions was higher with ^{18}F-DCFBC PET/CT compared to conventional imaging methods such as bone scanning and contrast-enhanced CT, with a sensitivity of 92% compared to 71%, respectively, in both hormone-naïve and castration-resistant patients [113]. Rowe et al. also investigated the utility of ^{18}F-DCFPyL PET/CT in patients with metastatic prostate cancer and reported superior performance of this tracer over conventional imaging modalities with regard to localizing sites of metastatic disease [114]. Rowe et al. in another study observed that ^{18}F-DCFPyL PET/CT could localize bone lesions with a far higher sensitivity (97.7%) than both ^{18}F-NaF PET/CT (43.8%) and ^{99m}TC-MDP bone scan (13.5%) [115]. Gorin et al. prospectively investigated the role of ^{18}F-DCFPyL PET/CT in preoperative staging of 25 patients with clinically localized PCa [116]. Results showed that ^{18}F-DCFPyL PET/CT detected sites of radiotracer avidity in prostate gland of all the studied patients. Also five out of seven (71.4%) patients, with otherwise clinically insignificant positive lymph nodes compared to histopathology reports, were correctly detected by ^{18}F-DCFPyL PET/CT (Fig. 13.2). Moreover, ^{18}F-DCFPyL PET/CT was able to localize sites of occult distant metastases in 12% of PCa patients [116].

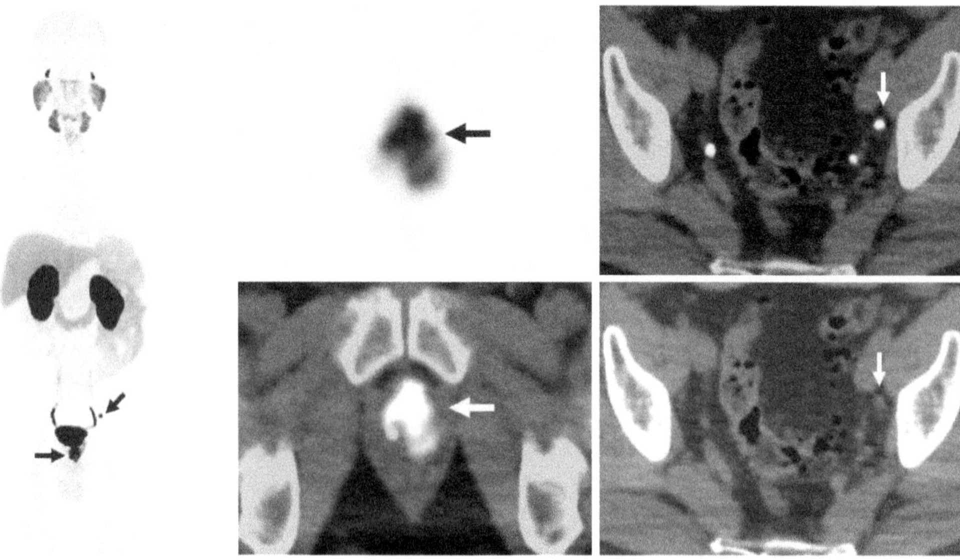

Fig. 13.2 58-year-old patient with newly diagnosed high-risk prostate cancer, Gleason 9, (4 + 5), *T2c* with PSA of 74.02 ng/mL. ^{18}F-DCFPyL PET/CT imaging, including maximal intensity projection, axial PET, fused PET/CT, and CT images, demonstrate a large intraprostatic DCFPyL focus involving the apical to base anterior transition and left peripheral zones of the prostate consistent with the biopsy-proven primary malignancy (arrows). Additional sub-centimeter size DCFPyL-avid left external iliac lymph node suspicious for nodal disease (white arrows). Of note that physiological uptake is noted in the bilateral ureters

13.6.6 Biochemical Recurrence

Mena and collaborators investigated the utility of ^{18}F-DCFBC PET/CT in the evaluation and management of biochemical recurrence PCa [117], reporting an overall lesion detection rate of 60.3%, with the detection rate being dependent on PSA values. ^{18}F-DCFBC PET/CT could detect tumor recurrence with high reliability when PSA values were greater than a threshold of 0.78 ng/mL. Moreover, positive results on ^{18}F-DCFBC PET/CT changed therapeutic management in 51.2% of patients [117]. Dietlein et al. compared the performance of ^{68}Ga-PSMA-11 PET/CT with ^{18}F-DCFPyL PET/CT in BCR PCa patients [109]. ^{18}F-DCFPyL PET/CT localized all the lesions that were detected by ^{68}Ga-PSMA-11 PET/CT. Moreover, additional lesions were identified by ^{18}F-DCFPyL PET/CT in three patients. For lesions with positive ^{18}F-DCFPyL PET/CT, a significantly higher average SUV_{max} was reported compared to ^{68}Ga-PSMA-11 PET/CT (14.5 vs. 12.2, $p = 0.025$). By considering the kidney, spleen, or parotid as reference organs, a significantly higher average tumor-to-background ratio was observed with ^{18}F-DCFPyL PET/CT compared to ^{68}Ga-PSMA-11 PET/CT. It was concluded that in view of the high image quality and superb sensitivity of ^{8}F-DCFPyL PET/CT imaging (Fig. 13.3), it could be an alternate for ^{68}Ga-PSMA-11 PET/CT in cases with biochemical recurrence [109].

^{18}F-PSMA-1007

The fluorine-based tracer ^{18}F-PSMA-1007 has been recently introduced [118]. As ^{18}F-PSMA-1007 has hepatobiliary excretion, it is advantageous in initial staging and evaluation of intraprostatic and locally recurrent PCa compared to other PSMA agents that are excreted via urinary tract [89, 119]. Kesch et al. assessed the value of ^{18}F-PSMA-1007 PET/CT for primary staging of PCa compared to mpMRI and histopathology of the prostatectomy specimens. Comparable accuracy was observed for mpMRI and ^{18}F-PSMA-1007 PET/CT. In comparison with histopathology, ^{18}F-PSMA-1007 PET/CT showed promising results in correctly staging prostate cancer [120]. In another study, ^{18}F-PSMA-1007 PET/CT showed sensitivity of 95% for localizing nodal metastases, as small as 1 mm [119].

In the setting of biochemical recurrence, Giesel et al. [118] for the first time evaluated

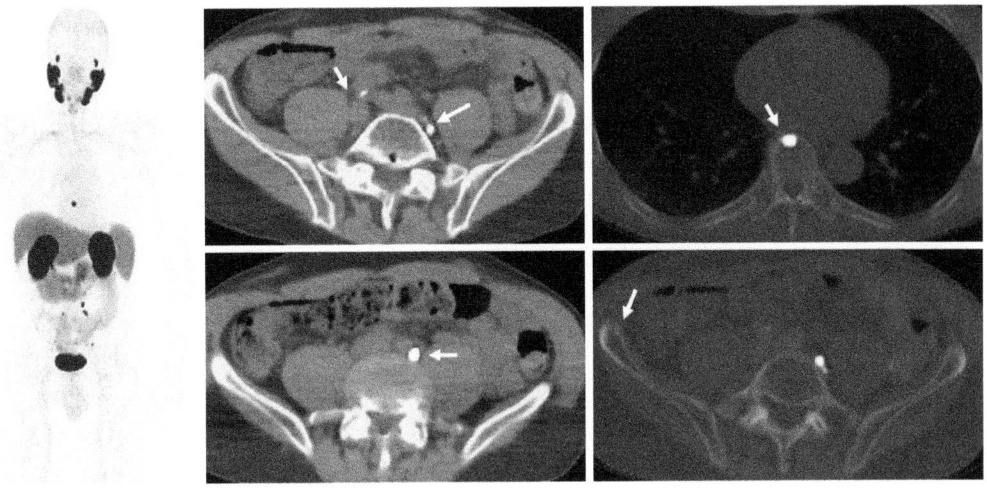

Fig. 13.3 70-year-old patient with a history of prostate cancer, Gleason 5 + 4 = 9, status post-definitive RT, and 2 years of ADT. Biochemical recurrence (PSA of 2.41 ng/mL) after 2 years from definitive treatment, with negative conventional imaging (CT and bone scan). Maximal intensity projection, and axial PET/CT fused images of ^{18}F-DCFPyL-PET/CT, demonstrate sub-centimeter bilateral pelvic nodes (arrows in middle column) and abnormal foci at the anterior right iliac bone and T9 vertebral body (arrows in the 3rd column). Following biopsy of the anterior right iliac bone lesion confirmed to have metastasis

^{18}F-PSMA-1007 PET/CT reporting high tumor detection rates for patients with lower PSA values: 61.5%, 74.5%, 90.9%, and 94.0% for PSA >0.2 to <0.5, 0.5 to <1.0, 1 to <2.0, and ≥2.0 ng/mL, respectively [118]. Seventeen lymph nodes showed increased ^{18}F-PSMA-1007 uptake at PSA values as low as 0.08 ng/mL, none of which were considered metastatic based on the Response Evaluation Criteria in Solid Tumors (RECIST) criteria. Therefore, ^{18}F-PSMA-1007 PET/CT showed a significant value in restaging PCa disease and planning the best therapeutic management. Paddubny et al. evaluated the utility of ^{18}F-PSMA-1007 PET/CT in BCR PCa patients. ^{18}F-PSMA-1007 PET/CT was able to identify biochemical recurrence not identifiable on mpMRI [121].

Thus, in addition to having the positive features of fluorinated PSMA agents, ^{18}F-PSMA-1007 has shown promising results in detection of very small sites of involvement in either primary or recurrent prostate cancer disease.

13.7 ^{18}F-NaF PET/CT

In prostate cancer, bone has shown to be the most prevalent site of distant metastasis, which involves up to 84% of patients with advanced prostate cancer [122]. Therefore, accurate detection of these lesions is of high clinical importance.

^{18}F-NaF is a positron emitter that attaches to foci of new bone formation and reflects osteoblastic activity [123]. It was first approved by FDA in 1972 to identify sites of abnormal osteogenic activity [124]. ^{18}F-NaF has a rapid blood clearance and considerably high bone-specific avidity, which facilitates acquiring images with enhanced spatial resolution and target-to-background ratio in comparison with ^{99m}Tc-labeled phosphonates [125]. Thus, the utility of ^{18}F-NaF PET/CT is solely limited to localization of bone metastases [3]. In spite of these benefits, this tracer was replaced with ^{99m}Tc-labeled phosphonates due to more availability of gamma cameras. With extensive accessibility of PET and PET/CT scanners during the past several years, ^{18}F-NaF has re-emerged as an advantageous tracer for bone imaging [126].

13.7.1 Staging

Some former studies have reported remarkable sensitivity and specificity for ^{18}F-NaF in the identification of bone lesions [127, 128]. Even-Sapir et al. prospectively studied 44 patients (25 newly diagnosed and 19 with BCR), comparing ^{18}F-fluoride PET/CT with 99mTc-MDP planar bone scintigraphy, SPECT, and ^{18}F-fluoride PET in detecting bone metastases [127]. Based on patient-based analysis, they reported sensitivity and specificity of 100% and 100% for ^{18}F-NaF PET/CT, respectively, 70% and 57% for planar bone scintigraphy, 92% and 82% for SPECT, and 100% and 62% for ^{18}F-NaF PET [127]. In another study, Apolo et al. reported that ^{18}F-NaF PET/CT could localize more bone metastases, earlier in the course of prostate cancer disease in comparison with ^{99m}Tc bone scintigraphy [129]. In addition, overall survival was reported to be significantly correlated with the number of detected lesions at the baseline and SUV changes in the follow-up ^{18}F-NaF PET/CT scans [129].

^{18}F-NaF PET/CT has shown better performance than ^{99m}Tc-phosphate-labeled bone scintigraphy; since ^{18}F-NaF uptake is associated with osteoblastic activity, both benign and malignant bone diseases show positive results on ^{18}F-NaF PET/CT [130]. A study by Poulsen et al. compared diagnostic accuracy of ^{18}F-NaF PET/CT with whole-body bone scintigraphy (WBS), ^{99m}Tc-MDP, and ^{18}F-fluoromethylcholine (FCH) PET/CT in detecting spinal metastases in patients with PCa, using MRI as the reference standard. A high sensitivity (93.1% vs. 50.8% for WBS) but a low specificity (54% vs. 82.2 for WBS) was reported for ^{18}F-NaF PET/CT [131]. The high false positivity was attributed to nonmalignant degenerative or inflammatory changes in older patients [131]. In a study by Muzahir et al., it was reported that by semi-quantitative analysis of lesions, i.e., SUV_{max} of ^{18}F-NaF PET/CT might be helpful in differentiating benign from malignant lesions, with SUV $_{max}$ >50 always indicating metastatic disease in castrate-resistant PCa patients [132].

13.7.2 Biochemical Recurrence

A limited number of studies have evaluated the value of ^{18}F-NaF in BCR prostate cancer. In a prospective study of 37 patients, Jadvar et al. compared the performance of ^{18}F-FDG and ^{18}F-NaF PET/CT in the evaluation of prostate cancer patients with BCR [41]. They reported that ^{18}F-NaF PET/CT was helpful in localizing occult bone metastases; however, ^{18}F-FDG PET/CT demonstrated a limited utility. In addition, in patients who had undergone prior radical prostatectomy, ^{18}F-NaF PET/CT positivity might correlate with increase in PSA values at the time of relapse, and ^{18}F-NaF might be positive for lower PSA values when conventional imaging methods are still negative [41].

To summarize, due to high efficiency in detecting occult bone metastases, ^{18}F-NaF PET/CT has the highest clinical utility in high-risk PCa patients, who have equivocal or negative findings on ^{99m}Tc bone scintigraphy.

References

1. Siegel RL, Miller KD, Jemal A. Cancer statistics, 2019. CA Cancer J Clin. 2019;69(1):7–34.
2. Wibmer AG, Burger IA, Sala E, Hricak H, Weber WA, Vargas HA. Molecular imaging of prostate cancer. Radiographics. 2015;36(1):142–59.
3. Bednarova S, Lindenberg ML, Vinsensia M, Zuiani C, Choyke PL, Turkbey B. Positron emission tomography (PET) in primary prostate cancer staging and risk assessment. Translational Androl Urol. 2017;6(3):413.
4. Kessler B, Albertsen P. The natural history of prostate cancer. Urol Clin. 2003;30(2):219–26.
5. Lindenberg L, Choyke P, Dahut W. Prostate cancer imaging with novel PET tracers. Curr Urol Rep. 2016;17(3):18.
6. Mazzone E, Preisser F, Nazzani S, Tian Z, Fossati N, Gandaglia G, et al. More extensive lymph node dissection improves survival benefit of radical cystectomy in metastatic urothelial carcinoma of the bladder. Clin Genitourin Cancer. 2019;17(2):105–13.e2. https://doi.org/10.1016/j.clgc.2018.11.003.
7. Keetch DW, Catalona WJ, Smith DS. Serial prostatic biopsies in men with persistently elevated serum prostate specific antigen values. J Urol. 1994;151(6):1571–4.
8. Hoeks CM, Barentsz JO, Hambrock T, Yakar D, Somford DM, Heijmink SW, et al. Prostate cancer: multiparametric MR imaging for detection, localization, and staging. Radiology. 2011;261(1):46–66.
9. Vargas HA, Wassberg C, Akin O, Hricak H. MR imaging of treated prostate cancer. Radiology. 2012;262(1):26–42.
10. Jadvar H. Molecular imaging of prostate cancer: PET radiotracers. Am J Roentgenol. 2012;199(2):278–91.
11. Vali R, Loidl W, Pirich C, Langesteger W, Beheshti M. Imaging of prostate cancer with PET/CT using 18F-Fluorocholine. Am J Nucl Med Mol Imaging. 2015;5(2):96.
12. Nabi HA, Zubeldia JM. Clinical applications of 18F-FDG in oncology. J Nucl Med Technol. 2002;30(1):3–9.
13. Tekade RK, Sun X. The Warburg effect and glucose-derived cancer theranostics. Drug Discov Today. 2017;22(11):1637–53.
14. Macheda ML, Rogers S, Best JD. Molecular and cellular regulation of glucose transporter (GLUT) proteins in cancer. J Cell Physiol. 2005;202(3):654–62.
15. Schuster DM, Nanni C, Fanti S. Editors. PET tracers beyond FDG in prostate cancer. Semin Nucl Med. 2016;46(6):507–21.
16. Jadvar H. PET of glucose metabolism and cellular proliferation in prostate cancer. J Nucl Med. 2016;57(Suppl 3):25S–9S.
17. Powles T, Murray I, Brock C, Oliver T, Avril N. Molecular positron emission tomography and PET/CT imaging in urological malignancies. Eur Urol. 2007;51(6):1511–21.
18. Backhaus B, Müller S, Matthies A, Palmedo H, Jaeger U, Biersack H, et al. Technical limits of PET/CT with 18FDG in prostate cancer. Aktuelle Urol. 2006;37(3):218–21.
19. Jadvar H. Molecular imaging of prostate cancer with 18 F-fluorodeoxyglucose PET. Nat Rev Urol. 2009;6(6):317.
20. Salminen E, Hogg A, Binns D, Frydenberg M, Hicks R. Investigations with FDG-PET scanning in prostate cancer show limited value for clinical practice. Acta Oncol. 2002;41(5):425–9.
21. Liu IJ, Zafar MB, Lai Y-H, Segall GM, Terris MK. Fluorodeoxyglucose positron emission tomography studies in diagnosis and staging of clinically organ-confined prostate cancer. Urology. 2001;57(1):108–11.
22. Hofer C, Laubenbacher C, Block T, Breul J, Hartung R, Schwaiger M. Fluorine-18-fluorodeoxyglucose positron emission tomography is useless for the detection of local recurrence after radical prostatectomy. Eur Urol. 1999;36(1):31–5.
23. Jadvar H. Prostate cancer: PET with 18F-FDG, 18F- or 11C-acetate, and 18F-or 11C-choline. J Nucl Med. 2011;52(1):81–9.
24. Meirelles GS, Schöder H, Ravizzini GC, Gönen M, Fox JJ, Humm J, et al. Prognostic value of baseline [18F] fluorodeoxyglucose positron emission tomography and 99mTc-MDP bone scan in progress-

ing metastatic prostate cancer. Clin Cancer Res. 2010;16(24):6093–9.
25. Jadvar H, Desai B, Ji L, Conti PS, Dorff TB, Groshen SG, et al. Baseline 18F-FDG PET/CT parameters as imaging biomarkers of overall survival in castrate-resistant metastatic prostate cancer. J Nucl Med. 2013;54(8):1195–201.
26. Beauregard J-M, Blouin A-C, Fradet V, Caron A, Fradet Y, Lemay C, et al. FDG-PET/CT for pre-operative staging and prognostic stratification of patients with high-grade prostate cancer at biopsy. Cancer Imaging. 2015;15(1):2.
27. Jadvar H. Imaging evaluation of prostate cancer with 18 F-fluorodeoxyglucose PET/CT: utility and limitations. Eur J Nucl Med Mol Imaging. 2013;40(1):5–10.
28. Minamimoto R, Uemura H, Sano F, Terao H, Nagashima Y, Yamanaka S, et al. The potential of FDG-PET/CT for detecting prostate cancer in patients with an elevated serum PSA level. Ann Nucl Med. 2011;25(1):21–7.
29. Liu Y. Diagnostic role of fluorodeoxyglucose positron emission tomography-computed tomography in prostate cancer. Oncol Lett. 2014;7(6):2013–8.
30. Minamimoto R, Senda M, Jinnouchi S, Terauchi T, Yoshida T, Murano T, et al. The current status of an FDG-PET cancer screening program in Japan, based on a 4-year (2006–2009) nationwide survey. Ann Nucl Med. 2013;27(1):46–57.
31. Bertagna F, Sadeghi R, Giovanella L, Treglia G. Incidental uptake of 18F-fluorodeoxyglucose in the prostate gland. Nuklearmedizin. 2014;53(06):249–58.
32. Kang PM, Seo WI, Lee SS, Bae SK, Kwak HS, Min K, et al. Incidental abnormal FDG uptake in the prostate on 18-fluoro-2-deoxyglucose positron emission tomography-computed tomography scans. Asian Pac J Cancer Prev. 2014;15(20):8699–703.
33. Reesink DJ, van de Putte EE F, Vegt E, De Jong J, van Werkhoven E, Mertens LS, et al. Clinical relevance of incidental prostatic lesions on fdg-positron emission tomography/computerized tomography—should patients receive further evaluation? J Urol. 2016;195(4 Part 1):907–12.
34. Sahin E, Elboga U, Kalender E, Basıbuyuk M, Demir HD, Celen YZ. Clinical significance of incidental FDG uptake in the prostate gland detected by PET/CT. Int J Clin Exp Med. 2015;8(7):10577–85. eCollection 2015
35. Brown AM, Lindenberg ML, Sankineni S, Shih JH, Johnson LM, Pruthy S, et al. Does focal incidental 18 F-FDG PET/CT uptake in the prostate have significance? Abdom Imaging. 2015;40(8):3222–9.
36. Kwon T, Jeong IG, You D, Hong JH, Ahn H, Kim C-S. Prevalence and clinical significance of incidental 18F-fluoro-2-deoxyglucose uptake in prostate. Korean J Urol. 2015;56(4):288–94.
37. Schöder H, Herrmann K, Gönen M, Hricak H, Eberhard S, Scardino P, et al. 2-[18F] fluoro-2-deoxyglucose positron emission tomography for the detection of disease in patients with prostate-specific antigen relapse after radical prostatectomy. Clin Cancer Res. 2005;11(13):4761–9.
38. Chang C-H, Wu H-C, Tsai JJ, Shen Y-Y, Changlai S-P, Kao A. Detecting metastatic pelvic lymph nodes by 18F-2-deoxyglucose positron emission tomography in patients with prostate-specific antigen relapse after treatment for localized prostate cancer. Urol Int. 2003;70(4):311–5.
39. Richter JA, Rodríguez M, Rioja J, Peñuelas I, Martí-Climent J, Garrastachu P, et al. Dual tracer 11 C-choline and FDG-PET in the diagnosis of biochemical prostate cancer relapse after radical treatment. Mol Imaging Biol. 2010;12(2):210–7.
40. Öztürk H, Karapolat İ. 18F-fluorodeoxyglucose PET/CT for detection of disease in patients with prostate-specific antigen relapse following radical treatment of a local-stage prostate cancer. Oncol Lett. 2016;11(1):316–22.
41. Jadvar H, Desai B, Ji L, Conti PS, Dorff TB, Groshen SG, et al. Prospective evaluation of 18F-NaF and 18F-FDG PET/CT in detection of occult metastatic disease in biochemical recurrence of prostate cancer. Clin Nucl Med. 2012;37(7):637.
42. Madigan AA, Rycyna KJ, Parwani AV, Datiri YJ, Basudan AM, Sobek KM, et al. Novel nuclear localization of fatty acid synthase correlates with prostate cancer aggressiveness. Am J Pathol. 2014;184(8):2156–62.
43. Mertan FV, Lindenberg L, Choyke PL, Turkbey B. PET imaging of recurrent and metastatic prostate cancer with novel tracers. Future Oncol. 2016;12(21):2463–77.
44. Seltzer MA, Jahan SA, Sparks R, Stout DB, Satyamurthy N, Dahlbom M, et al. Radiation dose estimates in humans for 11C-acetate whole-body PET. J Nucl Mee. 2004;45(7):1233–6.
45. Mena E, Turkbey B, Mani H, Adler S, Valera VA, Bernardo M, et al. 11C-Acetate PET/CT in localized prostate cancer: a study with MRI and histopathologic correlation. J Nucl Med. 2012;53(4):538–45.
46. Jambor I, Borra R, Kemppainen J, Lepomäki V, Parkkola R, Dean K, et al. Improved detection of localized prostate cancer using co-registered MRI and 11C-acetate PET/CT. Eur J Radiol. 2012;81(11):2966–72.
47. Mohsen B, Giorgio T, Rasoul ZS, Werner L, Ali GRM, Reza DKV, et al. Application of 11C-acetate positron-emission tomography (PET) imaging in prostate cancer: systematic review and meta-analysis of the literature. BJU Int. 2013;112(8):1062–72.
48. Oyama N, Akino H, Kanamaru H, Suzuki Y, Muramoto S, Yonekura Y, et al. 11C-acetate PET imaging of prostate cancer. J Nucl Med. 2002;43(2):181–6.
49. Liu J, Chen Z, Wang T, Liu L, Zhao L, Guo G, et al. Influence of four radiotracers in PET/CT on diagnostic accuracy for prostate cancer: a bivariate ran-

dom-effects meta-analysis. Cell Physiol Biochem. 2016;39(2):467–80.
50. Haseebuddin M, Dehdashti F, Siegel BA, Liu J, Roth EB, Nepple KG, et al. 11C-acetate PET/CT before radical prostatectomy: nodal staging and treatment failure prediction. J Nucl Med. 2013;54(5):699–706.
51. Schumacher MC, Radecka E, Hellström M, Jacobsson H, Sundin A. [11C] Acetate positron emission tomography-computed tomography imaging of prostate cancer lymph-node metastases correlated with histopathological findings after extended lymphadenectomy. Scandinavian J Urol. 2015;49(1):35–42.
52. Leisser A, Pruscha K, Ubl P, Wadsak W, Mayerhöfer M, Mitterhauser M, et al. Evaluation of fatty acid synthase in prostate cancer recurrence: SUV of [11C] acetate PET as a prognostic marker. Prostate. 2015;75(15):1760–7.
53. Dusing RW, Peng W, Lai S-M, Grado GL, Holzbeierlein JM, Thrasher JB, et al. Prostate-specific antigen and prostate-specific antigen velocity as threshold indicators in 11C-acetate PET/CTAC scanning for prostate cancer recurrence. Clin Nucl Med. 2014;39(9):777.
54. Almeida FD, Yen C-K, Scholz MC, Lam RY, Turner J, Bans LL, et al. Performance characteristics and relationship of PSA value/kinetics on carbon-11 acetate PET/CT imaging in biochemical relapse of prostate cancer. Am J Nucl Med Mol Imaging. 2017;7(1):1.
55. Regula N, Häggman M, Johansson S, Sörensen J. Malignant lipogenesis defined by 11 C-acetate PET/CT predicts prostate cancer-specific survival in patients with biochemical relapse after prostatectomy. Eur J Nucl Med Mol Imaging. 2016;43(12):2131–8.
56. Ackerstaff E, Pflug BR, Nelson JB, Bhujwalla ZM. Detection of increased choline compounds with proton nuclear magnetic resonance spectroscopy subsequent to malignant transformation of human prostatic epithelial cells. Cancer Res. 2001;61(9):3599–603.
57. Wallitt KL, Khan SR, Dubash S, Tam HH, Khan S, Barwick TD. Clinical PET imaging in prostate cancer. Radiographics. 2017;37(5):1512–36.
58. Krause BJ, Souvatzoglou M, Treiber U, editors. Imaging of prostate cancer with PET/CT and radioactively labeled choline derivates. Urolog Oncol Sem Orig Investig. 2013;31(4):427–35.
59. Bundschuh RA, Wendl CM, Weirich G, Eiber M, Souvatzoglou M, Treiber U, et al. Tumour volume delineation in prostate cancer assessed by [11 C] choline PET/CT: validation with surgical specimens. Eur J Nucl Med Mol Imaging. 2013;40(6):824–31.
60. Grosu A-L, Weirich G, Wendl C, Prokic V, Kirste S, Geinitz H, et al. 11 C-Choline PET/pathology image coregistration in primary localized prostate cancer. Eur J Nucl Med Mol Imaging. 2014;41(12):2242–8.
61. Pinaquy JB, De Clermont-Galleran H, Pasticier G, Rigou G, Alberti N, Hindie E, et al. Comparative effectiveness of [18F]-fluorocholine PET-CT and pelvic MRI with diffusion-weighted imaging for staging in patients with high-risk prostate cancer. Prostate. 2015;75(3):323–31.
62. Evangelista L, Guttilla A, Zattoni F, Muzzio PC, Zattoni F. Utility of choline positron emission tomography/computed tomography for lymph node involvement identification in intermediate-to high-risk prostate cancer: a systematic literature review and meta-analysis. Eur Urol. 2013;63(6):1040–8.
63. von Eyben FE, Kairemo K. Meta-analysis of 11C-choline and 18F-choline PET/CT for management of patients with prostate cancer. Nucl Med Comms. 2014;35(3):221–30.
64. Evangelista L, Cimitan M, Zattoni F, Guttilla A, Zattoni F, Saladini G. Comparison between conventional imaging (abdominal–pelvic computed tomography and bone scan) and [18F] choline positron emission tomography/computed tomography imaging for the initial staging of patients with intermediate- to high-risk prostate cancer: a retrospective analysis. Scandinavian J Urol. 2015;49(5):345–53.
65. Van den Bergh L, Lerut E, Haustermans K, Deroose CM, Oyen R, Isebaert S, et al. Final analysis of a prospective trial on functional imaging for nodal staging in patients with prostate cancer at high risk for lymph node involvement. Urol Oncol Sem Orig Investig. 2015:33(3):109.e23–109.e31.
66. Evangelista L, Briganti A, Fanti S, Joniau S, Reske S, Schiavina R, et al. New clinical indications for 18F/11C-choline, new tracers for positron emission tomography and a promising hybrid device for prostate cancer staging: a systematic review of the literature. Eur Urol. 2016;70(1):161–75.
67. Cimitan M, Evangelista L, Hodolič M, Mariani G, Baseric T, Bodanza V, et al. Gleason score at diagnosis predicts the rate of detection of 18F-choline PET/CT performed when biochemical evidence indicates recurrence of prostate cancer: experience with 1,000 patients. J Nucl Med. 2015;56(2):209–15.
68. García J, Cozar M, Soler M, Bassa P, Riera E, Ferrer J. Salvage radiotherapy in prostate cancer patients. Planning, treatment response and prognosis using 11C-choline PET/CT. Revista Española de Medicina Nuclear e Imagen Molecular (English Edition). 2016;35(4):238–45.
69. Goldstein J, Even-Sapir E, Ben-Haim S, Saad A, Spieler B, Davidson T, et al. Does choline PET/CT change the management of prostate cancer patients with biochemical failure? Am J Clin Oncol. 2017;40(3):256–9.
70. Incerti E, Fodor A, Mapelli P, Fiorino C, Alongi P, Kirienko M, et al. Radiation treatment of lymph node recurrence from prostate cancer: is 11C-choline PET/CT predictive of survival outcomes? J Nucl Med. 2015;56(12):1836–42.

71. Picchio M, Giovacchini G, Gianolli L, Suardi N, Abdollah F, Gandaglia G, et al. 930 [11C]Choline PET/CT predicts survival in hormone-naïve prostate cancer patients with biochemical failure after radical prostatectomy. Eur Urol Suppl. 2015;14(2):e930.
72. Giovacchini G, Picchio M, Garcia-Parra R, Briganti A, Abdollah F, Gianolli L, et al. 11C-choline PET/CT predicts prostate cancer–specific survival in patients with biochemical failure during androgen-deprivation therapy. J Nucl Med. 2014;55(2):233–41.
73. Leiblich A, Stevens D, Sooriakumaran P. The utility of molecular imaging in prostate cancer. Curr Urol Rep. 2016;17(3):26.
74. FDA Approves 11C-Choline for PET in Prostate Cancer. J Nucl Med. 2012;53(12):11N. PubMed PMID: 23203247.
75. Oka S, Hattori R, Kurosaki F, Toyama M, Williams LA, Yu W, et al. A preliminary study of anti-1-amino-3-18F-fluorocyclobutyl-1-carboxylic acid for the detection of prostate cancer. J Nucl Med. 2007;48(1):46–55.
76. McConathy J, Voll RJ, Yu W, Crowe RJ, Goodman MM. Improved synthesis of anti-[18F] FACBC: improved preparation of labeling precursor and automated radiosynthesis. Appl Radiat Isot. 2003;58(6):657–66.
77. Schuster DM, Taleghani PA, Nieh PT, Master VA, Amzat R, Savir-Baruch B, et al. Characterization of primary prostate carcinoma by anti-1-amino-2-[18F]-fluorocyclobutane-1-carboxylic acid (anti-3-[18F] FACBC) uptake. Am J Nucl Med Mol Imaging. 2013;3(1):85.
78. Turkbey B, Mena E, Shih J, Pinto PA, Merino MJ, Lindenberg ML, et al. Localized prostate cancer detection with 18F FACBC PET/CT: comparison with MR imaging and histopathologic analysis. Radiology. 2013;270(3):849–56.
79. Jambor I, Kuisma A, Kähkönen E, Kemppainen J, Merisaari H, Eskola O, et al. Prospective evaluation of 18 F-FACBC PET/CT and PET/MRI versus multiparametric MRI in intermediate-to high-risk prostate cancer patients (FLUCIPRO trial). Eur J Nucl Med Mol Imaging. 2018;45(3):355–64.
80. Kairemo K, Rasulova N, Partanen K, Joensuu T. Preliminary clinical experience of trans-1-Amino-3-(18) F-fluorocyclobutanecarboxylic Acid (anti-(18) F-FACBC) PET/CT imaging in prostate cancer patients. Biomed Res Int. 2014;2014:1.
81. Suzuki H, Inoue Y, Fujimoto H, Yonese J, Tanabe K, Fukasawa S, et al. Diagnostic performance and safety of NMK36 (trans-1-amino-3-[18F] fluorocyclobutanecarboxylic acid)-PET/CT in primary prostate cancer: multicenter phase IIb clinical trial. Japanese J Clin Oncol. 2016;46(2):152–62.
82. Parent EE, Schuster DM. Update on 18F-Fluciclovine PET for prostate cancer imaging. J Nucl Med. 2018;59(5):733–9.
83. Bach-Gansmo T, Nanni C, Nieh PT, Zanoni L, Bogsrud TV, Sletten H, et al. Multisite experience of the safety, detection rate and diagnostic performance of fluciclovine (18F) positron emission tomography/computerized tomography imaging in the staging of biochemically recurrent prostate cancer. J Urol. 2017;197(3 Part 1):676–83.
84. Odewole OA, Tade FI, Nieh PT, Savir-Baruch B, Jani AB, Master VA, et al. Recurrent prostate cancer detection with anti-3-[18 F] FACBC PET/CT: comparison with CT. Eur J Nucl Med Mol Imaging. 2016;43(10):1773–83.
85. Nanni C, Zanoni L, Pultrone C, Schiavina R, Brunocilla E, Lodi F, et al. 18 F-FACBC (anti1-amino-3-18 F-fluorocyclobutane-1-carboxylic acid) versus 11 C-choline PET/CT in prostate cancer relapse: results of a prospective trial. Eur J Nucl Med Mol Imaging. 2016;43(9):1601–10.
86. Schuster DM, Nieh PT, Jani AB, Amzat R, Bowman FD, Halkar RK, et al. Anti-3-[18F] FACBC positron emission tomography-computerized tomography and 111In-capromab pendetide single photon emission computerized tomography-computerized tomography for recurrent prostate carcinoma: results of a prospective clinical trial. J Urol. 2014;191(5):1446–53.
87. Ren J, Yuan L, Wen G, Yang J. The value of anti-1-amino-3-18F-fluorocyclobutane-1-carboxylic acid PET/CT in the diagnosis of recurrent prostate carcinoma: a meta-analysis. Acta Radiol. 2016;57(4):487–93.
88. Wright GL Jr, Haley C, Beckett ML, Schellhammer PF, editors. Expression of prostate-specific membrane antigen in normal, benign, and malignant prostate tissues. Urol Oncol Sem Orig Investig. 1995;1(1):18–28.
89. Czarniecki M, Mena E, Lindenberg L, Cacko M, Harmon S, Radtke JP, et al. Keeping up with the prostate-specific membrane antigens (PSMAs): an introduction to a new class of positron emission tomography (PET) imaging agents. Translational Androl Urol. 2018;7(5):831.
90. Demirci E, Sahin OE, Ocak M, Akovali B, Nematyazar J, Kabasakal L. Normal distribution pattern and physiological variants of 68Ga-PSMA-11 PET/CT imaging. Nucl Med Comms. 2016;37(11):1169–79.
91. Sweat SD, Pacelli A, Murphy GP, Bostwick DG. Prostate-specific membrane antigen expression is greatest in prostate adenocarcinoma and lymph node metastases. Urology. 1998;52(4):637–40.
92. Davis MI, Bennett MJ, Thomas LM, Bjorkman PJ. Crystal structure of prostate-specific membrane antigen, a tumor marker and peptidase. Proc Natl Acad Sci. 2005;102(17):5981–6.
93. Taneja SS. ProstaScint® scan: contemporary use in clinical practice. Rev Urol. 2004;6(Suppl 10):S19.
94. Eder M, Schäfer M, Bauder-Wüst U, Hull W-E, Wängler C, Mier W, et al. 68Ga-complex lipophi-

licity and the targeting property of a urea-based PSMA inhibitor for PET imaging. Bioconjug Chem. 2012;23(4):688–97.
95. Rauscher I, Maurer T, Fendler WP, Sommer WH, Schwaiger M, Eiber M. 68 Ga-PSMA ligand PET/CT in patients with prostate cancer: how we review and report. Cancer Imaging. 2016;16(1):14.
96. Afshar-Oromieh A, Malcher A, Eder M, Eisenhut M, Linhart H, Hadaschik B, et al. PET imaging with a [68 Ga] gallium-labelled PSMA ligand for the diagnosis of prostate cancer: biodistribution in humans and first evaluation of tumour lesions. Eur J Nucl Med Mol Imaging. 2013;40(4):486–95.
97. Eiber M, Weirich G, Holzapfel K, Souvatzoglou M, Haller B, Rauscher I, et al. Simultaneous 68Ga-PSMA HBED-CC PET/MRI improves the localization of primary prostate cancer. Eur Urol. 2016;70(5):829–36.
98. Herlemann A, Wenter V, Kretschmer A, Thierfelder KM, Bartenstein P, Faber C, et al. 68Ga-PSMA positron emission tomography/computed tomography provides accurate staging of lymph node regions prior to lymph node dissection in patients with prostate cancer. Eur Urol. 2016;70(4):553–7.
99. Budäus L, Leyh-Bannurah S-R, Salomon G, Michl U, Heinzer H, Huland H, et al. Initial experience of 68Ga-PSMA PET/CT imaging in high-risk prostate cancer patients prior to radical prostatectomy. Eur Urol. 2016;69(3):393–6.
100. Afshar-Oromieh A, Avtzi E, Giesel FL, Holland-Letz T, Linhart HG, Eder M, et al. The diagnostic value of PET/CT imaging with the 68 Ga-labelled PSMA ligand HBED-CC in the diagnosis of recurrent prostate cancer. Eur J Nucl Med Mol Imaging. 2015;42(2):197–209.
101. Perera M, Papa N, Christidis D, Wetherell D, Hofman MS, Murphy DG, et al. Sensitivity, specificity, and predictors of positive 68Ga–prostate-specific membrane antigen positron emission tomography in advanced prostate cancer: a systematic review and meta-analysis. Eur Urol. 2016;70(6):926–37.
102. Verburg FA, Pfister D, Heidenreich A, Vogg A, Drude NI, Vöö S, et al. Extent of disease in recurrent prostate cancer determined by [68 Ga] PSMA-HBED-CC PET/CT in relation to PSA levels, PSA doubling time and Gleason score. Eur J Nucl Med Mol Imaging. 2016;43(3):397–403.
103. Eiber M, Maurer T, Souvatzoglou M, Beer AJ, Ruffani A, Haller B, et al. Evaluation of hybrid 68Ga-PSMA ligand PET/CT in 248 patients with biochemical recurrence after radical prostatectomy. J Nucl Med. 2015;56(5):668–74.
104. Afshar-Oromieh A, Holland-Letz T, Giesel FL, Kratochwil C, Mier W, Haufe S, et al. Diagnostic performance of 68 Ga-PSMA-11 (HBED-CC) PET/CT in patients with recurrent prostate cancer: evaluation in 1007 patients. Eur J Nucl Med Mol Imaging. 2017;44(8):1258–68.
105. Morigi JJ, Stricker PD, van Leeuwen PJ, Tang R, Ho B, Nguyen Q, et al. Prospective comparison of 18F-fluoromethylcholine versus 68Ga-PSMA PET/CT in prostate cancer patients who have rising PSA after curative treatment and are being considered for targeted therapy. J Nucl Med. 2015;56(8):1185–90.
106. Fendler WP, Calais J, Eiber M, Flavell RR, Mishoe A, Feng FY, et al. Assessment of 68Ga-PSMA-11 PET accuracy in localizing recurrent prostate Cancer: a prospective single-arm clinical trial. JAMA Oncol. 2019;5(6):856–63.
107. Gorin MA, Pomper MG, Rowe SP. PSMA-targeted imaging of prostate cancer: the best is yet to come. BJU Int. 2016;117(5):715–6.
108. Sanchez-Crespo A. Comparison of Gallium-68 and Fluorine-18 imaging characteristics in positron emission tomography. Appl Radiat Isot. 2013;76:55–62.
109. Dietlein M, Kobe C, Kuhnert G, Stockter S, Fischer T, Schomäcker K, et al. Comparison of [18 F] DCFPyL and [68 Ga] Ga-PSMA-HBED-CC for PSMA-PET imaging in patients with relapsed prostate cancer. Mol Imaging Biol. 2015;17(4):575–84.
110. Szabo Z, Mena E, Rowe SP, Plyku D, Nidal R, Eisenberger MA, et al. Initial evaluation of [18 F] DCFPyL for prostate-specific membrane antigen (PSMA)-targeted PET imaging of prostate cancer. Mol Imaging Biol. 2015;17(4):565–74.
111. Rowe SP, Gage KL, Faraj SF, Macura KJ, Cornish TC, Gonzalez-Roibon N, et al. 18F-DCFBC PET/CT for PSMA-based detection and characterization of primary prostate cancer. J Nucl Med. 2015;56(7):1003–10.
112. Turkbey B, Mena E, Lindenberg L, Adler S, Bednarova S, Berman R, et al. 18F-DCFBC prostate-specific membrane antigen-targeted PET/CT imaging in localized prostate Cancer: correlation with multiparametric MRI and histopathology. Clin Nucl Med. 2017;42(10):735–40.
113. Rowe SP, Macura KJ, Ciarallo A, Mena E, Blackford A, Nadal R, et al. Comparison of prostate-specific membrane antigen–based 18F-DCFBC PET/CT to conventional imaging modalities for detection of hormone-naïve and castration-resistant metastatic prostate cancer. J Nucl Med. 2016;57(1):46–53.
114. Rowe SP, Macura KJ, Mena E, Blackford AL, Nadal R, Antonarakis ES, et al. PSMA-based [18 F] DCFPyL PET/CT is superior to conventional imaging for lesion detection in patients with metastatic prostate cancer. Mol Imaging Biol. 2016;18(3):411–9.
115. Rowe SP, Mana-Ay M, Javadi MS, Szabo Z, Leal JP, Pomper MG, et al. PSMA-based detection of prostate cancer bone lesions with 18F-DCFPyL PET/CT: a sensitive alternative to 99mTc-MDP bone scan and Na18F PET/CT? Clin Genitourin Cancer. 2016;14(1):e115–e8.
116. Gorin MA, Rowe SP, Patel HD, Vidal I, Mana-Ay M, Javadi MS, et al. Prostate specific membrane antigen targeted 18F-DCFPyL positron emission tomography/computerized tomography for the pre-

operative staging of high risk prostate cancer: results of a prospective, phase II, single center study. J Urol. 2018;199(1):126–32.
117. Mena E, Lindenberg ML, Shih JH, Adler S, Harmon S, Bergvall E, et al. Clinical impact of PSMA-based 18 F–DCFBC PET/CT imaging in patients with biochemically recurrent prostate cancer after primary local therapy. Eur J Nucl Med Mol Imaging. 2018;45(1):4–11.
118. Giesel FL, Cardinale J, Schäfer M, Neels O, Benešová M, Mier W, et al. 18 F-Labelled PSMA-1007 shows similarity in structure, biodistribution and tumour uptake to the theragnostic compound PSMA-617. Eur J Nucl Med Mol Imaging. 2016;43(10):1929–30.
119. Giesel FL, Hadaschik B, Cardinale J, Radtke J, Vinsensia M, Lehnert W, et al. F-18 labelled PSMA-1007: biodistribution, radiation dosimetry and histopathological validation of tumor lesions in prostate cancer patients. Eur J Nucl Med Mol Imaging. 2017;44(4):678–88.
120. Kesch C, Vinsensia M, Radtke JP, Schlemmer HP, Heller M, Ellert E, et al. Intraindividual comparison of 18F-PSMA-1007 PET/CT, multiparametric MRI, and radical prostatectomy Specimens in patients with primary prostate cancer: a retrospective, proof-of-concept study. J Nucl Med. 2017;58(11):1805–10.
121. Paddubny K, Freitag MT, Kratochwil C, Koerber S, Radtke JP, Sakovich R, et al. Fluorine-18 prostate-specific membrane antigen-1007 positron emission tomography/computed tomography and multiparametric magnetic resonance imaging in diagnostics of local recurrence in a prostate cancer patient after recent radical prostatectomy. Clin Genitourin Cancer. 2018;16(2):103–5.
122. Gandaglia G, Abdollah F, Schiffmann J, Trudeau V, Shariat SF, Kim SP, et al. Distribution of metastatic sites in patients with prostate cancer: a population-based analysis. Prostate. 2014;74(2):210–6.
123. Langsteger W, Rezaee A, Pirich C, Beheshti M, editors. 18F-NaF-PET/CT and 99mTc-MDP bone scintigraphy in the detection of bone metastases in prostate cancer. Semin Nucl Med. 2016;46(6):491–501.
124. Fraum TJ, Ludwig DR, Kim EH, Schroeder P, Hope TA, Ippolito JE. Prostate cancer PET tracers: essentials for the urologist. Can J Urol. 2018;25:9371–83.
125. Segall G, Delbeke D, Stabin MG, Even-Sapir E, Fair J, Sajdak R, et al. SNM practice guideline for sodium 18F-fluoride PET/CT bone scans 1.0. J Nucl Med. 2010;51(11):1813–20.
126. Bastawrous S, Bhargava P, Behnia F, Djang DS, Haseley DR. Newer PET application with an old tracer: role of 18F-NaF skeletal PET/CT in oncologic practice. Radiographics. 2014;34(5):1295–316.
127. Even-Sapir E, Metser U, Mishani E, Lievshitz G, Lerman H, Leibovitch I. The detection of bone metastases in patients with high-risk prostate cancer: 99mTc-MDP Planar bone scintigraphy, single- and multi-field-of-view SPECT, 18F-fluoride PET, and 18F-fluoride PET/CT. J Nucl Med. 2006;47(2):287–97.
128. Langsteger W, Balogova S, Huchet V, Beheshti M, Paycha F, Egrot C, et al. Fluorocholine (18F) and sodium fluoride (18F) PET/CT in the detection of prostate cancer: prospective comparison of diagnostic performance determined by masked reading. Q J Nucl Med Mol Imaging. 2011;55(4):448–57.
129. Apolo AB, Lindenberg L, Shih JH, Mena E, Kim JW, Park JC, et al. Prospective study evaluating Na18F PET/CT in predicting clinical outcomes and survival in advanced prostate cancer. J Nucl Med. 2016;57(6):886–92.
130. Edler von Eyben F, Kairemo K, Kiljunen T, Joensuu T. Planning of external beam radiotherapy for prostate cancer guided by PET/CT. Curr Radiopharm. 2015;8(1):19–31.
131. Poulsen MH, Petersen H, Høilund-Carlsen PF, Jakobsen JS, Gerke O, Karstoft J, et al. Spine metastases in prostate cancer: comparison of technetium-99m-MDP whole-body bone scintigraphy,[18 F] choline positron emission tomography (PET)/computed tomography (CT) and [18 F] NaF PET/CT. BJU Int. 2014;114(6):818–23.
132. Muzahir S, Jeraj R, Liu G, Hall LT, Del Rio AM, Perk T, et al. Differentiation of metastatic vs degenerative joint disease using semi-quantitative analysis with 18F-NaF PET/CT in castrate resistant prostate cancer patients. Am J Nucl Med Mol Imaging. 2015;5(2):162.

14 Pitfalls and Pearls of Prostate Imaging and Interpretation

Natasha E. Wehrli, Sunil Jeph, and Daniel J. A. Margolis

14.1 Introduction

Multiparametric prostate magnetic resonance imaging (mpMRI) has become a mainstay for the detection, characterization, staging, and monitoring of prostate cancer. While the technical specifications, appearance of the normal prostate, assessment (including staging), and reporting of mpMRI have become well documented and codified, reading mpMRI of the prostate is not trivial [1]. Fortunately, many of the "pitfalls and pearls" of mpMRI of the prostate are well documented [2].

Prostate carcinoma is the most common non-cutaneous carcinoma in men and remains a leading cause of cancer death worldwide [3]. Over the last decade, magnetic resonance imaging (MRI), and specifically multi-parametric MRI (mpMRI) of the prostate gland, in conjunction with digital rectal exam (DRE), serum prostate specific antigen (PSA), and transrectal ultrasound-guided (TRUS) biopsy, has become a mainstay in the management of prostate cancer [4]. While previously reserved for local staging and surgical planning of confirmed disease [5, 6], prostate MRI is now increasingly used for pre-biopsy work-up due to its ability to improve detection and localization of high-grade tumor [7–10] as well as identify candidates for either active surveillance [11, 12] or focal therapy [13].

It is incumbent upon diagnostic radiologists to be well versed in the normal imaging appearance and boundaries of the prostate zonal anatomy, including the anterior fibromuscular stroma, central zone, and surgical capsule as well as extraprostatic structures such as the neurovascular bundles, periprostatic venous plexus, ejaculatory ducts, and seminal vesicles [2, 14–16]. Radiologists should also be familiar with common abnormalities that may demonstrate overlapping imaging features with carcinoma, including stromal-rich BPH nodules, focal acute bacterial prostatitis, chronic granulomatous prostatitis, malakoplakia, calcification, biopsy-related hemorrhage, and changes in the appearance of the prostate gland related to prior focal therapy [16].

There are also pitfalls related to imaging acquisition and quality, perhaps the most important of which relate to diffusion-weighted imaging (DWI), which has become a key component of the PI-RADS scoring system, including its most recent iteration PI-RADS version 2.1 [1, 17]. Routine clinical DWI uses spin-echo

N. E. Wehrli · S. Jeph · D. J. A. Margolis (✉)
Weill Cornell Imaging/New York Presbyterian Hospital, Department of Radiology, New York, NY, USA
e-mail: naw9038@med.cornell.edu; suj9028@med.cornell.edu; djm9016@med.cornell.edu

T. Tirkes (ed.), *Prostate MRI Essentials*, https://doi.org/10.1007/978-3-030-45935-2_14

echo-planar imaging (EPI) which is acquired by rapidly switching strong magnetic gradients inducing eddy currents that make this sequence highly susceptible to geometric distortion in the phase-encoding direction [18]. Interfaces of materials with large susceptibility differences, such as air to soft tissue (i.e., rectal gas) and metal to tissue (i.e., femoral hardware), may therefore cause significant anatomic distortion which can affect the sensitivity of this sequence [19]. Finally, DWI relies on adequate suppression of normal benign tissue on high b-value imaging and proper windowing of the apparent diffusion coefficient (ADC) series to ensure adequate sensitivity for detection of pathology [2].

In this chapter, we will highlight the important pearls and pitfalls of interpreting prostate MRI, including attention to normal anatomic variants, common and uncommon pathology that may masquerade as tumor, and factors relating to image acquisition that may affect overall sensitivity of lesion detection.

14.2 Pitfalls

14.2.1 Category: Technical Challenges Related to Diffusion-Weighted Imaging

14.2.1.1 Anatomic Distortion of High B-Value Diffusion-Weighted Images and Motion Artifacts

In addition to characterizing the aggressiveness of a tumor, DWI has an important role in localizing the tumor in mpMRI. DWI is most commonly acquired by echo-planar technique. Rapid switching of strong magnetic gradients causes eddy currents. Unpredictable artifacts occur due to distortion of the magnetic field gradient caused by the magnetic field generated by the eddy currents. The artifact is more pronounced on high b-values resulting in anatomic distortion [2]. This geometric distortion is most pronounced in phase-encoding direction and pronounced by motion [20]. In addition to the geometric distortion, ghosting artifacts are more pronounced on 3 T MRI, as compared to 1.5 T MRI [21].

Geometric distortion artifacts can be reduced by reducing receiver bandwidth and parallel imaging reducing echo spacing, echo time, and echo train length [20]. It improves the localization for targeted biopsies and therapy at the cost of lesion characterization. Phase encoding in left-to-right direction reduces the artifact. Also, T2-weighted images are more useful for better localization and anatomic delineation [2, 20].

DWI techniques such as multi-shot based radially oriented parallel acquisition techniques significantly reduce the anatomic distortion, at the cost of reduced signal-to-noise ratio [22] (Fig. 14.1).

14.2.1.2 Lack of Suppression of Benign Prostate Tissue on Standard High B-Value Diffusion-Weighted Images

ADC map serves as a primary dataset for evaluation of DWI of the prostate. Increased DWI signal of the tumor relative to the background parenchyma is important for PI-RADS classification [23]. Qualitative analysis of DWI is enhanced by better signal suppression of benign prostate tissue by using higher b-values causing greater signal restriction in tumor lesions. In addition to poor suppression of benign prostate tissue, low b-value images ($b \leq 1000$ s/mm^2) obscure the tumor lesions by persistent T2 shine-through effect [24]. Higher b-values are associated with anatomical distortion. Computed DWI is derived mathematically using lower b-value images by applying standard mono-exponential fit. Exploiting lower b-values' higher SNR improves the tumor detection rate [25]. However, there is no overall improvement in diagnostic accuracy with the calculated DWI relative to the low b-value DWI. Increased sensitivity of tumor detection is undermined by the increasing false-positive findings on calculated DWI images [26] (Fig. 14.2).

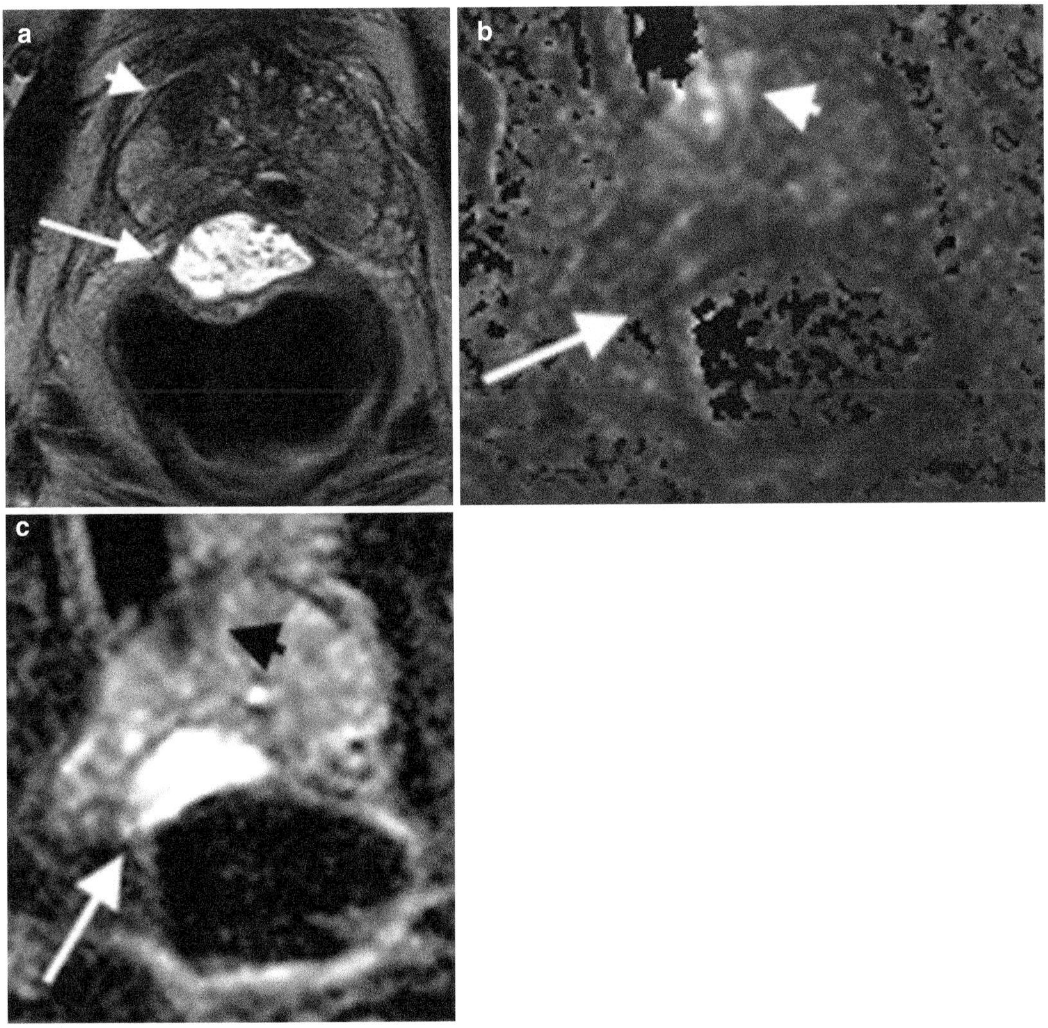

Fig. 14.1 Anatomic distortion of high b-value diffusion-weighted images. (**a**) Axial T2-weighted image showing a hypointense lesion with irregular margins in the right anterior peripheral zone (white arrowhead) and hyperintense rectal spacer hydrogel (white arrow). Also, noted gas-filled rectum. (**b**) Diffusion-weighted image at the same level is degraded due to susceptibility artifact from gas in the rectum and causing anatomic distortion of the position of hydrogel (white arrow) and the lesion (white arrowhead). (**c**) The corresponding ADC map at the same level shows the anatomic distortion with displaced position of hydrogel (white arrow) and the peripheral zone lesion (black arrowhead)

14.2.1.3 Suboptimal Windowing of the ADC Map

Stromal BPH involving the transition zone has low signal intensity on T2-weighted sequences and has an overlapping enhancement pattern with the transition zone tumor lesion. Tumors in the transition zone have a lower signal intensity on ADC maps compared to benign prostate tissue such as stromal hyperplasia [27]. The units of signal intensity have not been standardized across different MRI scanners and are not analogous to the Hounsfield units used for CT. This leads to a common pitfall by visual analysis of ADC due to variable default window settings across different MRI scanners

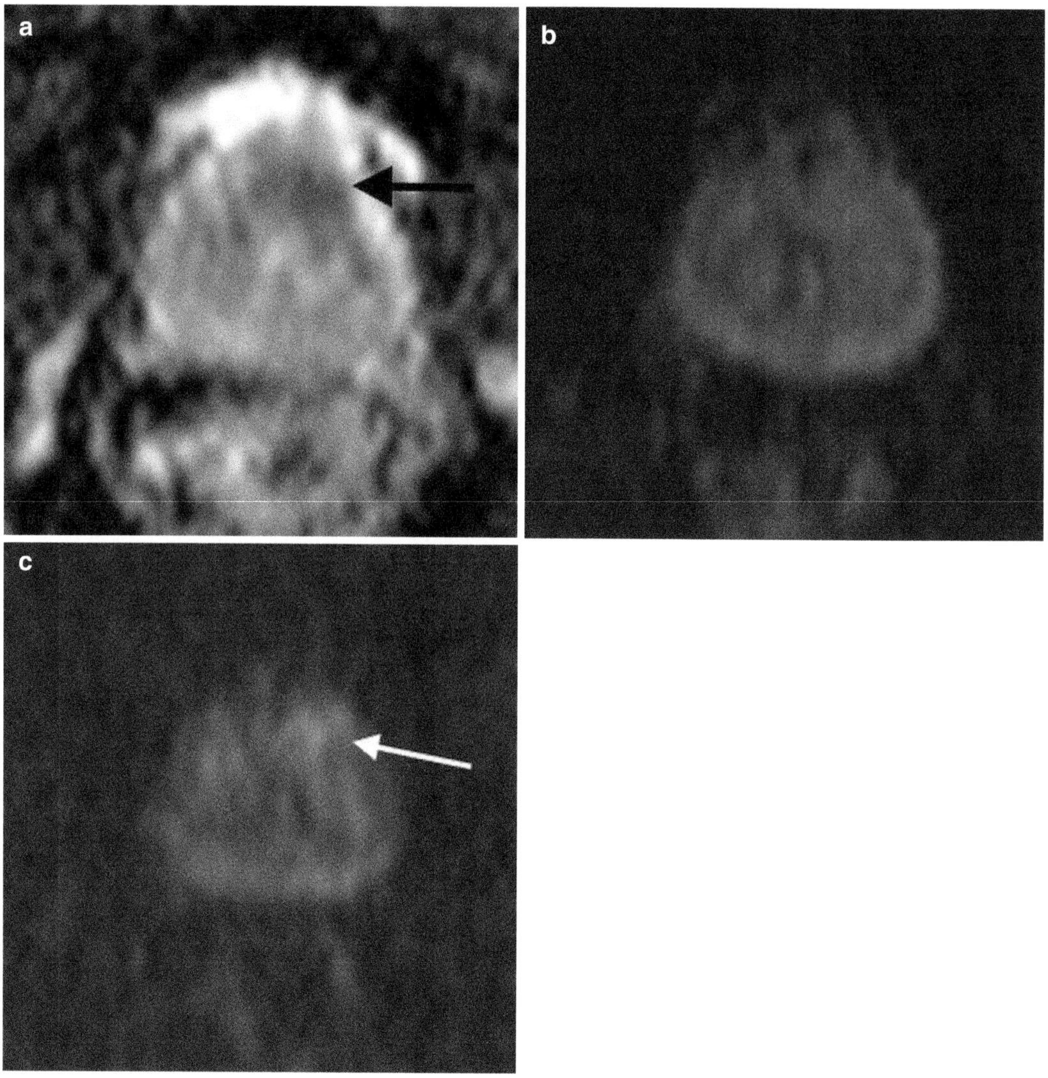

Fig. 14.2 Lack of suppression of benign prostate tissue on standard high b-value diffusion-weighted images. (**a**) ADC map showing hypointense lesion (black arrow) in the left anterior transition zone at the level of the mid-gland. (**b**) DWI image with a b-value of 800 s/mm2 at the same level shows inadequate suppression of the benign background parenchyma of the prostate making the lesion indistinguishable. (**c**) DWI image with a b-value of 1400 s/mm2 at the same level causes adequate suppression of the background benign prostate tissue and shows hyperintense lesion (white arrow) corresponding to the ADC map

that might not be optimal resulting in false-positive and false-negative outcomes. Window and width setting of 1.65 and 1.675 × 10–6 mm^2/s has been shown to consistently detect higher-grade tumors [28]. To improve the validity and prognostic value of ADC maps, the window width may be standardized for each MRI scanner within a practice with the help of an experienced radiologist (Fig. 14.3).

14.2.2 Category: Normal Anatomic Structures That May Be Mistaken for Tumor

14.2.2.1 Central Zone

Tumors arising from the central zone, although more aggressive, account for less than 5% of prostate cancers [29]. Asymmetric enlargement

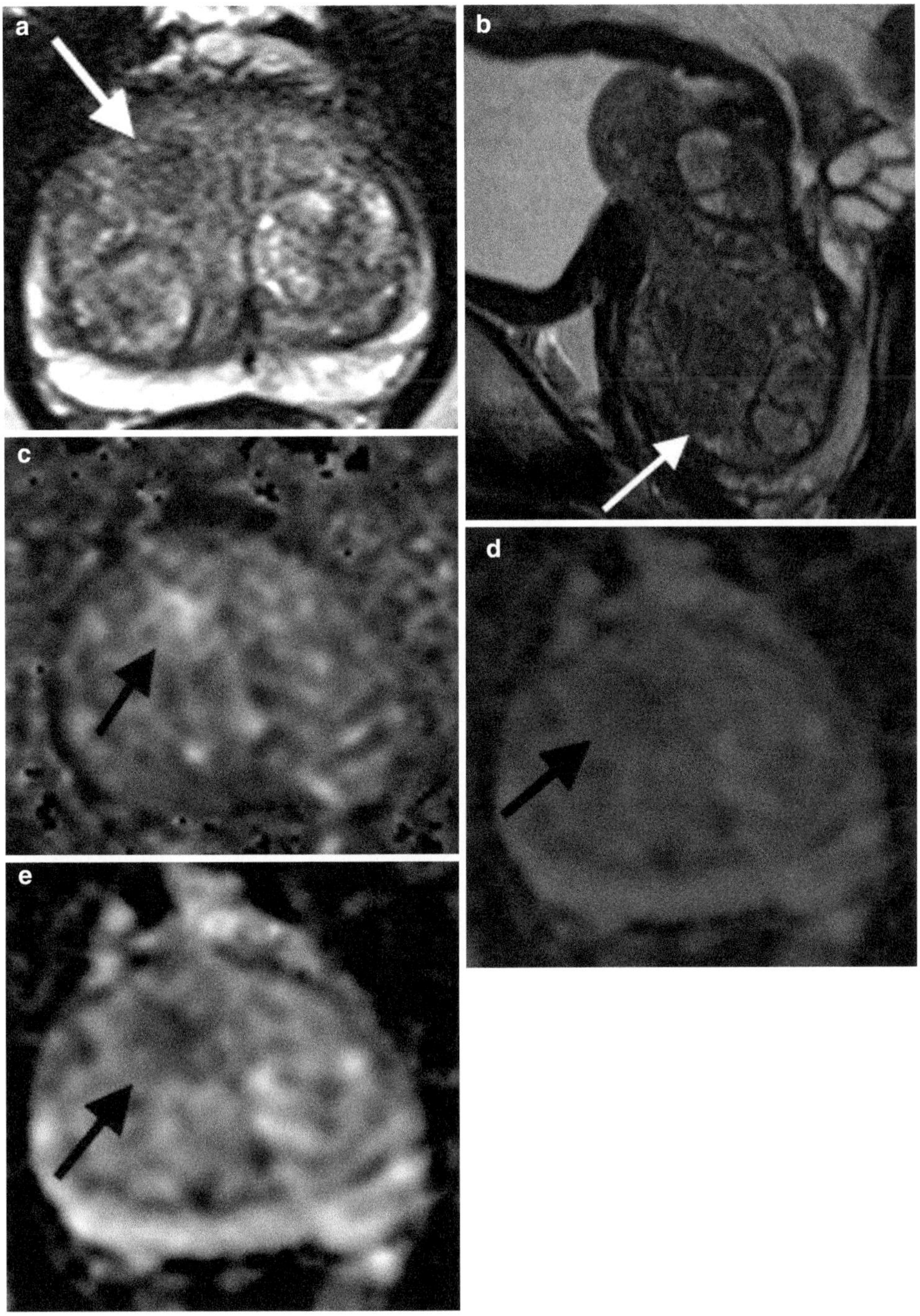

Fig. 14.3 Suboptimal windowing of the ADC map. (**a**) Axial T2-weighted image showing benign prostatic hyperplasia with scattered, benign, heterogeneous foci of low signal intensity. Circumscribed hypointense lesion is present in the right anterior transition zone (white arrow). (**b**) Sagittal T2-weighted image shows the lesion in apical transition zone (white arrow). (**c**) DWI image at the same level with high b-value shows the hyperintense transition zone lesion (black arrow) relative to the background benign prostate tissue. (**d**) ADC map with poor window setting at the same level shows the lesion with mild hypointense signal intensity (black arrow) consistent with PI-RADS 3 lesion. (**e**) ADC map with adequate window level and width setting shows the lesion darker with marked hypointense signal (black arrow), consistent with PI-RADS 4 lesion. The recommended window width/level settings of 1400/1400 have consistently shown to be useful in picking up clinically significant prostate lesions

of the heterogeneous transition zone due to BPH can efface the central zone, making it indistinguishable from the surrounding transition zone. Since the normal central zone is hypointense on ADC map and T2-weighted sequences, it can be easily misinterpreted as a dominated lesion arising from transition zone or peripheral zone [30]. The stereotypic location and lack of high signal on high b-value DWI and dynamic contrast-enhanced images confirm the benign nature of the central zone. Evaluation of coronal images to determine asymmetry or "tilting" of the prostate may also be useful.

14.2.2.2 Thickening of Surgical Capsule

Surgical capsule is a fibromuscular structure between the peripheral zone and transition zone, surrounding the transition zone. It is a thin, poorly defined structure in young men. In older men, there is reactive proliferation and thickening of the surgical capsule due to outward pressure caused by BPH of transition zone. Subsequently, it condenses into a distinct crescent band around the hypertrophied transition zone [31]. On MRI, it is hypointense on T2-weighted sequences and ADC map and can be misinterpreted as a focal tumor lesion. Anatomic knowledge about the expected location of surgical capsule and correlation of ADC maps with T2-weighted sequences on axial and coronals is helpful. It is normally low signal on high b-value DWI. Also, on DCE there is no corresponding rapid contrast enhancement with washout [32].

14.2.2.3 Periprostatic Venous Plexus and Neurovascular Bundle

Periprostatic neurovascular bundle courses along the outer margins of peripheral zone. Classically, the neurovascular bundles are believed to be located at 5 and 7 o'clock positions. But, in almost half of the cases, there is no discrete neurovascular bundle, and the nerve trunks and vessels are scattered along the outer margins of peripheral zone anteriorly and posteriorly. These nerves and vessels may appear round on en face axial sequences, and since they have decreased T2 and ADC signal density, they may be misinterpreted as tumors. This pitfall can be avoided by using the T2-weighted sequences, since they have a higher spatial resolution. The typical location, coursing along the outer margin of peripheral zone and the overall tubular appearance, as appreciated in different planes is useful in correctly identifying the neurovascular tissue (Fig. 14.4).

14.2.3 Category: Noncancerous Abnormalities That Can Mimic Tumor

14.2.3.1 Post-biopsy Hemorrhage

This is one of the first pitfalls identified well before the introduction of diffusion-weighted and dynamic contrast-enhanced imaging [33]. Blood products result in both T1 and T2 shortening, with the latter mimicking ill-defined cancer. The resulting inflammation may also result in changes on diffusion-weighted and dynamic contrast-enhanced (DCE) imaging, and the presence of inherently short T1 species compromises detection of enhancement on raw T1-weighted images. When hemorrhage is evident on precontrast T1-weighted images, subtraction or pharmacokinetic maps are crucial for the evaluation of enhancement, but even then, whether early enhancement is related to inflammation or neoplasia would be indeterminate. It is for this reason that waiting at least 6 weeks after biopsy for the resolution of hemorrhage is recommended [34]. On the other hand, some experts find the presence of hemorrhage reassuring in confirming the absence of cancer – the "hemorrhage exclusion sign" [35]. Normal prostate glands are enriched in citrate, a natural anticoagulant. Hemorrhage, therefore, is more common in the presence of healthy glands. However, this sign is considered unreliable and could obscure an underlying cancer adjacent to normal glands.

14.2.3.2 Stromal BPH Nodule

Benign prostatic hyperplasia (BPH) is a common condition in older men which nearly exclusively arises in the transition zone, although it can spread to adjacent zones. The origin can be glan-

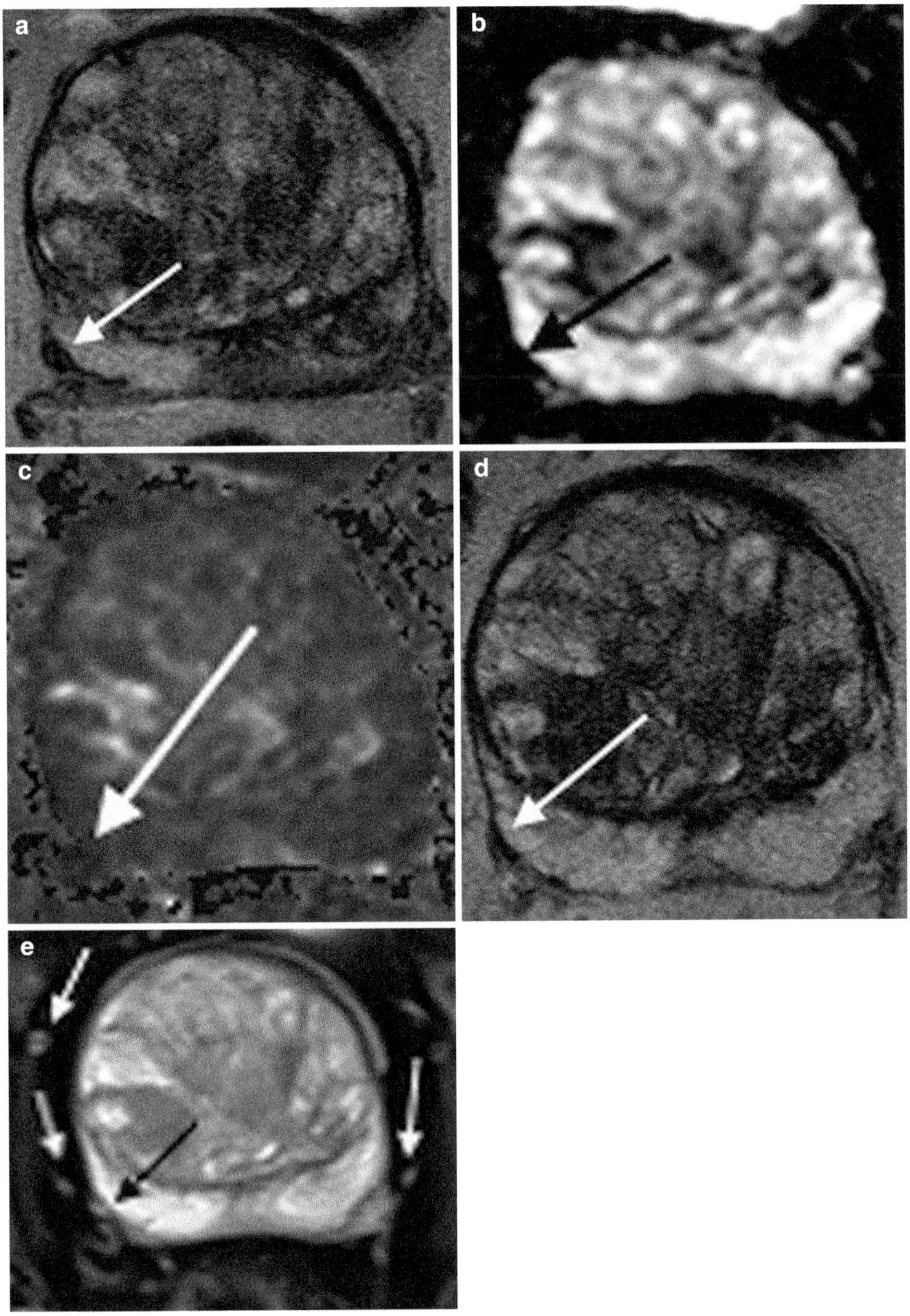

Fig. 14.4 Periprostatic venous plexus and neurovascular bundle. (**a**) Axial T2-weighted image showing well-circumscribed hypointense vessel in right posterolateral peripheral zone (white arrow) which can be misinterpreted as a lesion. (**b**) Corresponding area in the ADC map at the same level shows hypointense signal (black arrow). (**c**) DWI image shows no hyperintense signal in the corresponding region to suggest restricted diffusion. (**d**) Axial T2-weighted image level above shows a contiguous tubular structure (white arrow) consistent with a vessel. (**e**) Fat-suppressed T2-weighted image shows unsuppressed high signal in this vessel (black arrow) similar to other periprostatic vessels (white arrows)

dular or stromal, both of which are often nodular in character [16, 36]. One of the innovations in PI-RADS v2.1 was the recognition that, while glandular BPH common has long T2 and relatively unrestricted diffusion, stromal BPH contains less free water and therefore has shorter T2 and often low signal on the ADC map. These signal characteristics generally mimic those in cancer. However, these nodules are nearly uniformly circumscribed and commonly have a distinct "capsule" or a uniformly thin rim of compressed tissue which is low signal on T2-weighted imaging. While identification of this capsule allows for sufficient confidence to assign very low suspicion (PI-RADS v2.1 category 1), circumscribed or partially encapsulated nodules have features which overlap with cancer. Originally, these we all assigned PI-RADS v2 category 2: "low suspicion," on T2-weighted imaging and overall, and biopsy was not recommended. However, the degree of diffusion restriction in these nodules should not be dissimilar to other BPH in the same prostate. Therefore, if there is a greater degree of diffusion restriction – lower signal on the ADC map and higher signal on the high b-value DWI corresponding to PI-RADS v2.1 DWI categories 4 and 5 – there is sufficient suspicion that this could reflect neoplasia rather than hyperplasia. Although the majority of these nodules are likely to be benign, when the T2 appearance is of a circumscribed or partially encapsulated transition zone nodule (T2 category 2) but diffusion is highly restricted (diffusion category 4 or 5), these nodules are assigned an overall PI-RADS v2.1 category 3, equivocal suspicion.

14.2.3.3 Acute and Chronic Prostatitis and Post-inflammatory Scars and Atrophy

Inflammation in the peripheral gland, compared with other solid organs, can result in a paradoxical shortening of T2 and restrict diffusion – the inflammatory cells are smaller with less cytoplasm and free water motion compared with glandular cells – which can approach the appearance of cancer [37]. While the decrease in T2 and degree of diffusion restriction is generally less than that of significant cancer, these appearances overlap, at least in terms of absolute ADC value. However, the relative ADC compared with "normal" peripheral gland may show greater separation between inflammation and neoplasia. This was explicitly described in PI-RADS v2, but was removed from v2.1 for clarity and brevity: it is assumed because it is not mass-like, it would not be considered a discrete lesion. Another innovation in PI-RADS v2.1 over v2 is the harmonization of DWI categorization with T2 categorization of radial linear or wedge-shaped lesions in the peripheral zone. Post-inflammatory change often results in fibrosis along the course of the glandular channels, which are oriented in a radial linear or wedge-shaped fashion. Cancer, on the other hand, tends to be oval or "lenticular," oriented circumferentially [16].

14.2.3.4 Granulomatous Prostatitis

Similar to inflammation described in the above paragraph, granulomatous prostatitis was rapidly identified as a mimicker of cancer. Unlike common inflammation, granulomatous prostatitis was more commonly mass-like with markedly restricted diffusion – often greater than that seen in cancer [38]. Unfortunately, there is marked overlap in the appearance of cancer compared with granulomatous prostatitis, and while a history of exposure to intravesicular instillation of Bacillus Calmette-Guérin (BCG) or other agents that commonly produce a granulomatous response may raise this differential consideration, tissue diagnosis is often required to confirm the diagnosis, as these men generally also have risk factors for cancer, such as elevated serum PSA.

14.3 Pearls

14.3.1 Category: Differentiating Tumor from Benign or Normal Structures

14.3.1.1 Anterior Fibromuscular Stroma and Central Zone

Both anterior fibromuscular stroma and central zone have low T2 signal and low ADC map signal and can be misinterpreted as tumors.

The findings favoring benign etiology include midline location, symmetric appearance, well-defined margins, and absence of high signal intensity on high b-value images (true restriction). The anterior fibromuscular stroma shows benign type 1 progressive enhancement without any washout. The central zone shows type 1 and type 2 (early enhancement and plateau). They don't show type 3 enhancement kinetics [16] (Fig. 14.5).

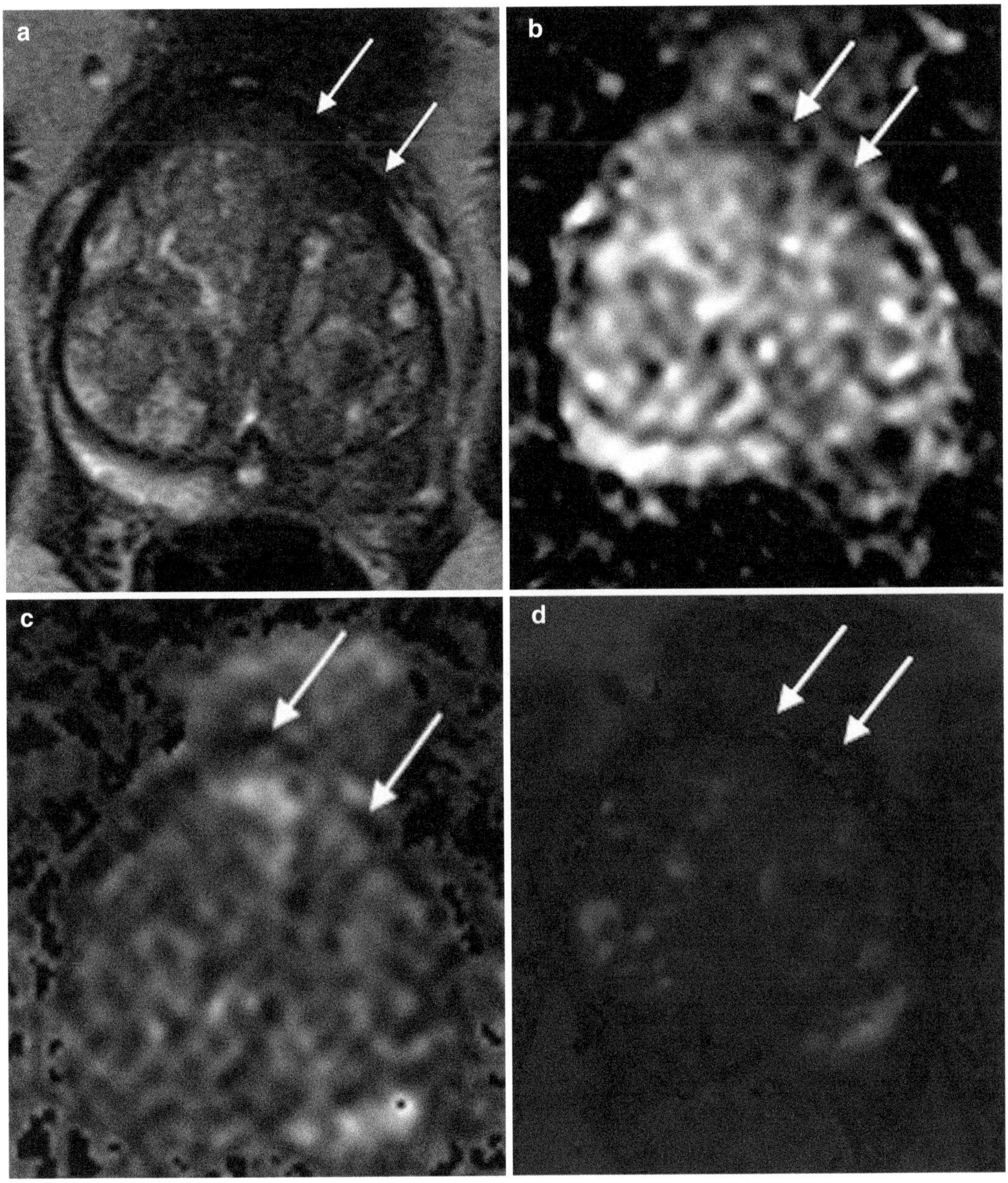

Fig. 14.5 Anterior fibromuscular stroma. (**a**) Axial T2-weighted image shows hypointense signal in the anterior fibromuscular stroma (white arrows). (**b**) The corresponding ADC map shows hypointense signal (white arrows). (**c**) DWI images show no restricted diffusion with hypointense signal (white arrows). (**d**) Pharmacokinetic K^{trans} map shows no corresponding abnormal enhancement

14.3.1.2 Volume Averaging of the Surgical Capsule at the Apex

The apex of prostate is known to be undersampled on routine, nontargeted TRUS biopsies and may contain clinically significant tumors [39]. The pseudocapsule is sparse at the apex, intermixed with supporting tissues, glands, and prostatic veins. Horizontal oblique orientation of the surgical capsule and veins with partial volume effect on axial images makes it difficult to delineate intra-prostatic from extra-prostatic structures. Examination of coronal and sagittal planes helps demonstrate continuity of these periprostatic structures. Also, axial images above and below the apex can be used to demonstrate the continuity of the surgical capsule and adjacent veins [16] (Fig. 14.6).

14.3.1.3 Ejaculatory Ducts

In patients with BPH, the anatomy of the central gland (central and transition zone) is distorted at the base of the prostate gland. Bilateral ejaculatory ducts help identify the central zone on coronal T2-weighted sequences as symmetric, well-defined, homogeneous, dark signal structure with smooth margins surrounding bilateral ejaculatory ducts. These may appear as a low signal triangular structure in the posterior midline peripheral zone with corresponding low ADC signal and intermediate high signal on high b-value DWI, possibly related to directionality in the direction of the fibers. However, no increased contrast enhancement would be associated. Conversely, prostate cancer is asymmetrical and hypointense with ill-defined margins [30].

14.3.2 Category: Suspicious Findings Not Explicit in PI-RADS Categorization

14.3.2.1 Tumors Are Homogeneous

Explicit in the PI-RADS v2.1 assessment criteria is that tumors tend to be more uniform than normal prostate glandular tissue, but are also more uniformed compared with the heterogeneity inherent in BPH [40, 41]. This is a welcome factor when evaluating the transition zone. The transition zone is normally much more heterogeneous than the peripheral zone with shorter T2, which is accentuated in BPH. While detecting the circumscribed or encapsulated margin of a BPH nodule can help to identify its nature, recognizing the internal heterogeneity adds an additional layer of comfort when trying to determine whether to "call" a nodule, especially when the diffusion could appear moderate or markedly restricted – therefore category 3 or 4 – depending on window-level settings. The heterogeneity applies to diffusion sequences as well: while a cancerous nodule may not show uniformly restricted diffusion, it will generally have a gradient rather than chaotic variation in its signal.

14.3.2.2 Dynamic Contrast As a Saving Grace

Interest in biparametric magnetic resonance imaging (bpMRI), or T2- and diffusion-weighted imaging without dynamic contrast-enhanced imaging (DCE), is gaining popularity, as its performance appears not significantly worse than truly mpMRI, with potential significant cost, time, and risk reduction [42]. DCE is only used to adjust the overall suspicion for lesions which are equivocal suspicion (category 3) on DWI in the peripheral gland, and even then, most category 3 lesions will undergo biopsy. However, there are a number of cases where contrast can be instrumental in the evaluation of prostate MRI, and often these cannot be predicted. In fact, this possibility was explicitly described in PI-RADS v2 and v2.1, where a table for both transition and peripheral zone lesions with inadequate DWI is provided using DCE to arrive at the overall category in both zones. While this is very common when evaluating patients with one or both hip prostheses, peristalsis, surgical clips, and surface coil displacement by redundant adipose can all severely compromise DWI. Additionally, in cases where diffusion may be evaluable but is distorted, limiting confidence in localizing

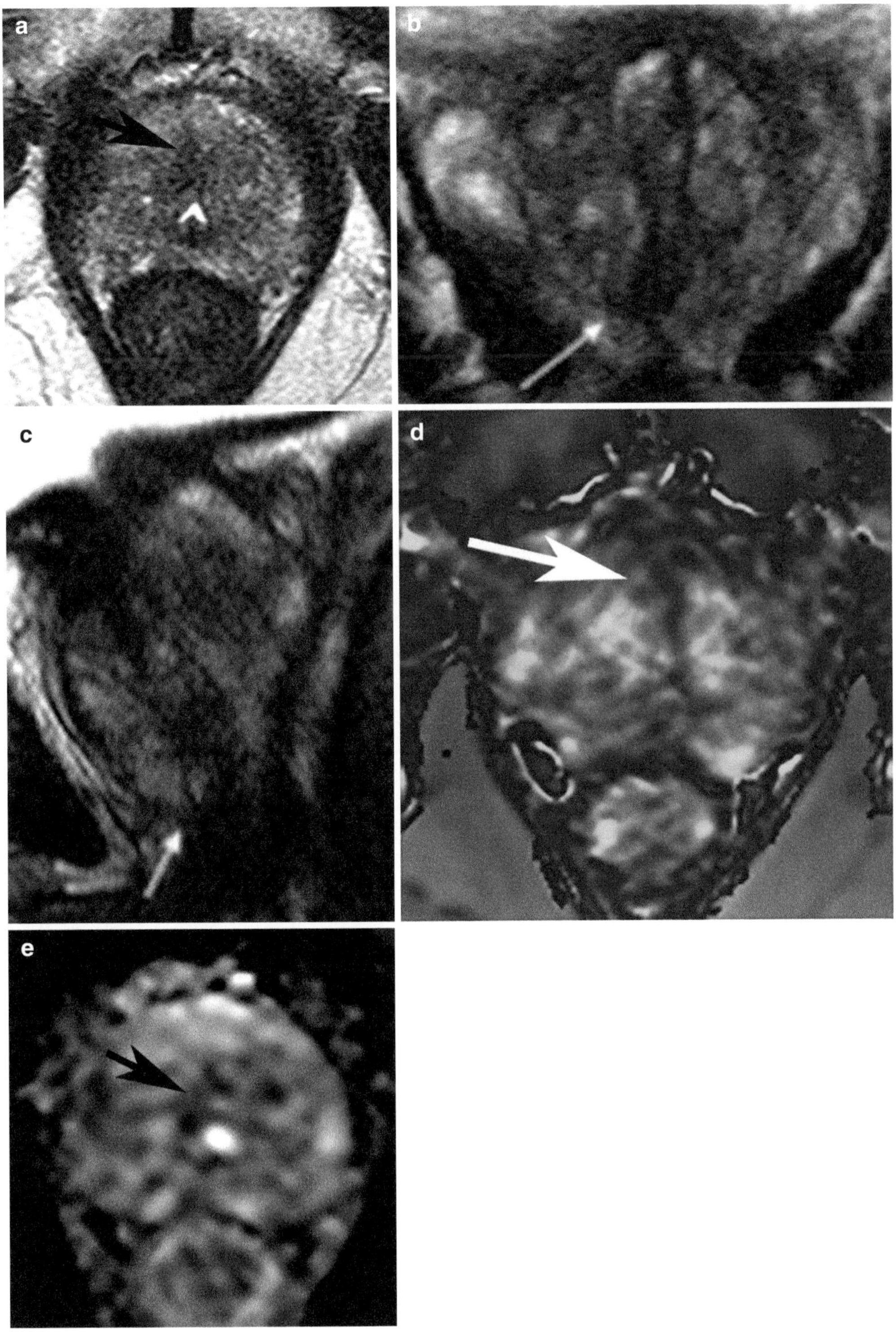

Fig. 14.6 Volume averaging of the surgical capsule at the apex. (**a**) Axial T2-weighted image at the level of apex showing indistinct surgical capsule with blurring due to volume averaging, resulting in a low signal ill-defined mass in the midline (black arrow). T2-weighted coronal (**b**) and sagittal (**c**) images showing surgical capsule (white arrows). Axial DCE map shows no enhancement (**d**), but there is corresponding low signal on the ADC map, which is normal for the fibrous surgical capsule (**e**)

abnormalities, DCE can provide an additional level of confidence in determining that a finding is focal or artifactual. Finally, when determining the overall size of a lesion, DCE has been shown to be the best correlate with size measured on the surgical specimen [43] (Fig. 14.7).

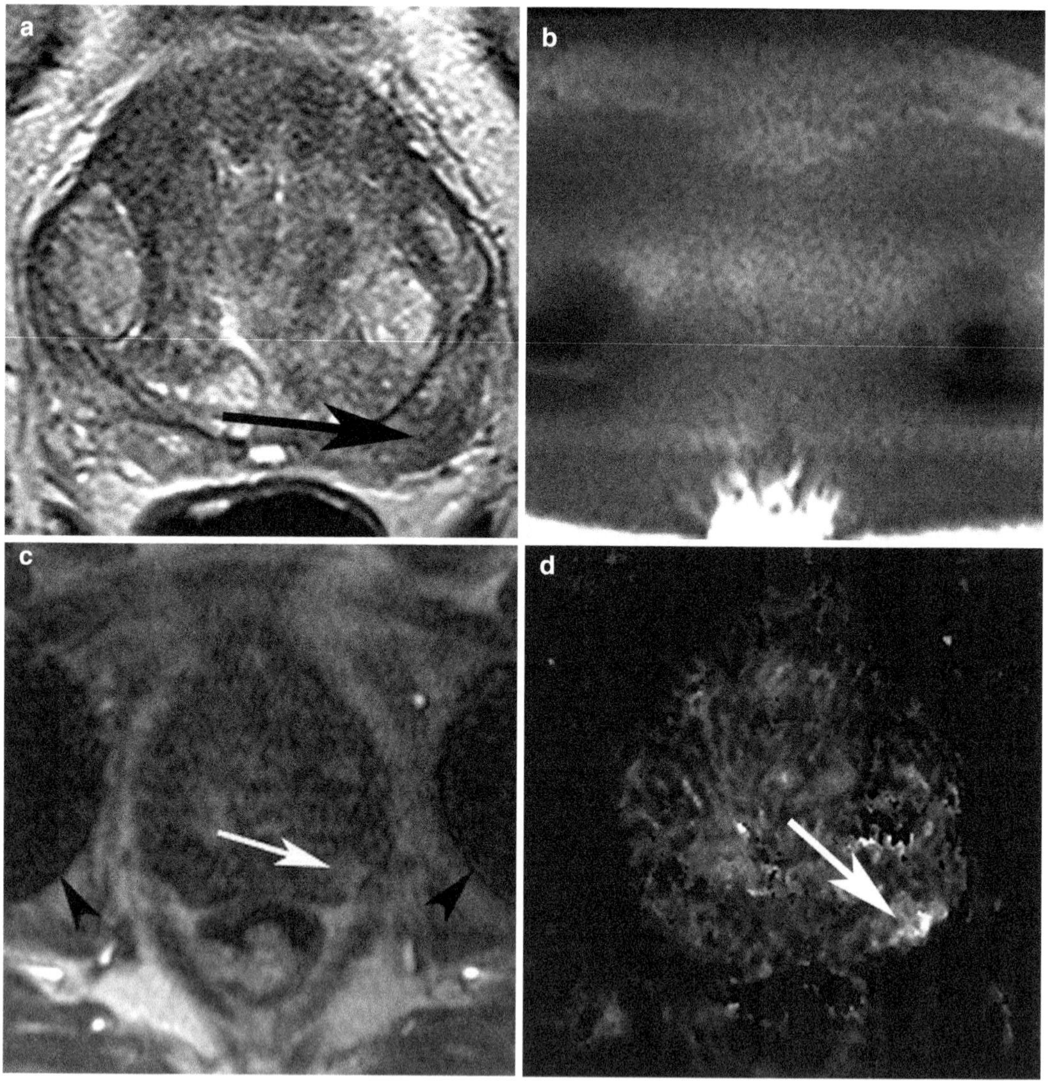

Fig. 14.7 Dynamic contrast as a saving grace. (**a**) Axial T2-weighted image showing a hypointense mass with irregular margins at the posterolateral left peripheral base (black arrow) with a moderate amount of image noise. (**b**) Diffusion-weighted image at the same level is obliterated by susceptibility artifact from bilateral hip prostheses. (**c**) Early enhancement T1-weighted image shows corresponding enhancement (white arrow) with susceptibility artifact (black arrowheads) not obscuring the prostate. (**d**) Pharmacokinetic K^{trans} map shows the focal enhancement more conspicuously (white arrow)

14.3.2.3 The Highly, Diffusely Heterogeneous Prostate and When to Find the Most Suspicious Area

Officially, the objective assessment of mpMRI of the prostate is done irrespective of clinical information. Practically, though, there are some cases which are more straightforward than others. One of the most challenging cases is the diffusely, highly heterogeneous prostate, sometimes called a "dirty MRI" because of the spotty nature of abnormal signal. Generally, this is chalked up to inflammatory changes (in the peripheral zone) and BPH (in the transition zone). However, these changes are often conspicuous not only on T2-weighted imaging but also on DWI and even DCE. This results in a quandary: Should one provide dozens of "targets," or none? This is where the clinical scenario can be useful. For patients with low suspicion, PSA density below 0.15 ng/mL^2, long doubling time/low PSA velocity, and favorable demographics and family history and especially when no one area is likely to be large enough for confident targeting using image fusion, it may be in the patient's best interest to give no target [44]. However, when there is an elevated suspicion, and especially in the face of prior negative nontargeted biopsies, identifying the most suspicious area may be useful, in that if targeted biopsy is negative, this provides increased confidence in surveillance. Generally, a combination of quantitative ADC to identify the site of greatest diffusion restriction, combined with T2 features, is the most useful to find the "most suspicious" area. However, this is another case where DCE may be a useful "tiebreaker."

14.3.2.4 How Wedge-Shaped Is "Wedge-Shaped"?

The inclusion of lesions which are "(radial) linear/wedge-shaped hypointense on ADC and/or hyperintense on high b-value DWI" for DWI category 2 in the peripheral gland allowed this assessment to harmonize with that already established for T2-weighted imaging. However, deciding whether a lesion is "linear" or "oval" may be difficult. One of the most useful components in making the determination is the appearance on T2-weighted imaging. While the assessment is made on DWI, the much higher spatial resolution of T2-weighted images, combined with the freedom from geometric distortion, allows for improved confidence in confirming the radial orientation of the lesion in question. Inflammation occurs along the course of the glands, which effectively point in a radial orientation to the urethra or verumontanum. Cancers are more commonly oriented circumferentially. Additionally, a "wedge-shaped" lesion should be widest at the periphery of the prostate, narrowing as it nears the surgical capsule (which separates the transition from peripheral zones). Linear lesions are generally uniformly thin; they should not appear bulbous in the middle or at either end (Fig. 14.8).

14.3.3 Category: Extra-Prostatic Structures

14.3.3.1 Bladder Inlet

The bladder mucosa is generally low signal on T2-weighted imaging as well as on DCE and high b-value DWI (although with greater signal than urine), similar to transition zone on ADC, similar to the anterior fibromuscular stroma. Because it may be caught at an angle, the uniformly low T2 signal may, at first glance, appear suspicious. However, its nature is generally readily apparent on sagittal and coronal images.

14.3.3.2 Seminal Vesicle Atrophy Versus Involvement

Seminal vesicles are fluid filled, with low signal intensity on T1-weighted images and high signal intensity on T2-weighted images. Radiation therapy and infection/inflammation in addition

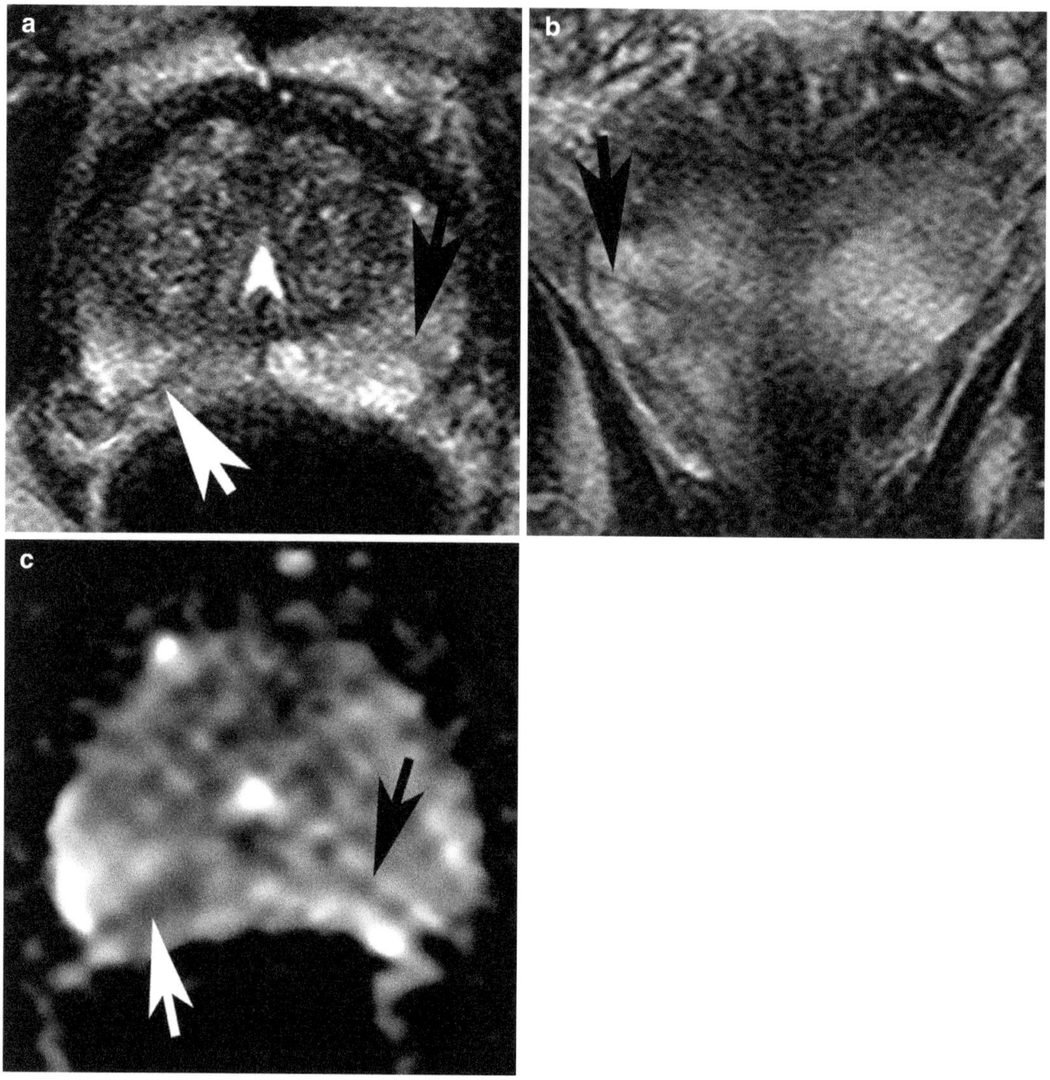

Fig. 14.8 How wedge-shaped is "wedge-shaped"? (**a**) Axial T2-weighted image shows right (white arrow) and left (black arrow) radially oriented linear hypointensities, although the latter is partially obscured. (**b**) Coronal T2-weighted image shows the right posterior linear hypointensity (black arrow) is oriented toward the verumontanum (not in the plane of this image). (**c**) Axial ADC map shows the same linear hypointensities (white, black arrows)

to the normal aging process ("andropause") can cause atrophy of the seminal vesicle secondary to reactive peritubular fibrosis. The fibrotic wall thickening from vesiculitis and radiation therapy can be indistinguishable from tumor invasion [45]. Granulomatous prostatitis involving periprostatic fat and seminal vesicles can mimic extra-prostatic tumor spread. Correct clinical history such as previous radiation therapy, BCG for bladder cancer, tuberculous prostatitis, or TURP can be helpful [46]. When the atrophic seminal vesicles are low signal on high b-value DWI and show no increased enhancement, they can generally be assumed to be uninvolved. However, histopathological confirmation is usually required when either of these is not true (Fig. 14.9).

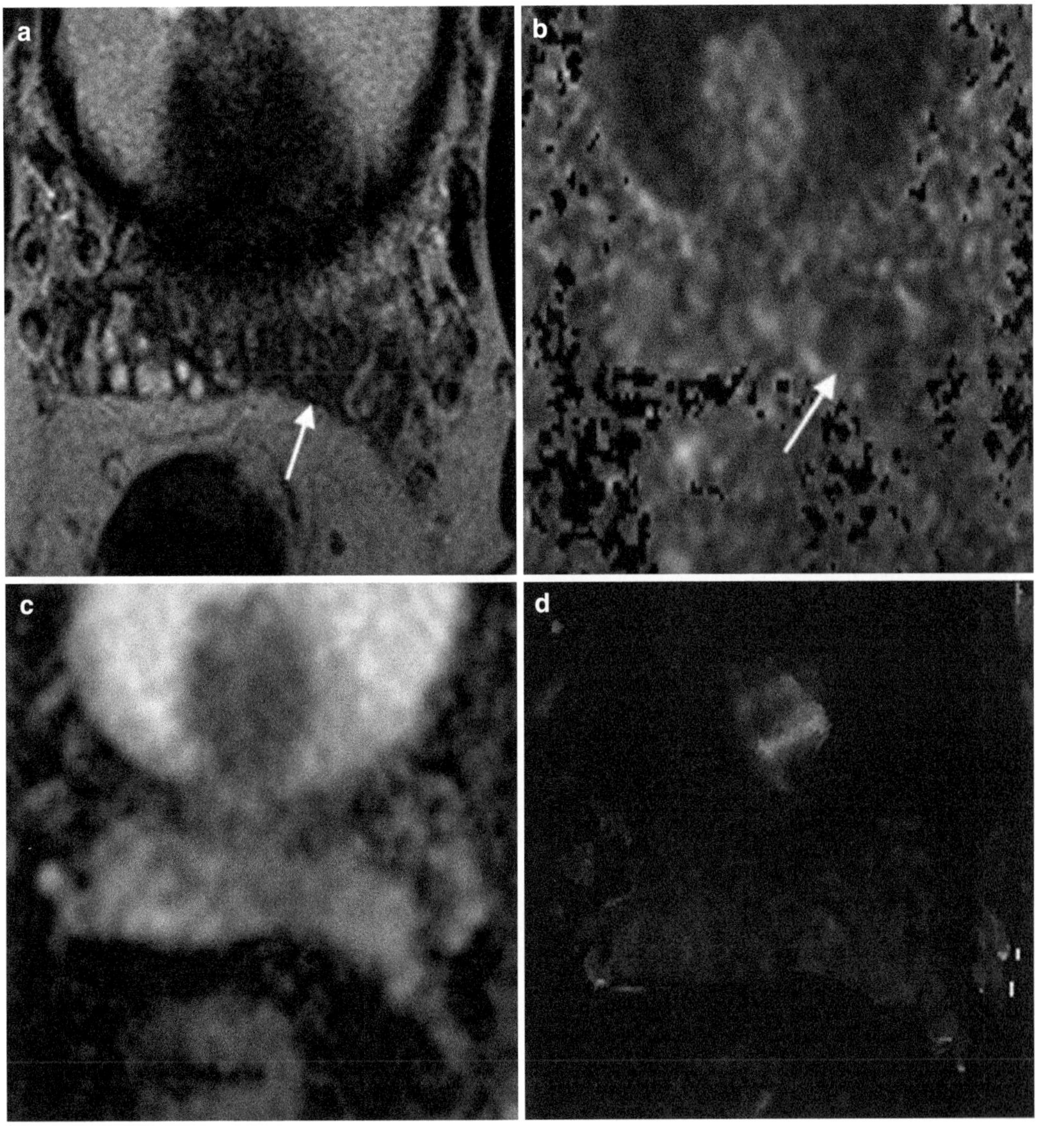

Fig. 14.9 Seminal vesicle atrophy versus involvement. (**a**) Axial T2-weighted image is showing benign, atrophic, left seminal vesicle with hypointense signal (white arrow). The right seminal vesicle is showing normal T2 hyperintense signal. (**b**) DWI images at the same level show hypointense signal (white arrow) in the atrophic left seminal vesicle with no evidence of restricted diffusion. (**c**) ADC map at the same level showing no signal abnormality in the atrophic left seminal vesicle. (**d**) Pharmacokinetic K^{trans} map shows no abnormal enhancement in the atrophic seminal vesicle

14.3.3.3 Other Cancers

An important consideration in the evaluation of the population of men that presents for prostate cancer detection is that, while prostate cancer is the most common non-cutaneous cancer in this population, it is certainly not the only cancer [3]. Just as one evaluates bones and lymph nodes for potential metastatic disease, the bladder, rectum, and other structures in the field of view should be scrutinized for suspicious abnormalities. Fortunately, these cancers will often also show increased perfusion on DCE and restricted diffusion on DWI, emphasizing the utility of these pulse sequences (Fig. 14.10).

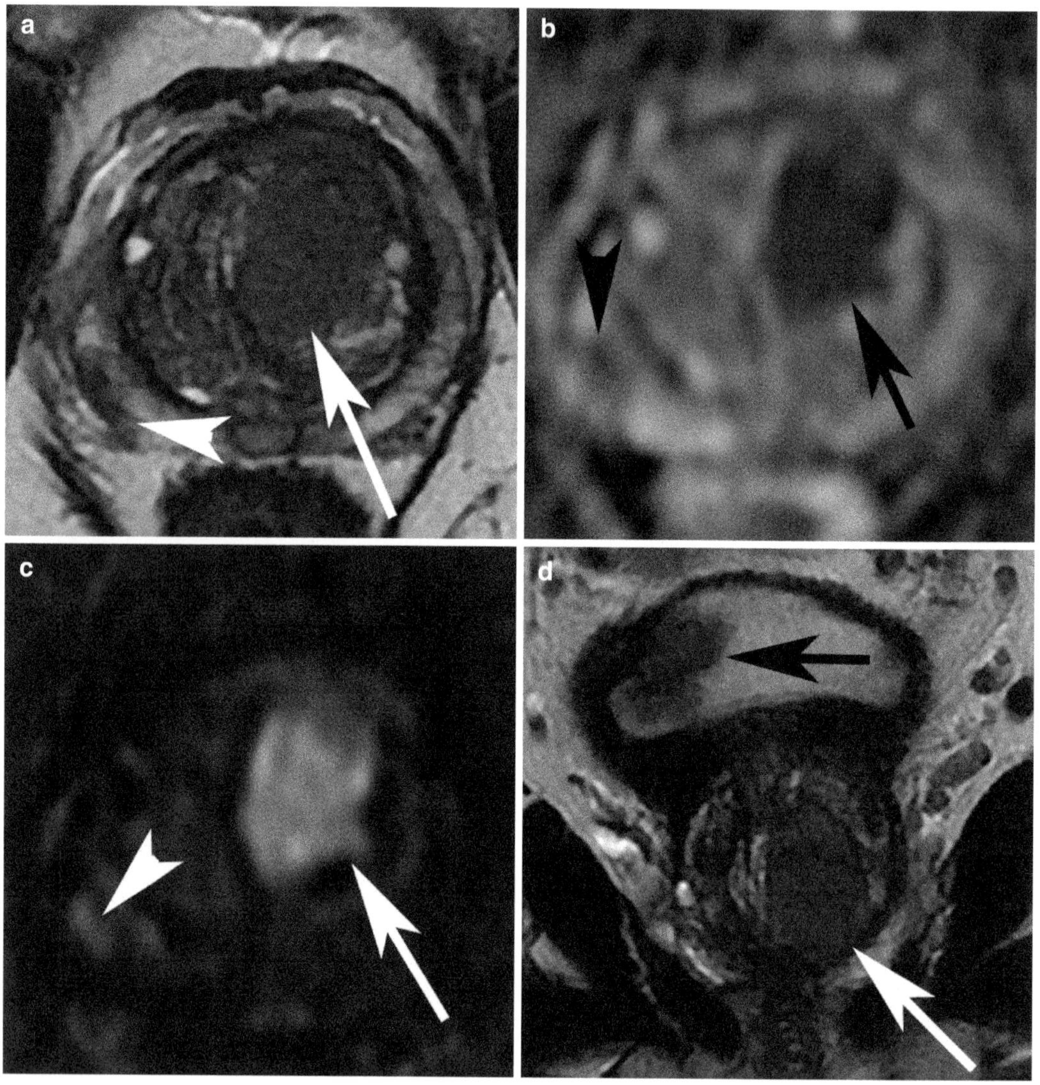

Fig. 14.10 Other cancers. (**a**) Axial T2-weighted image shows a large transition zone lesion with partially circumscribed and partially obscured borders in the left anterior transition zone (white arrow) and a smaller right posterolateral peripheral zone lesion with irregular borders (white arrowhead). (**b**) Corresponding ADC map shows markedly restricted diffusion in the transition zone lesion (arrow) and moderately restricted diffusion in the peripheral zone lesion (arrowhead). (**c**) High b-value DWI also shows markedly restricted diffusion in the transition zone lesion (arrow) and moderately restricted diffusion in the peripheral zone lesion (arrowhead). (**d**) Coronal T2-weighted image shows the transition zone lesion (white arrow) and an endophytic bladder mass (black arrow). (**e**) ADC map through the bladder shows two endophytic bladder lesions (arrows). (**f**) High b-value DWI also reveals endophytic bladder masses (arrows) without abnormal signal extending to the bladder wall. (**g**) Dynamic contrast-enhanced image through the bladder also shows enhancement of the endophytic bladder lesions (arrows) without extension to the bladder wall. Using VI-RADS, this is likely non-muscle-invasive bladder cancer [47]

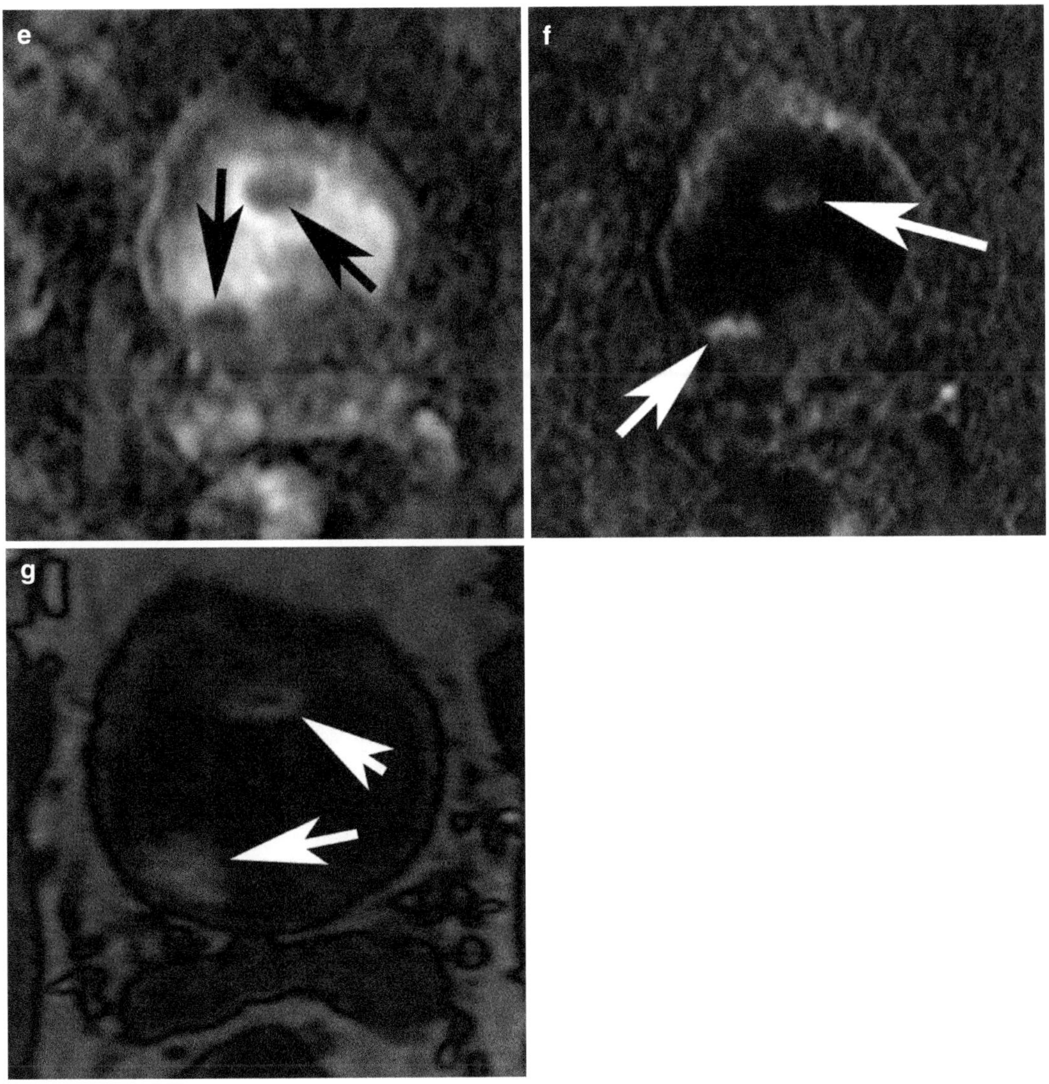

Fig. 14.10 (continued)

14.4 Conclusion

Multiparametric magnetic resonance imaging of the prostate is a challenging, but, ultimately, a rewarding clinical tool in the detection, characterization, and management of prostate cancer. By recognizing those idiosyncrasies inherent in its use, it becomes a reliable and valuable tool for the radiologist and referring practitioners. By grouping the potential pitfalls and pearls into their respective aspects, one can systematically interpret and report mpMRI of the prostate with confidence.

References

1. Turkbey B, Rosenkrantz AB, Haider MA, Padhani AR, Villeirs G, Macura KJ, et al. Prostate imaging reporting and data system version 2.1: 2019 update of prostate imaging reporting and data system version 2. Eur Urol. 2019;76(3):340–51.
2. Rosenkrantz AB, Taneja SS. Radiologist, be aware: ten pitfalls that confound the interpretation of multiparametric prostate MRI. AJR Am J Roentgenol. 2014;202(1):109–20.
3. Siegel RL, Miller KD, Jemal A. Cancer statistics, 2017. CA Cancer J Clin. 2017;67(1):7–30.
4. Murphy G, Haider M, Ghai S, Sreeharsha B. The expanding role of MRI in prostate cancer. AJR Am J Roentgenol. 2013;201(6):1229–38.
5. Gasser TC, Streule K, Nidecker A, Rist M. MRI and ultrasonography in staging prostate cancer. N Engl J Med. 1991;324(7):494–5.
6. Sumers EH. Staging prostate cancer with MR imaging. Radiology. 1993;187(3):875.
7. Park BK, Park JW, Park SY, Kim CK, Lee HM, Jeon SS, et al. Prospective evaluation of 3-T MRI performed before initial transrectal ultrasound-guided prostate biopsy in patients with high prostate-specific antigen and no previous biopsy. AJR Am J Roentgenol. 2011;197(5):W876–81.
8. Siddiqui MM, Rais-Bahrami S, Truong H, Stamatakis L, Vourganti S, Nix J, et al. Magnetic resonance imaging/ultrasound-fusion biopsy significantly upgrades prostate cancer versus systematic 12-core transrectal ultrasound biopsy. Eur Urol. 2013;64(5):713–9.
9. Porpiglia F, Manfredi M, Mele F, Cossu M, Bollito E, Veltri A, et al. Diagnostic pathway with multiparametric magnetic resonance imaging versus standard pathway: results from a randomized prospective study in biopsy-naive patients with suspected prostate cancer. Eur Urol. 2017;72(2):282–8.
10. Kasivisvanathan V, Rannikko AS, Borghi M, Panebianco V, Mynderse LA, Vaarala MH, et al. MRI-targeted or standard biopsy for prostate-cancer diagnosis. N Engl J Med. 2018;378(19):1767–77.
11. Stamatakis L, Siddiqui MM, Nix JW, Logan J, Rais-Bahrami S, Walton-Diaz A, et al. Accuracy of multiparametric magnetic resonance imaging in confirming eligibility for active surveillance for men with prostate cancer. Cancer. 2013;119(18):3359–66.
12. Barrett T, Haider MA. The emerging role of MRI in prostate cancer active surveillance and ongoing challenges. AJR Am J Roentgenol. 2017;208(1):131–9.
13. Calio B, Kasson M, Sugano D, Ortman M, Gaitonde K, Verma S, et al. Multiparametric MRI: an opportunity for focal therapy of prostate cancer. Semin Roentgenol. 2018;53(3):227–33.
14. McNeal JE. The zonal anatomy of the prostate. Prostate. 1981;2(1):35–49.
15. Hricak H, Dooms GC, McNeal JE, Mark AS, Marotti M, Avallone A, et al. MR imaging of the prostate gland: normal anatomy. AJR Am J Roentgenol. 1987;148(1):51–8.
16. Kitzing YX, Prando A, Varol C, Karczmar GS, Maclean F, Oto A. Benign conditions that mimic prostate carcinoma: MR imaging features with histopathologic correlation. Radiographics. 2016;36(1):162–75.
17. Barrett T, Rajesh A, Rosenkrantz AB, Choyke PL, Turkbey B. PI-RADS version 2.1: one small step for prostate MRI. Clin Radiol. 2019;74(11):841–52. doi: 10.1016.
18. Shen Y, Larkman DJ, Counsell S, Pu IM, Edwards D, Hajnal JV. Correction of high-order eddy current induced geometric distortion in diffusion-weighted echo-planar images. Magn Reson Med. 2004;52(5):1184–9.
19. Huang SY, Seethamraju RT, Patel P, Hahn PF, Kirsch JE, Guimaraes AR. Body MR imaging: artifacts, k-space, and solutions. Radiographics. 2015;35(5):1439–60.
20. Donato F Jr, Costa DN, Yuan Q, Rofsky NM, Lenkinski RE, Pedrosa I. Geometric distortion in diffusion-weighted MR imaging of the prostate-contributing factors and strategies for improvement. Acad Radiol. 2014;21(6):817–23.
21. Mazaheri Y, Vargas HA, Nyman G, Akin O, Hricak H. Image artifacts on prostate diffusion-weighted magnetic resonance imaging: trade-offs at 1.5 T and 3.0 T. Acad Radiol. 2013;20(8):1041–7.
22. Deng J, Omary RA, Larson AC. Multishot diffusion-weighted SPLICE PROPELLER MRI of the abdomen. Magn Reson Med. 2008;59(5):947–53.
23. Barentsz JO, Richenberg J, Clements R, Choyke P, Verma S, Villeirs G, et al. European Society of Urogenital Radiology.ESUR prostate MR guidelines 2012. Eur Radiol. 2012;22(4):746–57.
24. Rosenkrantz AB, Kong X, Niver BE, Berkman DS, Melamed J, Babb JS, et al. Prostate cancer: comparison of tumor visibility on trace diffusion-weighted images and the apparent diffusion coefficient map. AJR Am J Roentgenol. 2011;196(1):123–9.
25. Blackledge MD, Leach MO, Collins DJ, Koh DM. Computed diffusion-weighted MR imaging may improve tumor detection. Radiology. 2011;261(2):573–81.
26. Ning P, Shi D, Sonn GA, Vasanawala SS, Loening AM, Ghanouni P, et al. The impact of computed high b-value images on the diagnostic accuracy of DWI for prostate cancer: a receiver operating characteristics analysis. Sci Rep. 2018;8(1):3409.
27. Xiaohang L, Bingni Z, Liangping Z, Weijun P, Xiaoqun Y, Yong Z. Differentiation of prostate cancer and stromal hyperplasia in the transition zone with histogram analysis of the apparent diffusion coefficient. Acta Radiol. 2017;58(12):1528–34.
28. Haider MA, van der Kwast TH, Tanguay J, Evans AJ, Hashmi AT, Lockwood G, Trachtenberg J. Combined T2-weighted and diffusion-weighted

MRI for localization of prostate cancer. AJR Am J Roentgenol. 2007;189(2):323–8.
29. Vargas HA, Akin O, Franiel T, Goldman DA, Udo K, Touijer KA, et al. Normal central zone of the prostate and central zone involvement by prostate cancer: clinical and MR imaging implications. Radiology. 2012;262(3):894–902.
30. Panebianco V, Barchetti F, Barentsz J, Ciardi A, Cornud F, Futterer J, et al. Pitfalls in interpreting mp-MRI of the prostate: a pictorial review with pathologic correlation. Insights Imaging. 2015;6(6):611–30.
31. Semple JE. Surgical capsule of the benign enlargement of the prostate. Br Med J. 1963;1(5346):1640–3.
32. Yu J, Fulcher AS, Winks SG, Turner MA, Clayton RD, Brooks M, et al. Diagnosis of typical and atypical transition zone prostate cancer and its mimics at multiparametric prostate MRI. Br J Radiol. 2017;90(1073):20160693.
33. Qayyum A, Coakley FV, Lu Y, Olpin JD, Wu L, Yeh BM, et al. Organ-confined prostate cancer: effect of prior transrectal biopsy on endorectal MRI and MR spectroscopic imaging. AJR Am J Roentgenol. 2004;183(4):1079–83.
34. Rosenkrantz AB, Mussi TC, Hindman N, Lim RP, Kong MX, Babb JS, et al. Impact of delay after biopsy and post-biopsy haemorrhage on prostate cancer tumour detection using multi-parametric MRI: a multi-reader study. Clin Radiol. 2012;67(12):e83–90.
35. Purysko AS, Herts BR. Prostate MRI: the hemorrhage exclusion sign. J Urol. 2012;188(5):1946–7.
36. Chesnais AL, Niaf E, Bratan F, Mege-Lechevallier F, Roche S, Rabilloud M, et al. Differentiation of transitional zone prostate cancer from benign hyperplasia nodules: evaluation of discriminant criteria at multiparametric MRI. Clin Radiol. 2013;68(6): e323–30.
37. Ocak I, Bernardo M, Metzger G, Barrett T, Pinto P, Albert PS, et al. Dynamic contrast-enhanced MRI of prostate cancer at 3 T: a study of pharmacokinetic parameters. AJR Am J Roentgenol. 2007; 189(4):849.
38. Rais-Bahrami S, Nix JW, Turkbey B, Pietryga JA, Sanyal R, Thomas JV, et al. Clinical and multiparametric MRI signatures of granulomatous prostatitis. Abdom Radiol (NY). 2017;42(7):1956–62.
39. Bott SR, Young MP, Kellett MJ, Parkinson MC. Anterior prostate cancer: is it more difficult to diagnose? BJU Int. 2002;89(9):886–9.
40. Vignati A, Mazzetti S, Giannini V, Russo F, Bollito E, Porpiglia F, et al. Texture features on T2-weighted magnetic resonance imaging: new potential biomarkers for prostate cancer aggressiveness. Phys Med Biol. 2015;60(7):2685–701.
41. Wibmer A, Hricak H, Gondo T, Matsumoto K, Veeraraghavan H, Fehr D, et al. Haralick texture analysis of prostate MRI: utility for differentiating non-cancerous prostate from prostate cancer and differentiating prostate cancers with different Gleason scores. Eur Radiol. 2015;25(10):2840–50.
42. Choi MH, Kim CK, Lee YJ, Jung SE. Prebiopsy Biparametric MRI for clinically significant prostate cancer detection with PI-RADS version 2: a multicenter study. AJR Am J Roentgenol. 2019;212(4):839–46.
43. Sun C, Chatterjee A, Yousuf A, Antic T, Eggener S, Karczmar GS, et al. Comparison of T2-weighted imaging, DWI, and dynamic contrast-enhanced MRI for calculation of prostate cancer index lesion volume: correlation with whole-mount pathology. AJR Am J Roentgenol. 2019;212(2):351–6.
44. Abdi H, Zargar H, Goldenberg SL, Walshe T, Pourmalek F, Eddy C, et al. Multiparametric magnetic resonance imaging-targeted biopsy for the detection of prostate cancer in patients with prior negative biopsy results. Urol Oncol. 2015;33(4):165. e1–7.
45. Reddy MN, Verma S. Lesions of the seminal vesicles and their MRI characteristics. J Clin Imaging Sci. 2014;4:61.
46. Quon JS, Moosavi B, Khanna M, Flood TA, Lim CS, Schieda N. False positive and false negative diagnoses of prostate cancer at multi-parametric prostate MRI in active surveillance. Insights Imaging. 2015;6(4):449–63.
47. Panebianco V, Narumi Y, Altun E, Bochner BH, Efstathiou JA, Hafeez S, et al. Multiparametric magnetic resonance imaging for bladder cancer: development of VI-RADS (vesical imaging-reporting and data system). Eur Urol. 2018;74(3):294–306.

Index

T. Tirkes (ed.), *Prostate MRI Essentials*, https://doi.org/10.1007/978-3-030-45935-2